医学基础化学实验(双语版)

(第二版)

主　　编　冯　清　刘　敏
副 主 编　李海玲　赵云斌
参　　编　刘　文　吕雅娟　李　宝
　　　　　齐　伟　熊必金　刘奕静
　　　　　张　建　李桂玲　袁红玲
　　　　　胡国志　万　宏　刘　嵩

华中科技大学出版社
中国·武汉

内 容 提 要

本书主要内容分为两大板块:中文板块和英文板块。各板块自成体系,通过灵活取舍分别供中文实验教学、全英文实验教学和双语实验教学使用。各板块的内容均包括基础化学实验须知和基础化学实验部分。基础化学实验部分内容由浅入深,循序渐进,逐步提高,分为四个层次:基本技能训练实验、应用技能训练实验、综合性技能训练实验和设计性技能训练实验。另外,本书充分利用移动互联网和数字信息技术手段,设置了数字化的预习系统和实验操作视频,方便学生学习。

图书在版编目(CIP)数据

医学基础化学实验:双语版:英汉对照/冯清,刘敏主编.—2 版.—武汉:华中科技大学出版社,2021.8
ISBN 978-7-5680-7333-2

Ⅰ. ①医… Ⅱ. ①冯… ②刘… Ⅲ. ①医用化学-化学实验-医药院校-教材-英、汉 Ⅳ. ①R313-33

中国版本图书馆 CIP 数据核字(2021)第 147937 号

医学基础化学实验(双语版)(第二版) 冯 清 刘 敏 主编
Yixue Jichu Huaxue Shiyan(Shuangyu Ban)(Di-er Ban)

策划编辑:王新华
责任编辑:丁 平
封面设计:原色设计
责任校对:李 琴
责任监印:周治超
出版发行:华中科技大学出版社(中国·武汉)　　电话:(027)81321913
　　　　　武汉市东湖新技术开发区华工科技园　　邮编:430223
录　排:华中科技大学惠友文印中心
印　刷:武汉市洪林印务有限公司
开　本:710mm×1000mm　1/16
印　张:21.5
字　数:430 千字
版　次:2021 年 8 月第 2 版第 1 次印刷
定　价:48.00 元

网络增值服务使用说明

欢迎使用华中科技大学出版社医学资源网yixue.hustp.com

1.教师使用流程

（1）登录网址：http://yixue.hustp.com （注册时请选择教师用户）

（2）审核通过后，您可以在网站使用以下功能：

管理学生

建立课程　　　　　　　　布置作业

下载教学资源　　　教师　　　查询学生学习记录等

2.学员使用流程

建议学员在PC端完成注册、登录、完善个人信息的操作。

（1）PC端学员操作步骤

①登录网址：http://yixue.hustp.com （注册时请选择普通用户）

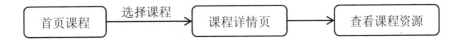

②查看课程资源

如有学习码，请在个人中心-学习码验证中先验证，再进行操作。

```
首页课程  --选择课程-->  课程详情页  -->  查看课程资源
```

（2）手机端扫码操作步骤

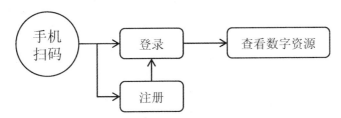

前　　言

　　医学基础化学实验是医学生的一门重要实验课,对培养学生科学核心素养、思维方法、综合能力、创新意识,养成规范操作习惯和严谨求实作风、树立医德具有重要意义。

　　为进一步推进医学基础化学实验教学的改革和发展,体现高阶性、创新性和挑战度的"两性一度"的金课建设要求,满足线上、线下混合式教学模式需要,本书根据教育部有关医药院校和生命科学相关专业基础化学、无机化学和分析化学的教学规划,结合编者多年基础化学实验教学改革、双语教学实践,借鉴和吸收国内外相应教材的优点编写而成。本书旨在通过两大板块和四个层次,建立一个将知识、能力和素质培养为一体的二段式四层次的实验技能训练模式,即以基础知识为主的基本知识与技能训练和以能力为主的综合性、设计性应用技能训练,使学生熟练地掌握有关无机化合物的合成、组分的定性和定量分析及常用理化常数测定等实验技能;结合 PBL 教学法开设"设计性实验",使学生的动手能力、创新思维、科学素养等综合素质得到全面培养。本书具有下列特点。

　　1.本书主要内容分为两大板块——中文板块和全英文板块。各板块自成体系,通过灵活取舍分别供中文实验教学、全英文实验教学和双语实验教学使用。在我校多年的实验课程双语教学和全国英语教学实践中,该体系对构建数字化、信息化和外语教学的平台,提高学生的科技英语水平,起到了良好的效果。

　　2.实验内容的安排是以加强实验技能的综合训练和素质能力培养为主线,实验内容由浅入深,循序渐进,逐步提高,分为四个层次:基本技能训练实验、应用性技能训练实验、综合性技能训练实验和设计性技能训练实验。基本技能训练实验重在夯实学生基础知识和培训学生基本技能,培养学生良好的实验素养、严谨的科学态度和思维方法;应用性技能训练实验注重对学生社会责任感、实践能力、创新精神的综合培养;而综合性技能训练实验和设计性技能训练实验着力打造实验教学的高阶性、创新性和挑战度。

　　3.设计性实验具有研究性、探索性、创造性等特点,在形式和内容设计上对学生有一定的挑战,没有预定的实验方案,需要学生预先查阅资料,对相关知识进行深度了解,实验小组成员协作配合,制订科学合理的实验方案,线上提交方案;线下课堂交互分享和探讨实验路径,在教师点评和学生自我修改完善的基础上,最终完成实验。设计性实验将极大地激发学生的学习兴趣和主观能动性,同时培养参与者的批判性思维,挖掘学生的思维潜能。

4.充分利用移动互联网和数字信息技术手段,设置了数字化的预习系统。通过在教材纸质内容的标题处设置的二维码,学生可在实验前使用手机、平板电脑扫描二维码,随时随地通过互联网访问实验预习系统,并完成自主学习。实验预习系统提供了实验原理、在线测试、理论视频、现象释疑、实验引入、操作过程、实验过程、实验花絮等相关教学内容。

5.增加了现代仪器分析部分实验,以满足学生未来科研工作需要。

本书在整个筹划编写过程中得到华中科技大学化学与化工学院全体同仁的大力支持和帮助,实验室的刘芳、汪志慧、曹灿灿和王文云四位教师为学生录制本书实验视频做了大量准备工作,在此一并表示衷心的感谢。

尽管在本书的编写过程中,我们力求做到选材恰当,翻译准确,但由于编者学识水平有限,书中难免存在欠妥甚至错误之处,恳请同行专家及读者批评指正。

编　者

目　　录

上篇　中文部分

下篇　英文部分

上 篇

中文部分

第一章　基础化学实验须知

第一节　实 验 守 则

【实验目的】

  化学是一门以实验为基础的学科,是医学和生物学等相关专业重要的基础课程。科学实验是培养人才的重要手段。开设医学基础化学实验课程,总的来说是为使学生得到科学研究所需的基本操作和基本技能的全面训练,培养学生严肃、求实的科学态度,准确、细致、严谨、整洁等良好的科学素养,让学生意识到为医者就要德才兼备,实验是否严谨细致可以造成"一刀成佛,一刀成魔"的天壤之别;逐步掌握科学研究的基本方法。具体目的有三。一是配合课堂教学,验证和巩固课堂讲授的基本理论和基本知识,在不断学习和解决问题的过程中,推进知识与技能的深度学习,为以后的学习和工作打下扎实的基础。二是学习科学实验方法,展开实验设计,将基本操作和技能训练与生产、生活实际相结合,提高分析、解决问题的能力,学以致用,激发创新能力。三是掌握正确的实验操作方法,明确地树立起"量"的概念;正确的操作才能得出准确的数据和结果,准确的数据和结果是正确结论的主要依据。

【实验室规则】

  为了保证实验的顺利进行和培养学生良好的实验作风,学生做实验时必须遵守下列实验室规则。

  (1) 实验前要做好准备工作,包括预习实验内容及写好预习报告。若准备工作未做好,不得进入实验室。进入实验室后首先了解实验室的各项规章制度,熟悉实验室的环境、布置及各种设施(水电阀门、急救箱、消防用具等)的位置。

  (2) 进入实验室需穿实验服。实验前清点仪器,如发现有破损或缺少的情况,应立即报告,按规定手续向实验预备室补领。实验时仪器如有损坏,要立即办理登记手续,以便及时补发。未经教师同意,不得使用其他实验台上的仪器或试剂。

  (3) 实验时保持安静,集中精力,认真操作,仔细观察现象,积极思考问题,如实记录结果,不做与实验无关的事情。实验时不得迟到、外出或早退。

  (4) 应保持实验室整洁,做到仪器、桌面、地面和水槽均保持干净,废纸和火柴梗等固体废物应放入指定的地方,不得扔在地上或水槽中。废酸和废碱应小心地倒入废液缸内。待用的仪器和试剂应摆放得井然有序。

(5) 公用试剂和仪器应在指定地点使用,用完后及时放回原处并使其保持整洁。防止试剂的浪费和相互污染,试剂应按规定量取用,取用固体试剂时,注意勿使其散落;试剂自瓶中取出后,不应再倒回原瓶中,以免带入杂质而引起瓶中试剂变质;试剂瓶用完后,应立即盖上瓶塞,放回原处,以免和其他瓶塞搞混;实验完毕,需回收的试剂应倒入回收瓶中。实验时要爱护仪器设备,使用精密仪器时,必须严格按照操作规程进行,要谨慎、细致。如发现仪器有故障,应立即停止使用,并及时报告指导教师。

(6) 实验记录须经教师审核。每次做完实验后,应写好实验报告,交指导教师批阅。

(7) 实验完毕,及时将玻璃仪器洗刷干净,擦净实验台,锁好实验柜,最后检查电源开关和水龙头是否关好。得到教师许可后,才能离开实验室。严禁将实验室的物品带出实验室。

(8) 学生轮流值日,值日生应负责整理公用仪器和试剂,打扫实验室,清理公共实验桌面、水槽和废物缸,检查水、电、气,关好门窗。

【实验方法】

1. 预习

预习是做好实验的前提和保证。为了避免盲目性并获得良好的实验效果,在进行实验前必须认真阅读实验教材,明确实验目的、内容、有关原理、方法、步骤(认真阅读实验技术和有关仪器的使用方法)及注意事项等,查找有关实验数据,并初步估计实验中每一步的预期结果,根据不同实验及指导教师的要求写出预习报告。

2. 实验

实验中应做到"看""想""做""记""论"。认真操作,按照操作规程和实验步骤进行实验,仔细观察实验现象("看");遇到疑难问题或异常现象,应积极思考("想");主动提出新的见解或建议,但要改变实验步骤或试剂规格及用量时,应先请示指导教师,获准后方可进行("做");及时、如实、完整地记录实验现象与数据("记"),实验记录作为原始依据,不能随便涂改;实验时相互讨论("论"),从而提高每次实验的效果。

3. 实验报告

实验报告是实验的总结。撰写实验报告是把感性认识上升到理性认识的关键环节,是培养学生思维能力、书写能力和总结能力的有效方法。实验报告应简明扼要、书写整齐规范、结果真实、结论明确。实验报告内容包括以下几个方面:

(1) 实验名称(实验日期);

（2）实验目的（写明对本实验的要求）；

（3）实验原理（简述实验的基本原理及反应方程式）；

（4）实验步骤（可结合箭头、方框、表格等形式简洁明了地表达实验进行的过程）；

（5）实验结果（包括实验数据的处理及结果表达）；

（6）实验讨论（包括对实验条件与结果进行讨论,分析实验误差产生的原因,以及回答实验教材中所附的思考题等）。

【实验室的安全】

化学实验中的试剂很多是易燃、易爆、有腐蚀性或有毒的,所用的仪器大部分是玻璃制品,如果使用不当,就有可能发生着火、爆炸、烧伤、割伤或中毒等事故。必须高度重视、敏锐洞察实验过程中的潜在危险,在实验前充分了解安全事项,在实验过程中遵守操作规程,并采取适当的预防措施,避免事故的发生。

（一）实验事故的预防

1.着火的预防

（1）水、电、气使用完毕后应立即关闭。使用酒精灯时,应随用随点,不用时盖上灯罩。不能用酒精灯直接点燃其他的酒精灯,避免酒精溢出而发生火灾。

（2）取用易燃物质（如乙醇、乙醚、丙酮等）或做涉及易燃、易挥发物质的实验时,应远离明火,并尽可能在通风橱中进行。

（3）钾、钠和白磷等暴露在空气中易燃烧,因此钾、钠应保存在煤油中,白磷应保存在水中,且取用时应用镊子夹取。

（4）易燃及易挥发物质不得倒入废物缸内,应按要求倒入指定的地方,经有关人员专门处理。

2.爆炸的预防

（1）常压操作时,切勿在密闭系统内进行加热或反应,否则体系压力增加,从而导致爆炸。

（2）强氧化剂（如氯酸钾）及其混合物（如氯酸钾与红磷、炭、硫等的混合物）不能研磨,否则易发生爆炸。

（3）氢气遇火易爆炸,操作时必须严禁接近烟火。银氨溶液不能长期保存,因久置后也易爆炸。

（4）高压气体钢瓶的主要危险是可能引发爆炸和泄漏,因此必须严格按操作规程进行操作。高压气体钢瓶应存放在阴凉、干燥的地方,远离热源,最好能存放于单独的小屋中,通过导管将气体引入实验装置。高压气体钢瓶的种类可由其颜色加以辨认（表1-1）。

表 1-1　高压气体钢瓶的标示

气体名称	瓶体颜色	字样	字样颜色	横条颜色
氧气	天蓝	氧	黑	—
氢气	深绿	氢	红	红
氮气	黑	氮	黄	棕
二氧化碳	黑	二氧化碳	黄	—
压缩空气	黑	压缩空气	白	—
硫化氢	白	硫化氢	红	红
二氧化硫	黑	二氧化硫	白	黄
石油气	灰	石油气	红	—
氩气	灰	氩	绿	—

3.中毒的预防

(1) 切勿让化学试剂沾在皮肤上,尤其是剧毒的试剂。称量任何试剂都应使用工具,不得用手直接接触,特别注意防止毒品溅入口、眼、鼻等敏感部位或接触伤口。取用有腐蚀性的化学试剂时可戴橡皮手套和防护眼镜。实验完毕要及时、认真洗手。

(2) 实验室应通风良好,尽量避免吸入化学试剂的烟雾和蒸气。如需感受物质的气味,应用手轻拂气体,将少量气体拂向自己后再嗅。处理有毒或有腐蚀性、刺激性的物质时,应在通风橱中进行,防止有毒气体在实验室内扩散。

(3) 金属汞易挥发,人吸入后易引起慢性中毒。一旦把汞洒落在桌面或地面上,应尽可能收集起来,并将硫黄粉覆盖在汞洒落的地方,使汞变成不挥发的硫化汞。液汞应保存在水中,不能将汞温度计当作玻棒使用。

(4) 不得用口尝试任何化学试剂,严禁在实验室内进食。

(5) 剧毒试剂应由专人负责,使用者必须遵守操作规程。含有毒试剂(如重铬酸钾、砷和汞的化合物、氰化物、镉盐和铅盐等)的废液不能随便倒入下水道,应统一回收后由专人处理。

4.玻璃割伤的预防

(1) 玻璃管切割后,断面应在火上烧熔以消除棱角。

(2) 将玻璃管(或温度计)插入橡皮管、橡皮塞或软木塞时,应先用水或甘油润湿玻璃管插入的一端,然后一手持橡皮管、橡皮塞或软木塞,另一手捏着玻璃管,均匀用力将其逐渐插入。应当注意的是,插入或拔出玻璃管时,手指捏住玻璃管的位置与塞子(或橡皮管)的距离不可太远,一般为 2～3 cm。插入弯形玻璃管时,不能把弯曲处当成旋柄来用力。正确方法如图 1-1 所示。

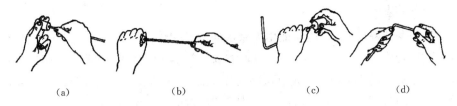

(a)　　　　　　(b)　　　　　　(c)　　　　　　(d)

图 1-1　玻璃管(或温度计)插入橡皮管、橡皮塞的方法

(a)正确;(b)不正确;(c)正确;(d)不正确

(二) 实验事故的处理

1. 着火

一旦发生着火事故,首先应立即关闭附近所有的火源,切断电源,迅速移去着火现场周围的易燃物质。用石棉布、干沙或适当的灭火器材灭火。常用灭火器的适用范围见表 1-2。有机溶剂着火时,在大多数情况下,严禁用水灭火,应用沙土覆盖。因为有机溶剂一般比水轻,燃着的液体会在水面上蔓延开来,使燃烧面积扩大。

如果实验者衣服着火,切勿惊慌乱跑,以免因空气的扰动而使火势扩大。可迅速脱下衣服或用石棉布、厚外套覆盖着火处,将火闷熄。情况危急时应就地卧倒打滚,以免火焰烧向头部。

如果着火面积较大,在尽力扑救的同时及时拨打"119"报警。

表 1-2　实验室常用灭火器及其适用范围

灭火器类型	成　分	适 用 范 围
酸碱式	H_2SO_4 和 $NaHCO_3$	非油类和电器的一般初起火灾
泡沫灭火器	$Al_2(SO_4)_3$ 和 $NaHCO_3$	油类起火
二氧化碳灭火器	液态 CO_2	电器设备、小范围油类及忌水化学物品的失火
四氯化碳灭火器	液态 CCl_4	电器设备、小范围汽油、丙酮等的失火,不能用于活泼金属钾、钠的失火(否则会因强烈分解而发生爆炸)
干粉灭火器	$NaHCO_3$、硬脂酸铝、云母粉、滑石粉等	油类、可燃性气体、精密仪器和遇水易燃物品的初起火灾
1211 灭火器	CF_2ClBr 液化气体	特别适用于油类、有机溶剂、精密仪器、高压设备的失火

2. 烫伤

切记用自来水冲洗。轻伤者可用 $KMnO_4$ 或苦味酸溶液涂于烫伤处,再搽上凡士林或烫伤膏(如万花油、氧化锌软膏等);重伤者应涂以烫伤膏,而后立即送医院治疗。

3.化学灼伤

皮肤被酸或碱灼伤时,应立即用大量水冲洗。酸灼伤用5％ $NaHCO_3$ 溶液(或肥皂水)洗,碱灼伤则用1％乙酸(或5％硼酸)洗,然后用水冲洗。若是氢氟酸灼伤,则应在水冲洗后用稀 Na_2CO_3 溶液中和,然后浸泡在冷的 $MgSO_4$ 饱和溶液中半小时,最后敷上特制药膏(20％ $MgSO_4$ 、18％甘油、1.2％盐酸普鲁卡因、水)。

皮肤被溴灼伤时,伤处立即用石油醚或乙醇冲洗,然后用2％ $Na_2S_2O_3$ 溶液清洗,最后用蘸有甘油的棉花擦干并敷上烫伤膏。

眼睛被试剂灼伤时,应立即用大量水冲洗,快速送往医院治疗,不允许用其他试剂进行中和。

4.玻璃割伤

一般轻伤,应立即挤出污血,用消毒过的镊子取出玻璃碎片,用洁净水洗净伤口,涂上碘酒,再用绷带包扎。如果为大伤口,应立即用绷带扎紧伤口上部进行止血,然后送医院治疗。

5.中毒

在进行有毒物质的实验时最好戴口罩。如果有毒物质不幸进入口中,首先应用大量水漱口,饮用大量清水后用手指伸入咽喉处,促使呕吐(若是腐蚀剂中毒则不宜采用此法,可服用牛奶、蛋清或植物油等),然后立即送医院治疗。

吸入 Br_2 蒸气或 Cl_2 蒸气时,可通过吸入少量乙醇和乙醚的混合蒸气以解毒。吸入 H_2S 气体而感到头晕时,应到室外呼吸新鲜空气,必要时尽快送医院治疗。

6.触电

遇到触电事件时,首先要拉开电闸以切断电源,并尽快用绝缘物(干燥的木棒、竹竿等)将触电者与电源隔离,必要时进行人工呼吸并迅速将伤者送医院救治。

【实验室三废处理】

化学实验室的"三废"即废气、废液和废渣,若"三废"排放到空气或下水道中,将对环境造成污染,威胁人们的健康。如 Cl_2 、 SO_2 等气体对人的呼吸道有强烈的刺激作用,对植物也有伤害作用;As、Pb、Hg 等的化合物进入人体后,不易分解和排出,长期积累会引起胃痛、皮下出血、肾功能损伤等;氯仿、 CCl_4 等能导致肝癌;多环芳烃导致皮肤病和膀胱癌。因此,要治理这些环境污染,从根本上来讲,实现化学实验教学的环保化是唯一途径。目前,一方面,要大力推广微型实验,从节约试剂、减少污染物的产生方面入手;另一方面,必须对实验过程中产生的有毒、有害物质进行必要的处理。

1.常用的废气处理方法

(1)溶液吸收法。溶液吸收法是用适当的液体吸收剂处理气体混合物,从而除去其中的有害气体的方法。常用的液体吸收剂有水、碱性溶液、酸性溶液、氧化剂溶液和有机溶液,它们可用于净化含有 Cl_2、HCl、HF、NH_3、SO_2、NO_x、酸雾和各种有机物蒸气等的废气。

(2)固体吸收法。固体吸收法是使废气与固体吸收剂接触,废气中的污染物吸附在吸收剂表面从而被分离出来的方法。常用的固体吸收剂有活性炭、活性氧化铝、硅胶和分子筛等。

2.常用的废水处理方法

(1)中和法。对于酸含量为 $3\%\sim5\%$ 或更低的酸性废水或碱含量为 $1\%\sim3\%$ 或更低的碱性废水,常采用中和法进行处理。

(2)化学沉淀法。在废水中加入某种化学试剂,使其与其中的污染物发生化学反应,生成沉淀而被分离,如氢氧化物沉淀法和硫化物沉淀法等。该法适用于除去废水中的重金属离子、碱土金属离子及某些非金属等。

(3)氧化还原法。水中溶解的有害无机物或有机物,可通过化学反应将其氧化或还原,转化成无害的新物质或易从水中分离除去的形态。常用的氧化剂有漂白粉等,常用的还原剂有 $FeSO_4$、Na_2SO_3、铁屑、锌粒等。

此外,还有吸附法、萃取法、离子交换法、电化学净化法等。而对于有机溶剂废液,可经蒸馏、分馏后分类回收,循环使用。

3.常用的废渣处理方法

废渣处理主要采用掩埋法。有毒废渣必须先进行化学处理后深埋在远离居民区的指定地点。

第二节 基 本 知 识

【基础化学实验常用仪器】

基础化学实验常用仪器如图 1-2 所示。

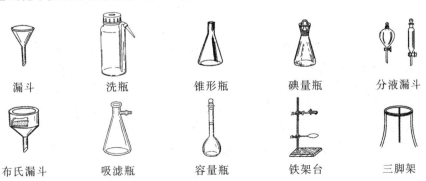

| 漏斗 | 洗瓶 | 锥形瓶 | 碘量瓶 | 分液漏斗 |

| 布氏漏斗 | 吸滤瓶 | 容量瓶 | 铁架台 | 三脚架 |

图 1-2　基础化学实验常用仪器

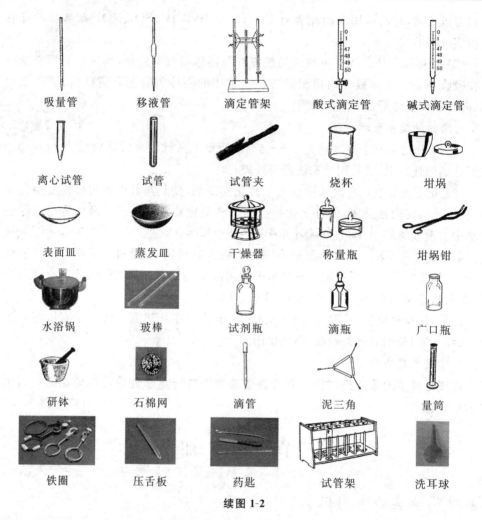

续图 1-2

【常用玻璃仪器的洗涤与干燥】

1.洗涤

化学实验必须在干净的容器中进行,才能得到正确、可靠的结果。因此,在开始实验之前,必须将仪器洗涤干净。

洗涤仪器的方法很多,应根据实验的要求、污物的性质和沾污的程度来选用。一般来说,附着在仪器上的污物既有可溶性物质,也有尘土或其他不溶性物质,如油污等。针对这种情况,可以分别采用下列洗涤方法。

(1) 水刷洗。用毛刷刷洗,可洗去可溶性物质和尘土,但往往洗不去油污和有机物质。

(2) 去污粉或合成洗涤剂洗。去污粉中含有 Na_2CO_3,合成洗涤剂中含有表面活性剂,它们都能除去仪器上的油污。

（3）铬酸洗液洗。对于口径细小的仪器,如容量瓶、移液管、吸量管、滴定管等,很难用上述方法洗涤,可用铬酸洗液洗。

铬酸洗液的配制:4 g 重铬酸钾溶解在 100 mL 温热的浓 H_2SO_4 溶液中。铬酸洗液具有很强的氧化性,对有机物和油污的去除能力特别强。

洗涤时,在仪器中加入少量洗液,倾斜仪器,来回旋转,使器壁全部被洗液润湿,稍等片刻,待洗液与污物充分作用,然后把洗液倒回原瓶,再用自来水把残留洗液冲洗干净。如果用洗液将仪器浸泡一段时间,或用热的洗液洗,则效果更好。

使用洗液时必须注意以下几点。

① 尽量把待洗仪器内的积水除去后,再注入洗液,以免洗液被稀释。

② 使用后的洗液应倒回原瓶,可以反复使用至失效为止（失效的洗液呈绿色,为重铬酸钾被还原后的硫酸铬的颜色）。

③ 绝不允许将毛刷放入洗液中刷洗。

④ 洗液具有很强的腐蚀性,会灼伤皮肤和损坏衣物。若不慎把洗液洒在皮肤、衣物或实验桌上,应立即用水冲洗。

⑤ Cr(Ⅵ)有毒,其残液排入下水道中会污染环境,造成公害,因此要尽量避免使用。

（4）碱液。NaOH 的乙醇溶液可用于洗涤油脂或一些有机酸等。

（5）有机溶剂洗涤。当胶状或焦油状的有机污垢用上述方法不能洗去时,可选用丙酮浸泡,并加盖以免丙酮挥发,然后用清水洗净。

（6）超声波清洗。有机合成实验中常用超声波清洗器来洗涤玻璃仪器,该法省时、方便。把用过的玻璃仪器放在配有洗涤剂的溶液中,用超声波清洗,即可达到清洗仪器的目的。

（7）特殊物质的去除。根据沾在器壁上的污物的性质,采取"对症下药"的方法进行处理。如 MnO_2 或碳酸盐可用 HCl 溶液或草酸溶液洗净,AgCl 沉淀可用氨水处理,难溶的硫化物沉淀可用王水溶解。

已洗净的仪器,可以被水润湿,将水倒出后将仪器倒置,可观察到仪器透明,器壁不挂水珠,否则仪器尚未洗净。

2.干燥

玻璃仪器洗净后,可用自然晾干、电吹风吹干或电热鼓风干燥箱烘干后保存。

（1）晾干。不急用的、要求一般干燥的仪器,可将洗净后的仪器倒置在干净的实验柜内或仪器架上,任其自然晾干。

（2）烤干。烧杯、蒸发皿等可以放在石棉网上用小火烤干。试管可直接在酒精灯的火焰上烤干,但试管口应稍向下倾斜,从底部烤起,无水珠时再使试管口向上,以便把水汽赶净。

（3）吹干。急用的仪器或不能用烘干方法干燥的仪器可以吹干。方法是先倒出水分,再用电吹风吹干,先冷风吹 1～2 min,再热风吹至接近干燥,最后冷风吹干。

(4) 烘干。实验室中常用的是电热鼓风干燥箱,温度可以控制在 50～300 ℃。其主要用来干燥玻璃仪器或无腐蚀性、加热时不分解的试剂。

【实验室用水的规格】

我国已建立了实验室用水规格的国家标准(GB/T 6682—2008),该标准规定了实验室用水的技术指标、制备方法及检验方法。实验室用水的级别及主要技术指标如表1-3所示。

表 1-3　实验室用水的级别和主要技术指标

指 标 名 称	一级	二级	三级
pH 值范围(25 ℃)	—	—	5.0～7.5
电导率(25 ℃)/(μS · m^{-1})	≤10	≤100	≤500
吸光度(254 nm,1 cm 光程)	≤0.001	≤0.01	—
可溶性硅(以 SiO_2 计)/(mg · L^{-1})	<0.01	<0.02	—

实验室常用的蒸馏水、去离子水和电导水在 25 ℃时的电导率与三级水的指标相近。纯水必须严格保持纯净,为了防止污染,在储存、运输过程中可选用聚乙烯容器。一级水一般在使用前临时制取。

1. 纯水的制备

(1) 蒸馏水。将自来水在蒸馏装置中加热汽化、冷却,即得到蒸馏水。此法能除去水中的非挥发性杂质,但不能完全除去水中溶解的气体杂质。此外,一般蒸馏装置所用的材料是不锈钢、纯铝或玻璃,所以可能会带入金属离子。

(2) 去离子水。将自来水依次通过阳离子树脂交换柱、阴离子树脂交换柱及两者混合的交换柱后所得的水即为去离子水。离子树脂交换柱除去离子的效果好,去离子水的纯度比蒸馏水高。但此法不能除去非离子型杂质,因此去离子水中常含微生物和少量有机物。

(3) 电导水。在第一套蒸馏器(最好是石英制的,其次是硬质玻璃制的)中装入蒸馏水,加入少量高锰酸钾固体,经蒸馏除去水中的有机物,得重蒸水。再将重蒸水注入第二套蒸馏器(最好也是石英制的)中,加入少许硫酸钡和硫酸氢钾固体,进行蒸馏。弃去馏头、馏后各 10 mL,收集中间馏分。电导水应保存在带有碱石灰吸收管的硬质玻璃瓶内,放置时间不能太长,一般在两周以内。

(4) 三级水。采用蒸馏法或离子交换法制备。

(5) 二级水。将三级水再次蒸馏后制得,可能含有微量的无机、有机或胶态杂质。

(6) 一级水。将二级水经进一步处理后制得。如将二级水用石英蒸馏器再次蒸馏,制得的水基本上不含胶态杂质及有机物。

2.水纯度的检验

由表 1-3 可知,纯水质量的主要指标是电导率,可用电导率仪(最小量程为 0.02 $\mu S \cdot m^{-1}$)来测定。

【固体样品的干燥方法和干燥器的使用】

1.自然干燥

自然干燥适用于在空气中稳定、不吸潮的固体。将样品在干燥、洁净的表面皿、滤纸或其他敞口容器中摊开,上面覆盖透气物体以防灰尘落入,任其在空气中通风晾干。此法最简便、经济。

2.加热干燥

加热干燥适用于熔点较高且遇热不分解的固体。将样品置于表面皿或蒸发皿中,用电热鼓风干燥箱或红外灯烘干,注意加热温度必须低于样品的熔点。在较高温度下易分解的样品宜用真空恒温干燥箱于较低温度下烘干。

3.干燥器干燥

干燥器干燥适用于易吸潮、分解或升华的物质。干燥器由厚质玻璃制成,上面是一个带磨口边的盖子(盖子的磨口边上一般涂有凡士林),底部放有干燥的氯化钙或变色硅胶等干燥剂,干燥剂的上面放一个带孔的圆形瓷盘,可承放需干燥或保持干燥的物品。

操作时,用左手扶住干燥器的底部,右手沿水平方向移动盖子,即可将干燥器打开(图 1-3(a))。盖子打开后,将盖子翻过来放在桌子上(不要使涂有凡士林的磨口边触及桌面)。放入或取出物品后,必须将盖子盖好,此时也应将盖子沿水平方向推移,使盖子的磨口边与干燥器口吻合。

搬动干燥器时,必须用两手的大拇指将盖子按住(图 1-3(b)),以防盖子滑落而打碎。

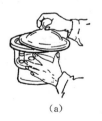
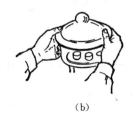

(a)　　　　　　　　　　　(b)

图 1-3　干燥器的使用

(a)打开干燥器的方法;(b)搬动干燥器的方法

使用干燥器时应注意下列事项。

(1) 干燥器应保持清洁,不得存放很潮湿的物品。温度很高的物品必须冷却至接近室温后,方可放入干燥器内。否则,干燥器内空气受热膨胀,可能将盖子冲开,即使盖子能盖好,也往往因冷却后,干燥器内空气压力降低,致使盖子很难打开。

(2) 干燥器只在需要用时打开,东西取出或放入后,应立即盖上盖子,以免干燥剂受潮。

(3) 放在底部的干燥剂,不得高于底部的 1/2 处,以防沾污被干燥的物品。

(4) 应经常观察干燥剂是否失效,一旦失效应更换新的干燥剂。

干燥器长期不用后(尤其在冬天),磨口边的凡士林因凝固而难以打开,可以用湿的热毛巾或电吹风热风吹干燥器的边缘,使凡士林融化,再打开盖子。

【温度计和停表的使用】

1. 温度计的使用

实验室最常用的是膨胀式温度计。它是用玻璃毛细管制成的,毛细管内充有水银、酒精或甲苯。普通毛细管温度计有不同的规格,可以测至 0.1 ℃;刻度为 0.1 ℃ 的温度计比较精确,可测至 0.01 ℃。

测量液体的温度时要选用适当量程的温度计,使用时将水银球完全浸没在液体中,但不能使水银球接触容器的底部或器壁。使用温度计时要轻拿轻放,温度计水银球部位的玻璃很薄,容易打破,温度计不能当作玻棒搅拌液体。刚测量高温的温度计不能立即用冷水冲洗或测低温液体,否则会使液柱快速缩回导致液柱断开。不能把温度计长时间放在高温的液体中,否则会使水银球变形而导致读数不准。温度计用后应悬挂在铁架台上让它慢慢冷却,冷却后洗净抹干保存。

2. 停表的使用

实验室常用的停表是秒表和定时钟。使用时应首先检查各部件和各旋钮是否齐全,然后向下按动表侧面的开关,再用拇指按下表顶端的柄头,表针便走动,第二次按下柄头,表针停止,即可读出时间,第三次按下柄头,表针回复原位(零点)。测量过程中若需暂停,可向上推动表侧面的开关,表针便停止,再向下按表侧面的开关,表针继续走动。

使用停表前应先检查零点(表针指在零刻度)。若不在零点,可记下差距,最后校准。停表不能碰撞或敲打,要保持其干燥和清洁。

【试剂及其取用】

1. 化学试剂的规格

世界各国对化学试剂的分类和分级的标准不尽一致,都有自己国家、行业及学会的标准。国际标准化组织(ISO)近年来已经陆续颁布了许多种化学试剂的国际标准。国际纯粹与应用化学联合会(IUPAC)将化学标准物质分为五级,其中 C 级和 D 级为滴定分析标准试剂,E 级为一般试剂。我国的化学试剂标准有国家标准(GB)、化工部标准(HG)及企业标准(QB)三级。我国常用试剂等级的划分参见表 1-4。

表 1-4　我国的试剂规格及适用范围

等　　级	一级品	二级品	三级品	四级品
名称	优级纯	分析纯	化学纯	生物试剂
英文名称	guarantee reagent	analytical reagent	chemically pure	biological reagent
表示的符号	GR	AR	CP	BR
适用范围	精密分析及科研工作	一般的分析及科研工作	一般定性及化学制备	—
标签标志	绿色	红色	蓝色	黄色或其他颜色

除上述四个等级外,还根据特殊需要而定出相应的纯度规格,如供光谱分析用的光谱纯(高纯试剂)、供核试验及其分析用的核纯等。

此外,化学试剂中的指示剂,其纯度往往不太明确。生物化学中使用的特殊试剂纯度的表示方法与化学试剂也有所不同,如蛋白质类试剂的纯度常以含量表示,而酶试剂则以酶的活力来表示。

不同的试剂具有不同的纯度标准。总的来说,优级纯试剂杂质含量最低,实验试剂杂质含量较高。选用适当等级的试剂应根据实际工作的需要,既要满足工作要求,又要避免浪费。

2.化学试剂的保管

由于化学试剂种类繁多,性质各异,有些试剂会因保管不当而变质失效,严重的会导致实验失败甚至发生事故,因此,化学试剂的保管十分重要,一般应注意如下几点。

(1)剧毒试剂:如氰化物和含砷、汞的化合物及 HF 等,要有严格的领用登记制度。

(2)见光易分解及易被空气氧化的试剂:如 H_2O_2、$AgNO_3$ 和 $SnCl_2$、$FeSO_4$ 等,要用棕色瓶存放,并置冷暗处。

(3)吸水性强的试剂:如无水 Na_2CO_3、Na_2O_2 等,应严格密封保存于干燥器中。

(4)易腐蚀玻璃的试剂:如 NaOH、HF 等,要用塑料瓶存放。

(5)易相互反应的试剂:如氧化剂和还原剂,要分开存放。

(6)易挥发的试剂:如有机溶剂等,要存放在有通风设备的专用试剂柜中。

3.化学试剂的取用

所有化学试剂瓶都应有标签,标明试剂的名称、规格及配制日期。无标签的试剂在未确定品种和规格前不能取用。

瓶盖(塞)取下后应将顶部朝下放在干净的桌面上,还原时要对号入座,以免交叉沾污。

除校验 pH 计的标准缓冲溶液外,任何已取出试剂瓶的试剂均不得再倒回原瓶内。

(1)固体试剂的取用。在实验室中,固体试剂一般放在广口瓶中,常用药匙取用,专匙专用。药匙的两端一头大、一头小,大头端取用大量固体,小头端取用少量固体。取用时,如果瓶塞顶是扁平的,瓶塞取出后可倒置桌上;如果瓶塞顶不平,可用食指和中指(或中指和无名指)将瓶塞夹住或放在清洁的表面皿上,绝不可将它横置桌上。一般的固体试剂可放在干燥的纸上称量,具有腐蚀性或易潮解的固体应放在表面皿或玻璃容器内称量;固体颗粒较大时,可在清洁干燥的研钵中研碎。有毒试剂要在教师指导下取用。向试管中加入固体试剂时,应先将试管平放,用药匙或干净的对折纸片装上固体试剂后伸进试管距管口约 2/3 处,将试管慢慢竖直,使固体试剂沿管壁慢慢滑下,以免碰破管底。

(2)液体试剂的取用。在实验室中,液体试剂一般放在细口瓶或滴瓶中。取用细口瓶中的液体试剂时,用右手掌心向着标签处握住试剂瓶,瓶口紧靠盛接容器边缘慢慢倾倒(图 1-4(a)),直至所需量。倒完后,将试剂瓶在盛接容器口上靠一下,再将瓶竖起,盖上瓶盖。向烧杯中倒液体时,则左手持一玻棒,其下端紧靠烧杯内壁,斜搁于烧杯中,试剂瓶口紧靠玻棒慢慢倾倒液体,使液体沿玻棒流入烧杯,如图 1-4(b)所示。

从滴瓶中取液体试剂时,要使用滴瓶中的滴管,注意保持滴管垂直,避免倾斜,尤忌倒立,以防试剂流入乳胶头内弄脏乳胶头。使用时提起滴管,使管口离开液面,用手指紧捏滴管上部乳胶头,赶出空气,然后伸入滴瓶中,放开手指,吸入试剂。将试剂滴入试管中时,必须将它悬空地放在靠近试管口的上方,然后挤捏乳胶头,使试剂滴入试管中(图 1-4(c))。绝不可将滴管伸入试管中,否则,滴管口易沾有试管壁上的其他液体,如果再将此滴管放入滴瓶中,则会沾污该瓶试剂。滴瓶中的滴管,使用后应立即插回原来的滴瓶中。

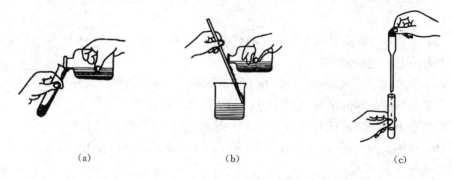

(a)　　　　　　(b)　　　　　　(c)

图 1-4　从试剂瓶中取出液体试剂

(a)向试管中倒入液体试剂;(b)往烧杯中倒入液体试剂;(c)用滴管滴加液体试剂的正确操作

定量取用液体试剂时,可用量筒或移液管。用量筒量取液体时,应左手持量筒,并以大拇指指示所需体积的刻度处。右手持试剂瓶(标签应在手心处),瓶口紧靠量筒口边缘,慢慢注入液体(图1-5(a))到所指刻度。读取刻度时,视线应与液面在同一水平面上(图1-5(b))。如果不谨慎,倾出了过多的液体,多取的试剂不能倒回原瓶,应将其弃去或及时给他人使用。对于1 mL、2 mL等少量试剂的量取可用滴管滴加(1 mL为20~25滴)。

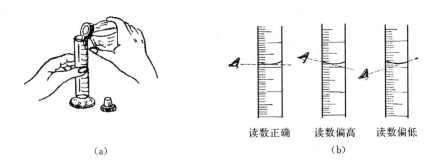

(a)

读数正确　　读数偏高　　读数偏低

(b)

图1-5　量筒的使用

(a)量筒量取液体的操作;(b)量筒的读数方法

试剂取用后,必须立即将瓶塞盖好。实验室中试剂瓶的摆放,一般均有一定的次序和位置,不得任意变动。取用浓酸、浓碱等腐蚀性试剂时,要防止沾到眼睛、皮肤或洒在衣服上。如果酸、碱等洒在桌上,应立即用湿布擦去;如果沾到眼睛或皮肤,要立即用大量清水冲洗(参见实验室意外事故的处理)。

【加热和冷却】

(一)加热

1.常用加热仪器

(1)酒精灯。酒精灯一般是玻璃制的,由灯帽、灯芯、灯壶三个部分组成。其灯焰温度通常可达400~500 ℃,外焰温度最高,内焰次之,焰心最低。酒精灯常用于温度不需太高的实验。切勿用点燃的酒精灯直接点火;添加酒精时,必须将火焰熄灭且加入的量不能超过灯壶容量的2/3;熄灭酒精灯时必须用灯罩罩熄,切勿用嘴吹灭。

(2)电炉。电炉是一种用电热丝将电能转化为热能的装置。其温度的高低可通过调节电阻来控制。使用时,容器和电炉之间要添加石棉网,以使受热均匀。

(3)数显恒温水浴锅。数显恒温水浴锅有两孔、四孔、六孔等不同规格。水浴锅恒温范围一般为37~100 ℃,用于蒸发和恒温加热。

(4)马弗炉。马弗炉一般可以加热到1 000 ℃以上,并适用于某一温度下长时间加热。

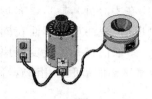

图1-6　电加热套

(5) 电加热套。电加热套是由玻璃纤维包裹着电热丝制成的碗状半球形加热器(图1-6),可以密切地贴合在烧瓶的周围,因而加热较为均匀。电加热套有可调控温度装置,可以提供100 ℃以上的温度,加热迅速,使用安全,适用范围较广,但必须注意不可用来加热空烧瓶,否则会烧坏电加热套。

(6)电吹风。电吹风(图1-7(a))有两个热风挡和一个冷风挡。电吹风使用完后须悬挂在铁圈上直至喷口冷却(图1-7(b))。电吹风主要用于玻璃仪器的快速干燥和薄层分析中。

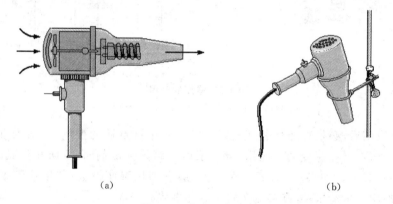

(a)　　　　　　　　　　　　　　　　　　(b)

图1-7　电吹风的使用

(a) 电吹风；(b)电吹风的放置

升降台是一种升降稳定性好、适用范围广的物体举升设备。它主要用于调节加热套和水浴锅的高度以适应已经装配好的反应装置(图1-8)。

2.加热方法

(1) 直接加热。在加热前必须将容器外壁擦干。在火焰上加热试管时,试管内的液体量不得超过试管容量的1/3,应使用试管夹夹住试管的中上部,试管与桌面成约60°的角(图1-9(a))。如果加热液体,应先加

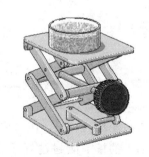

图1-8　升降台

热液体的中上部,慢慢移动试管,加热下部,然后不时上下移动或摇荡试管,务必使各部分液体受热均匀,以免管内液体因受热不均匀而骤然溅出。

如果加热潮湿的或加热后有水产生的固体,应将试管口稍微向下倾斜,使管口略低于底部(图1-9(b)),以免在试管口冷凝的水流向灼热的管底,使试管破裂。

加热烧杯中的液体时,液体量不应超过烧杯容量的1/2,烧杯应放在石棉网上加热,使之受热均匀,如图1-9(c)所示。同时,还需适当搅拌,以防烧杯内液体暴沸。

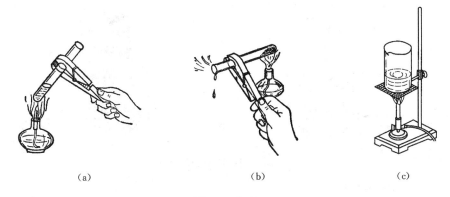

图 1-9　加热

(a)加热试管中的液体;(b)加热试管中的固体;(c)加热烧杯中的液体

(2)水浴加热。当被加热物要求受热均匀,而温度又不能超过 100 ℃时,用水浴加热(常在数显恒温水浴锅、一般水浴锅或烧杯中进行,如图 1-10 所示)。如果需要加热到 100 ℃,可用沸水浴或蒸汽浴的方式。同时应注意,水浴锅内存水量应保持在总体积的 2/3 左右。离心试管由于管底玻璃较薄,不宜直接加热,应在水浴中加热。

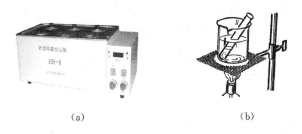

图 1-10　水浴加热装置

(a)数显恒温水浴锅;(b)烧杯代替水浴锅加热

(3)油浴加热。加热温度若需为 100～250 ℃,可用油浴方式。容器内反应物的温度一般要比油浴温度低 20 ℃左右。油浴锅一般以玻璃缸、不锈钢锅为宜。油浴中应悬挂温度计,并用调压器随时调控油浴温度,当油的冒烟情况严重时,应停止加热。常用的油类有液体石蜡、植物油(如棉籽油)、硬化油(如氢化棉籽油)、硅油等。植物油加热后因部分分解而冒烟,故不宜超过 200 ℃;液体石蜡过热虽不分解,但易冒烟和燃烧,只可加热到 220 ℃左右;硬化油可加热到 250 ℃左右;硅油在 250 ℃仍稳定,不冒烟,透明度好,只是价格较高。水浴和油浴的优点是受热均匀,易控制,比较安全。

(4)沙浴加热。采用沙浴方式时,可加热到 350 ℃。将清洁而又干燥的细沙平铺于铁盘上,把盛有液体的容器埋入沙中,容器底部沙层稍薄,便于受热;容器周围的沙层要厚,以利于保温(图 1-11)。沙浴的缺点是沙的传热能力较差,温度分布不

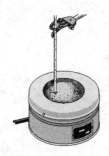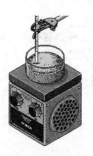

图 1-11 沙浴加热

均匀,散热较快,不易控制。

(二)冷却

有些化学反应需要在低温下进行,一些制备操作如结晶、液态物质的凝固等也需要低温冷却。可根据所要求的温度条件,选择不同的冷却剂。

水可使温度降到接近室温,冰水制冷剂可得到 0 ℃的温度。若需要将温度降到0 ℃以下,可用碎冰和某些无机盐按一定比例混合后作为制冷剂。有机溶剂制冷剂,如干冰、丙酮等溶剂以适当比例混合,可以冷却到 -78 ℃。液氮可冷却到 -196 ℃,而液态氦可冷却到 -268.9 ℃。常用制冷剂及其最低制冷温度如表 1-5 所示。

表 1-5 常见制冷剂及其最低制冷温度

制 冷 剂	最低制冷温度/℃	制 冷 剂	最低制冷温度/℃
冰-水	0	$CaCl_2 \cdot 6H_2O$-碎冰(1.25:1)	-40.3
NaCl-碎冰(1:3)	-20	液氨	-33
NaCl-碎冰(1:1)	-22	干冰	-78.5
NH_4Cl-碎冰(1:4)	-15	液态甲烷	-161.4
NH_4Cl-碎冰(1:2)	-17	液氧	-183.0
$CaCl_2$-碎冰(1:1)	-29	液氮	-195.8

当操作温度低于 -38 ℃时,不可再使用水银温度计,而应使用低温温度计(内装甲苯、正戊烷等有机溶剂)。此外,使用低温冷浴时,为防止外界热量的传入,冷浴锅外壁应用隔热材料包裹覆盖。

【溶解、蒸发和结晶】

1.固体的溶解

物质的溶解在烧杯、烧瓶或试管中进行。若固体的颗粒较大,应先在洁净、干燥的研钵中研碎。溶解固体时,常用搅拌、加热等方法以加快溶解的速度,但要注意根据被加热固体的热稳定性,有针对性地选用不同的加热方法。

2.蒸发与浓缩

当需从稀溶液中析出晶体时,需要进行蒸发、浓缩、结晶的操作。将稀溶液放入蒸发皿中,缓慢加热并不断搅拌,溶液中的水分便不断蒸发,溶液不断浓缩,当蒸发至一定程度后,放置冷却即可析出晶体。溶液浓缩的程度与被结晶物质的溶解度大小及溶解度随温度的变化情况等因素有关。若被结晶物质的溶解度较小或随温度变化较大,则蒸发至出现晶膜即可;若被结晶物质的溶解度随温度变化不大,则蒸发至稀粥状后再冷却。若希望得到大颗粒的晶体,则不宜浓缩得太浓。

在实验室中,蒸发、浓缩的过程是在蒸发皿中完成的,蒸发皿中所盛放的溶液量不可超过其容量的 2/3。一般当物质的热稳定性较好时,可将蒸发皿直接放在石棉网上加热蒸发,否则需用水浴间接加热蒸发。

3.结晶与重结晶

当溶液浓缩到一定程度(饱和)时,冷却后就有晶体析出,此过程称为结晶。晶体析出的颗粒大小和结晶的条件有关,溶液浓缩得较浓、溶解度随温度变化较大、快速冷却、搅拌溶液都会使晶体的颗粒较小;反之,会使晶体长成较大的颗粒。晶体颗粒的大小也与晶体的纯度有关。若晶体颗粒太小且大小不均匀,易形成糊状物,夹带母液较多,从而影响纯度。缓慢长成的大晶体,在生长过程中也易包裹母液,影响纯度。因此,颗粒大小适中、均匀的晶体纯度高。

若一次结晶所得晶体的纯度不符合要求,可进行重结晶。重结晶是提纯固体物质常用、有效的方法之一,它适用于溶解度随温度变化较大、杂质含量小于 5% 、被提纯物与杂质间溶解度相差较大的一类化合物的提纯。重结晶的操作一般如下:加适量的水(或其他溶剂)于被提纯物中,加热溶解并蒸发溶液至饱和,趁热过滤,除去不溶性杂质,滤液经冷却后,析出被提纯物,杂质留在母液中,通过过滤、洗涤,可得到纯度较高的晶体。若一次重结晶达不到纯度要求,可再次重结晶。

【沉淀的分离和洗涤】

沉淀(晶体)与溶液的分离方法一般有三种:倾析法、过滤法和离心分离法。

1.倾析法

当沉淀的密度较大或结晶颗粒较大,静置后能较快沉降至容器底部时,常用倾析法进行沉淀的分离和洗涤。该方法是把沉淀上部的清液沿玻棒小心倾入另一容器内(图 1-12),然后向盛沉淀的容器内加入少量洗涤剂,充分搅拌后,让沉淀下沉,倾去洗涤剂。重复操作三次,即能将沉淀洗净。

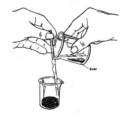

图 1-12　倾析法

2.过滤法

过滤法是最常用的固液分离方法,常用的过滤法有常压过滤、减压过滤和热过滤三种。

(1) 常压过滤。在常压下,使用普通漏斗过滤的方法称为常压过滤。此法简便、常用,适合颗粒较小的沉淀的过滤,但过滤速度较慢。常用的滤器是贴有滤纸的漏斗。先将滤纸对折两次(若滤纸不是圆形的,此时应剪成圆形),拨开一层即成圆锥形,内角为60°(标准的漏斗内角为60°,若漏斗角度不标准,应适当改变滤纸折叠的角度,使其能配合所用漏斗),一边是三层,另一边是一层,在三层的一边撕去一个小角(图 1-13(a))。再把圆锥形滤纸平整地放入干净的漏斗中,使滤纸与漏斗壁靠紧。用左手食指按住滤纸,右手持洗瓶挤水(或加入溶剂)使滤纸湿润,然后用清洁的手指(或玻棒)轻压,使之紧贴在漏斗壁上,此时滤纸与漏斗密合,其间不留气泡。一般滤纸边缘应低于漏斗边缘 3～5 mm。将漏斗放在漏斗架上,下面放置接收滤液的容器,漏斗颈口长的一边紧靠容器壁,使滤液沿容器壁流下,不致溅出。过滤时一般采用倾析法,即将沉淀上面的清液小心地倾入滤纸上,尽可能让沉淀留在烧杯内。倾析时,溶液沿着玻棒流入漏斗中,如图 1-13(b)所示。玻棒的下端靠着三层滤纸的一边。随着溶液的倾入,将玻棒逐渐提高,以免触及液面,待漏斗中液面离滤纸边缘约5 mm 时,暂时停止倾注,以免少量沉淀因毛细作用越过滤纸上缘,造成损失。暂停倾注时,应将烧杯嘴沿玻棒向上提,并逐渐竖直烧杯,避免烧杯嘴上的液滴流到烧杯外壁,再将玻棒放回烧杯中。注意玻棒绝对不可放在桌上,也不可放在烧杯嘴处,以免使沾在玻棒上的少量沉淀损失和污染。如此进行,至沉淀上的清液几乎全部倾入漏斗中为止。杯中沉淀的洗涤:用滴管将洗涤液(约需 10 mL)沿杯壁四周淋洗,使沾在杯壁的沉淀集中到烧杯底部,用玻棒搅动沉淀,充分洗涤,待沉淀下沉后,将上层清液以倾析法过滤。初步洗涤若干次后,可将沉淀转移到滤纸上。转移的方法:在盛有沉淀的烧杯中加入少量洗涤液并搅动,然后立即按上述方法将悬浮液转移到滤

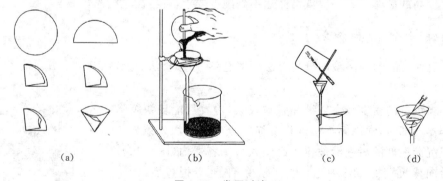

图 1-13　常压过滤

(a)滤纸的折法;(b)常压过滤;(c)沉淀的转移;(d)漏斗中沉淀的洗涤

纸上,再向烧杯中加入少量洗涤液并转移。如此重复几次,一般可将大部分沉淀转移到滤纸上。最后少量沉淀的转移可按图 1-13(c)所示的方法进行,即将烧杯倾斜放在漏斗上方,烧杯嘴朝着漏斗,将玻棒架在烧杯嘴上,玻棒下端对着三层滤纸处,用洗涤液冲洗烧杯内壁,沉淀连同溶液一起流入漏斗中。重复上述步骤,至沉淀完全转移为止。沉淀全部转移到滤纸上后,需进行最后的洗涤,方法是用洗涤液冲洗滤纸边缘稍下一些的部位,按螺旋形向下移动,如图 1-13(d)所示,使沉淀集中于滤纸底部。重复上述步骤,直至沉淀洗净。洗涤沉淀时应遵循"少量多次"的原则。如果需过滤的混合物中含有能与滤纸作用的物质(如浓 H_2SO_4 溶液),则可用石棉或玻璃丝在漏斗中铺成薄层作为滤器。

(2) 减压过滤(抽吸或抽气过滤)。过滤装置由吸滤瓶、布氏漏斗、安全瓶和抽气泵(水泵)四个部分组成,如图 1-14 所示。减压过滤的原理是利用玻璃抽气管把吸滤瓶中的空气抽出,造成部分真空,而使过滤速度大大加快。安全瓶的作用是防止抽气管中的水倒流进吸滤瓶中。减压过滤的特点是快速、沉淀易被抽干。但颗粒太小的沉淀和胶体沉淀,不适宜用此法过滤。减压过滤的基本操作:先取一张滤纸覆于布氏漏斗内,滤纸的大小略小于布氏漏斗的内径且能盖住所有的瓷孔;用少量溶剂(水)润湿滤纸,安装布氏漏斗和吸滤瓶,使布氏漏斗出口处的斜面对准吸滤瓶的抽气支管;开启抽气阀门使滤纸紧贴布氏漏斗的瓷板,沿玻棒将溶液慢慢倒入布氏漏斗内,每次倒入的量不得超过布氏漏斗容积的 2/3;待溶液倒完再将沉淀转移至布氏漏斗,抽干。若需洗涤沉淀,应先停止抽滤,待加入的洗涤液与沉淀充分接触后再抽滤至干。在抽滤过程中,吸滤瓶中滤液液面不应超过支管口。抽滤完毕,应先拔下吸滤瓶支管上的橡皮管,再关水泵,不然,易造成水泵中的水倒吸。

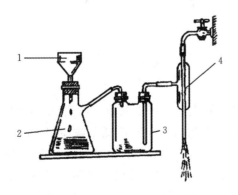

图 1-14　减压过滤

1.布氏漏斗;2.吸滤瓶;3.安全瓶;4.水泵

布氏漏斗内沉淀的取出方法:用玻棒轻轻揭起滤纸边,取下滤纸和沉淀;也可将漏斗倒置,轻轻敲打漏斗边缘或用气吹漏斗口,将沉淀和滤纸一同吹出。滤液应从吸滤瓶的上口倒出,同时,吸滤瓶的支管必须向上,切不可从吸滤瓶的支管口倒出。如过滤的固、液体具有强氧化性、强酸性或强碱性,则不能用滤纸过滤,可用石棉纤维代替滤纸,或用玻璃漏斗代替布氏漏斗。

(3)热过滤。如果溶液冷却后会析出溶质,而又不希望这些溶质留在滤纸上,就需要进行热过滤(图 1-15(b))。过滤时,把玻璃漏斗(应选用短颈玻璃漏斗)放在装有热水的保温漏斗中。保温漏斗是一个用铜皮制作的双层漏斗,使用时在夹层中注入热水,将其安放在铁圈上,将玻璃三角漏斗连同伞形滤纸放入其中,在支管端部加热,至水沸腾后过滤,在热过滤过程中漏斗和滤纸始终保持在近 100 ℃。为了加快过滤速度,滤纸应折叠成折叠滤纸(亦称伞形滤纸):取一张大小合适的圆形滤纸对折成半圆形(Ⅰ),再对折成 90°的扇形(Ⅱ),继续向内对折(Ⅲ),再把半圆分成八等份(Ⅳ),最后在八个等份的各小格中间向相反方向对折,即得 16 等份的折扇形(Ⅴ)。将其打开,外形如(Ⅵ)所示,再在 1 和 2 两处各向内对折一次,展开后如(Ⅶ)所示,即为折叠滤纸(图 1-15(a))。靠近滤纸中心处折纹密集,在折叠过程中不宜用力推压,以免在过滤时破裂。

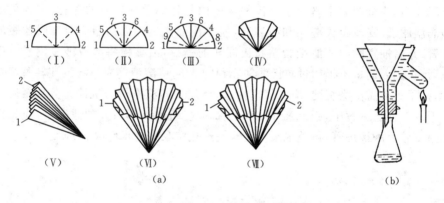

图 1-15　热过滤

(a)折叠滤纸的折法;(b)热过滤装置图

在过滤前应把漏斗放在电热鼓风干燥箱中预热,待过滤时才取出放在保温漏斗中,迅速放入伞形滤纸,伞形滤纸的上沿应低于滤斗口,并使其棱边紧贴漏斗壁;用少许热溶剂润湿滤纸,倒入热溶液后应迅速盖上表面皿,以减少溶剂挥发。如果热溶液较多,一次不能完全倒入漏斗中,则剩余的部分应继续加热保温。过滤时若操作合适,在滤纸上仅有少量晶体析出。若漏斗未预热或虽已预热,但操作过慢,则往往有较多晶体在滤纸上析出,这时必须仔细地将滤纸和结晶一起放回原来的瓶中,加入适量的溶剂重新溶解,再进行热过滤。

3.离心分离法

少量溶液与沉淀的混合物可用离心机进行离心分离以代替过滤,操作简单、迅速。

　　离心机是实验室固、液分离的常用设备,外形有圆筒形(图 1-16(a))和方形等多种。离心机由一电动机带动,按其转速可分为普通离心机、高速离心机和超速离心机等,常规的为 4 000 r·min^{-1},而超速离心机则每分钟可达数万至数十万转。

　　离心机的使用程序:开启电源开关,将盛有沉淀和溶液的离心试管放入离心机的试管套内(离心试管内盛放溶液的量不能超过其容量的 2/3),为保持平衡,在与此对称的另一试管套内也放一支盛有等体积水的离心试管,盖上离心机盖子,将离心机变速器旋转至最低挡开动,再逐渐加速,结晶形的紧密沉淀的转速一般为 1 000 r·min^{-1},无定形的疏松沉淀的转速以 2 000 r·min^{-1} 为宜。结晶形沉淀的离心时间为 1～2 min,无定形沉淀的离心时间为 5～10 min。停止离心时,应逐挡减速,待其自然减速至停止。离心完毕,关闭电源,打开盖子,取出离心试管,并盖好盖子。

　　分离离心试管中的沉淀和溶液的具体操作如下:取一捏瘪了乳胶头的滴管,轻轻插入斜置的离心试管中,沿液面慢慢放松乳胶头吸出上层清液(图 1-16(b)),至全部溶液被吸出为止。注意滴管管尖不能触及沉淀。若需洗涤沉淀,可加少量洗涤液于沉淀中,充分搅拌后,离心沉降,吸出上层清液。一般洗涤 2～3 次即可。第一次的洗涤液并入原离心液中,第二、三次的洗涤液可弃去。

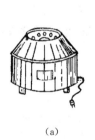　　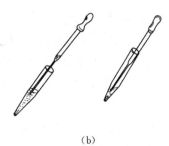

(a)　　　　　　　　　　　　　　　　　　　(b)

图 1-16　离心机的使用

(a)电动离心机;(b)溶液与沉淀分离

　　离心机在使用中要注意:离心机的转动必须保持平衡,运转时如发生反常的振动或响声,应立即停止,查明原因;不可用普通试管进行离心操作,而必须使用离心试管;不能用手按住离心机的轴强制其停止,以免损坏离心机,也可避免意外的发生。

【数字式电子电位差计的使用】

1.校准

　　校准零点,功能选择至"外标"位置,"外标"接口短接。将电动势拨挡拨到电动势指示零,按"校准"按钮,平衡指示即为零。

　　标准电池接在"外标",功能选择拨至"外标"位置,将电动势拨挡拨到电动势指示为标准电池的电势值。按"校准"按钮,平衡指示即为零。

2.测量

功能选择拨至"测量"位置,连接待测电池至"测量",调节电动势拨挡直到平衡指示接近于零,稳定时读数为所测"电动势"(图1-17)。

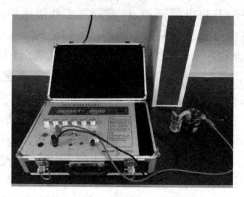

图 1-17　数字式电子电位差计

【试纸的使用】

实验室中经常需要用试纸来证实某些物质的存在及相应的性质。常用的试纸有红色和蓝色石蕊试纸、广泛和精密 pH 试纸、乙酸铅试纸、碘化钾-淀粉试纸等。

(1) pH 试纸用于检验溶液的 pH 值,一般有两类:一类是广泛 pH 试纸,变色范围为 pH=1~14;另一类是精密 pH 试纸,该试纸在 pH 值变化较小时就有颜色变化,其变色范围有 pH=2.7~4.7、3.8~5.4、5.4~7.0、6.8~8.4、8.2~10.0、9.5~13.0 等。pH 试纸的使用方法:先将 pH 试纸剪成小块,放在干燥的表面皿(或点滴板)上,用干净的玻棒蘸取待测液,点在试纸的中央润湿试纸,试纸变色后立即将其与标准色阶板比较,与试纸颜色相似色阶的 pH 值即为溶液的 pH 值(注意:不要将待测液倾倒在试纸上,更不能将试纸浸泡在待测液中,以免影响与色阶的比较)。各种 pH 试纸有配套的色阶板,不能混用。

(2) 乙酸铅试纸是用乙酸铅溶液浸泡过而又经干燥的试纸,可根据是否生成黑褐色的硫化铅沉淀斑点来检验 H_2S 气体的存在。

(3) 碘化钾-淀粉试纸上浸有碘化钾和淀粉的混合物,用于确定 Cl_2、Br_2 等强氧化性气体的存在。当氧化性气体与湿润的试纸接触后,能将试纸上的 I^- 氧化为 I_2,I_2 遇淀粉变蓝。当氧化性气体量较多且氧化性很强时,会使 I_2 进一步转化为 I_3^-,将会使已变蓝的试纸又变成无色,因此应注意观察。

各种试纸在使用时都要注意节约,每次用一小块即可。所用试纸应避免受到实验室中气体的污染而失效。现在,各种新型专用试纸不断面世,如体温试纸、可卡因专用试纸等,需要我们及时掌握。

第三节 基 本 技 能

【称量】

台秤和天平都是根据杠杆原理设计制成的,如图 1-18 所示。AC 表示等臂的天平梁,B 为支点,位于天平梁中央,被称物体的质量为 P,砝码的质量为 Q。根据杠杆原理,当天平梁处于平衡状态时,力矩相等,即 $P \times \overline{CB} = Q \times \overline{AB}$。因为天平梁两臂是等距离的,即 $\overline{AB} = \overline{CB}$,所以 $P = Q$。由此可知,天平平衡时,砝码的质量等于被称物体的质量。

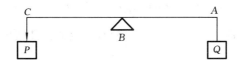

图 1-18 天平的工作原理示意图

电子天平是新一代的天平,是根据电磁学原理制成的:当把通电导线放在磁场中时,导线将产生磁力,当磁场强度不变时,力的大小与流过线圈中的电流成正比;如物体的重力方向向下,电磁力方向向上,两者相平衡,则通过导线的电流与被称物体的质量成正比。故该天平在使用时,要随使用地的纬度、海拔高度随时校准其 g 值,方可获取准确的质量。电子天平有顶部承载式和底部承载式两种类型。一般的电子天平都装有单片机,具有数字显示、自动调零、自动校准、扣除皮重、输出打印等功能,有些产品还具备数据储存与处理功能。电子天平操作简便、称量快速,广泛应用于实验中。

目前,实验室中用于称量的天平主要分为两大类:第一类是托盘天平和常规使用的 DT/DTA 系列电子天平,可准确到 $0.01 \sim 0.1$ g;第二类为分析天平,主要包括双盘电光分析天平(全机械加码的 TG-328A 型和半机械加码的 TG-328B 型两种)和电子分析天平(BSA 系列电子天平),可准确到 $0.01 \sim 0.1$ mg。

(一)DT/DTA 系列电子天平

DT/DTA 系列电子天平(图 1-19)用于精确度不高的称量,一般能准确到 0.01 g。DT/DTA系列电子天平的基本操作方法如下。

(1)天平开机。接通电源,打开开关,显示窗显示"0.0 g",通电预热 15 min。如果在空称情况下的显示偏离零点,应按去皮键 T 使显示回归零点。

(2)天平校准。先按去皮键 T,再按校准键 C,显示窗显示"CAL",进入校准状态,再把相对应的校准砝码放在秤盘上,待稳定后天平显示校准砝码的质量值即校

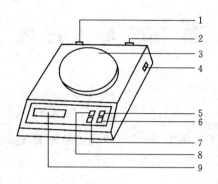

图 1-19 DT/DTA 系列电子天平

1.数据输出口;2.电源插座(带保险丝);3.秤盘;4.开关;5.计数键(P);

6.去皮键(T);7.量值转换键(F);8.校准键(C);9.显示窗

准完毕,可以进行正常称量(200~1 000 g 配有相应的校准砝码)。去除砝码,按去皮键 T,天平显示"0.0 g"。

(3)称量样品。将容器轻放在已进入称量模式的秤盘上(如果是直接称量可记录此时的数据)。按去皮键 T 把秤盘上被称物体的质量清零,天平显示"0.0 g"。然后取下容器,向其中加入试样,再次将盛有试样的容器放在秤盘上,记录的质量为加入试样的量。如被称物体的质量超出天平的称量范围,天平将显示"H"以示警告。

电子天平的注意事项如下。

(1)电子天平为精密仪器,称量时物体要小心轻放,尤其不能人为地对秤盘瞬间加压,这样容易损坏天平。

(2)电子天平不应放在有振动、电源干扰、气流、热辐射及含有腐蚀性气体的环境中,必须保证天平电源接地良好。

(二)BSA 系列电子天平

BSA 系列电子天平(图 1-20)用于精确度较高的称量。一般能准确到 0.1 mg。BSA 系列电子天平基本操作方法如下。

1.准备

称量前取下防尘布罩,叠好后放在电子天平右后方的台面上。

2.调节水平

调节水平调整脚,将水准器调到水平位置。

3.开机操作

将电源线插头插到 220 V 交流电源上;打开天平开关,按开机键,天平显示全亮并扫描,稳定后显示"0.0000 g"。天平开机后应有 30 min 的预热时间。

显示区域及操作键

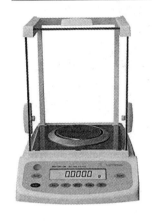
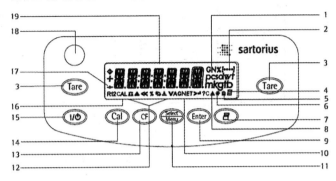

图 1-20　BSA 系列电子天平

1.重量单位；2.菜单层次指示器；3.去皮；4.“GLP 打印模式启动”符合；5.“打印模式启动”符合；6.“应用程序启动”符合；7.数据输出（按压此键，向内置的数据接口发送读出值）；8.计算值指示器（不是称量值）；9.启动应用程序；10.符合：毛重或净重值；11.选择应用程序|打开操作菜单；12.应用程序符合（▷◁, ▲▲, %, ▥, ⊥, A, C）；13.删除（清除功能），此键一般用来撤销以下功能，如退出应用程序，撤销校正/调整程序|退出操作菜单；14.启动校正/调整程序；15.开关键；16.校正/调整符合；17.零范围符号（仅用于校验型号）；18.水平仪；19.显示屏上用所选质量单位的质量值符号含义：≪ 为保存设置，退出操作菜单；< 为上一级菜单；V 为滚动显示菜单选项；> 为当前菜单水平上的下一项；」为选择一个参数设定状态

4.天平的校准

空盘按去皮键 Tare，天平显示"0.0000 g"。按校准键 Cal，天平显示"－200.0000 g"，将 200 g 校准砝码放在秤盘上，待天平显示"CAL. END"，校准完毕。

5.称量样品（差减法）

从干燥器中用纸条取出盛有适量试样的称量瓶（图 1-21（a）），轻放在已进入称量模式的秤盘中央（如果是直接称量可记录此时的数据）。按 Tare 键，秤盘上被称物体的质量显示"0.0000 g"。然后取出称量瓶，将称量瓶倾斜放在盛取出试样的容器上方，用瓶盖轻轻敲瓶口上部，使试样慢慢落入容器中（图 1-21（b））。当取出的试样已接近所需的量时，慢慢地将瓶抬起，再用瓶盖轻敲瓶口上部，使沾在瓶口的试样落下，然后盖上瓶盖，放回称盘中。此时取出被称物体，则显示负值，表示取出物体的质量值。如果是向称量瓶中加入试样，此时加入被称物体，则显示正值，表示加入物体的质量值。

6.天平读数

当天平显示的数值已稳定时，可以进行读数，读数准确到 0.1 mg。

7.整理

使用完天平后，取下被称物体或容器，关好天平。检查天平上下是否清洁，若有脏物，用毛刷清扫干净。罩好防尘布罩，切断电源，填写天平使用登记簿后方可离开

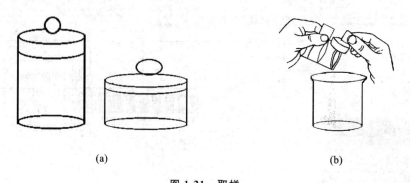

图 1-21 取样

(a)称量瓶;(b)从称量瓶中取出样品

天平室。

8.分析天平使用规则

分析天平是一种精密而贵重的仪器,为了爱护国家财产及使称量获得准确的结果,使用时应遵守下列各项规则。

(1)一切操作都要细心,要轻拿轻放,轻开轻关。

(2)在称量时,必须把天平门关好,否则,称量的结果会不准确。

(3)绝不能使天平载重超过限度(一般为 200 g)。不能在天平上称热的或散发腐蚀性气体的物质;具有腐蚀性蒸气或吸湿性的物体,必须放在密闭容器内称量。

(4)禁止用手拿砝码,一定要用镊子取放,完成称量后必须放回盒中原来的位置。两盒砝码不可混用。

(5)为了减少称量误差,做同一实验中的各次称量时,均要用同一架天平和同一组砝码。

【滴定分析仪器及其基本操作】

(一)滴定管及滴定操作

1.滴定管

滴定管是滴定时用来精确量取液体的量器,分酸式滴定管和碱式滴定管两种类型。酸式滴定管具有玻璃活塞开关(图 1-22(a)),碱式滴定管下端连有软橡皮管(管内放一玻璃珠,以控制液体的流速),橡皮管的下端连有尖嘴玻璃管(图 1-22(b))。

酸式滴定管可用来装酸性和氧化性溶液;碱式滴定管可用来装碱性溶液,不能用来装能与橡皮起作用的溶液,如 $KMnO_4$、I_2、$AgNO_3$ 溶液等。

(1)洗涤。滴定管可用自来水冲洗,或用细长刷子蘸肥皂水刷洗(不能用去污粉)。如有油污,可在酸式滴定管中倒入铬酸洗液浸洗,油污严重时,可用热的洗液浸泡一段时间后再洗，每次加入约 10 mL，将滴定管平持，并不断转动，至洗液布满全管为止。对于碱式滴定管，则要拔去橡皮管，接上一乳胶头，倒入洗液浸洗，再用水冲洗，最后用少量蒸馏水润洗三次。洗净的滴定管，其内壁应完全被水润湿且不挂水珠。

（2）查漏。将已洗净的滴定管装满水，夹在滴定管架上，观察 2 min，如无水滴滴下，缝隙中无水渗出，则将活塞转动 180°或挤捏玻璃珠旁的橡皮管，再观察 2 min，仍然无水滴滴下，缝隙中也无水渗出，则表明滴定管不漏水。

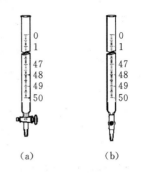

图 1-22 滴定管

(a)酸式滴定管；(b)碱式滴定管

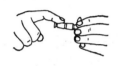

图 1-23 涂凡士林

酸式滴定管漏水时需涂凡士林。其涂法如下（图 1-23）：先将活塞取下，用滤纸或纱布擦干活塞及活塞槽，然后在活塞的两端涂上一层薄薄的凡士林（不要涂到中间有孔处，以免凡士林堵住活塞孔），把活塞插入活塞槽内，并转动整个活塞，直到从外面观察时全部透明为止。涂完后，检查是否漏水。

碱式滴定管漏水时可将橡皮管中的玻璃珠略微移动位置。这样处理后若仍然漏水，则需更换玻璃珠或橡皮管。

（3）装液。为了使装入滴定管的溶液浓度不被滴定管内残留的水所稀释，需先用待装溶液润洗滴定管，每次注入约 10 mL 待装溶液，将滴定管平持，慢慢转动，使溶液流遍全管。打开滴定管的活塞或挤捏玻璃珠旁的橡皮管，使润洗液从管口下端流出。润洗 2～3 次后，即可装入溶液。

（4）排气泡。溶液装入滴定管后，应检查活塞附近及橡皮管内有无气泡，如有气泡，应排出。酸式滴定管：用右手拿住滴定管，使之成约 30°的倾斜，左手迅速打开活塞使溶液冲出（下接一烧杯）将气泡排出。碱式滴定管：将橡皮管弯曲向上，挤捏玻璃珠旁的橡皮管，气泡即被溶液压出（图 1-24）。

图 1-24 碱式滴定管排气泡

气泡排出后，加入标准溶液至"0"刻度以上，再转动活塞或挤捏玻璃珠旁的橡皮管，把液面调节到 0.00 mL 刻度处或略低于"0"刻度处。

（5）读数。读数时，滴定管应处于竖直位置，注入溶液或放出溶液后需等 1～2 s 方可读数。对于无色液体或浅色溶液，读数时，视线应与弯月面下缘的最低点保持在同一水平面上，否则，由于眼睛的位置不同会得到不同的读数（图 1-25(a)）；有的滴定管刻度背面有一"蓝带"，无色溶液装在这种滴定管中，有两个弯月面相交于滴定管蓝线的某一点，读数时，视线应与此点在同一水平面上（图 1-25(b)）；如为有色溶液，应使视线与液面两侧的最高点相切，为了使读数清晰，也可在滴定管后衬一张纸片为背景，形成较深颜色的弯月面，读取弯月面下缘的最低点（图 1-25(c)）。

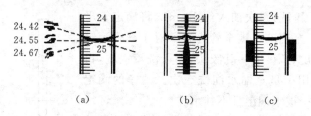

图 1-25 滴定管的读数

(a)读数时视线的位置;(b)乳白板蓝线;(c)读数卡

此外,为便于读数和计算,并消除因上下刻度不均匀而引起的误差,每次滴定时最好均从 0.00 mL 或从接近"0"的某一刻度开始。读数必须准确读至小数点后第二位,如读数为 24.55 mL。

2.滴定操作

滴定开始前,先把悬挂在滴定管尖端的液滴除去。滴定时,左手操纵活塞(或挤捏玻璃珠),右手的大拇指、食指和中指拿住锥形瓶颈(瓶口应接近滴定管尖端,滴定管下端伸入瓶口约 1 cm),沿同一方向按圆周摇动锥形瓶,不要前后摇动。边滴边摇,使溶液混合均匀。

左手控制酸式滴定管活塞的方法:左手从中间向右伸出,大拇指在管前活塞柄中央处,食指及中指在管后活塞柄两端控制活塞,手心握空,旋转活塞的同时稍稍向内(左方)用力,以使活塞与活塞槽保持密合,防止活塞松动,溶液漏出。必须学会慢慢地旋开活塞以控制溶液的流速(图 1-26)。使用带有磨口玻璃塞的碘量瓶进行滴定时,玻璃塞应夹在右手(即拿锥形瓶的手)的中指与无名指之间(图1-27)。

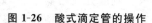
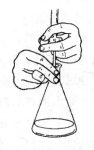

图 1-26 酸式滴定管的操作　　　　　　　　**图 1-27 滴定操作**

使用碱式滴定管时,不要按住玻璃珠以下的地方,否则易使空气进入而形成气泡。

开始滴定时,液滴流出的速度可以快一些,但必须成滴而不能成线状流出,滴定速度一般控制为每秒 3~4 滴,注意观察锥形瓶中颜色的变化。当接近终点时,颜色消失较慢,这时就应逐滴加入,最后应控制液滴悬在滴定管尖上而不落下,用锥形瓶的内壁把液滴靠下来(这时加入的是半滴溶液),用洗瓶中的蒸馏水冲洗锥形瓶的内壁,摇匀。如此重复操作直到颜色变化在 30 s 内不消失为止,即可认为到达滴定终点。滴定完毕,倒去管内剩余的溶液,用蒸馏水冲洗数次,并倒立夹在滴定管架上,便于下次使用。

(二) 移液管与吸量管

移液管是中间有一膨大部分(称为球部)的玻璃管(图 1-28(a)),可准确移取一定体积的液体。球部上下较细,下部尖端为出口,接近管颈口部刻有一标线,球部标刻有容量和温度,当吸取液体至弯月面与标线相切后,让液体自然放出,此时所放出液体的体积即等于管上所标刻的容量。常用的移液管有 5 mL、10 mL、25 mL 等规格。

吸量管是具有分刻度的玻璃管(图 1-28(b)),可准确量取液体。常用的吸量管有 1 mL、2 mL、5 mL、10 mL 等规格。

移液管和吸量管的洗涤方法除按一般玻璃仪器的洗涤方法(即铬酸洗液浸洗,自来水冲洗,蒸馏水润洗)外,吸取时还必须用待取溶液润洗 2～3 次,确保待取溶液的浓度不变。

使用移液管时,右手的大拇指和中指夹持住管颈标线上方,将管尖插入待取溶液的液面之下(不可太深,以免管的外壁黏附的溶液太多;也不能太浅,防止空气突然吸入管中;更不能把管尖搁在容器的底部,因为这样不仅不易吸上来,且易碰损管尖),左手拿洗耳球,先把球内空气压出,然后把球的尖端插入移液管口,慢慢松开左

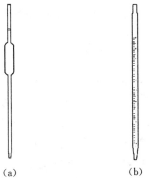

图 1-28　移液管和吸量管
(a)移液管;(b)吸量管

手,使溶液吸入管内(图 1-29(a))。当液面升到"0"刻度以上时,移去洗耳球,立即用右手食指按住管口(图 1-29(b)),使管中液体不致流出。将已吸满液体的移液管提高到与眼睛在同一水平线上(左手拿着盛溶液的容器跟着上升),再将移液管提离液面,管的末端仍靠在容器的内壁上,略为放松食指,不断转动移液管管身,使液面平稳下降,直到溶液的弯月面与所需体积的刻度标线相切时,立即用食指压紧管口,取出移液管,插入承接溶液的容器中,管的末端仍靠在容器内壁上。此时移液管应垂直,承接的容器稍稍倾斜,松开食指,让管内溶液自然地全部沿器壁流下(图 1-29(c)),再等待 10～15 s,拿下移液管即可。此时残留于管尖内的溶液不必用洗耳球吹出,因移液管的容量只计算自由流出的液体的体积,刻制标线时已把留在管尖内的液滴考虑在内(图 1-29(d))。一种血清学实验专用的标有"吹"字的刻度吸管,则属例外。

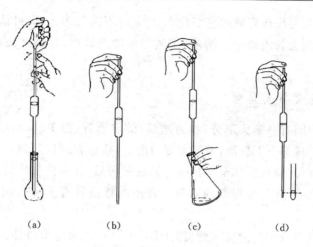

图 1-29　吸取溶液的操作

(a)吸取溶液;(b)移液管拿法;(c)放出溶液;(d)管尖溶液的处理

(三) 容量瓶

容量瓶是一种细颈、梨形的平底玻璃瓶,带有玻璃磨口塞或塑料塞,如图 1-30 (a)所示。颈上有一标线,一般表示在 20 ℃时,液体充满至标线时的容量。它主要用于配制标准溶液或试样溶液。常用的容量瓶有 50 mL、100 mL、250 mL 等规格。容量瓶的洗涤与滴定管相同。

使用前应检查瓶塞是否漏水。向容量瓶内加水,塞好瓶塞,左手拿瓶,右手顶住瓶塞,将瓶倒立,瓶塞无漏水现象后方能使用。为了避免打破瓶塞,要用细绳(或橡皮筋)把塞子系在瓶颈上。

如用固体物质配制溶液,要先在烧杯里将固体溶解,再将其溶液倾入相应容量的容量瓶中(图 1-30(b)),然后用蒸馏水(或相应溶剂)洗涤烧杯 3~4 次,将每次洗涤的液体并入容量瓶中,以保证溶质全部转移。当加水(或相应溶剂)至容量瓶容积

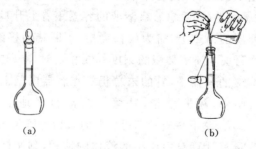

图 1-30　容量瓶的使用

(a)容量瓶;(b)溶液转移至容量瓶中

的 3/4 时,应将容量瓶内的溶液初步混匀。最后快到容量瓶颈部的刻度标线时,改用滴管滴加水(或相应溶剂)到弯月面恰与标线相切,塞紧瓶塞,将容量瓶倒转,反复振荡,使溶液混合均匀。按照同样的方法,可将一定量的溶液稀释到一定体积。

容量瓶不能加热,热溶液冷却至室温后,才能注入容量瓶中,否则会造成体积误差。装有碱液如 NaOH 溶液的容量瓶,不可使用玻璃塞;装有 $KMnO_4$、$AgNO_3$、I_2 溶液的容量瓶,不可使用橡皮塞或软木塞,以免橡皮塞或软木塞被腐蚀。

【酸度计】

酸度计(亦称 pH 计)是实验室用来测量溶液 pH 值的常用仪器,除测量溶液的 pH 值外,还可以测量电池的电动势。实验室的 pH 计虽然型号较多、结构各异,但它们的基本原理相同。

1. 基本原理

酸度计测量 pH 值的方法是电位分析法。酸度计主要由参比电极(饱和甘汞电极)、指示电极(玻璃电极)和精密电位计三个部分组成。

测量时用玻璃电极作指示电极,饱和甘汞电极(SCE)作参比电极,组成电池:

(一)玻璃电极|待测溶液|SCE(+)

饱和甘汞电极的电极电位不随溶液的 pH 值变化,在一定温度下为一定值,而玻璃电极的电极电位随溶液 pH 值的变化而改变,所以它们组成的原电池的电动势只随溶液的 pH 值而变化。

玻璃电极(图 1-31)由 Ag-AgCl 电极、HCl 溶液和特制的球形玻璃膜构成。将它插入待测溶液中,其电极电位 φ 与溶液的 pH 值有下列关系:

$$\varphi_G = \varphi_G^{\ominus} - \frac{2.303RT}{F}pH$$

式中:$\varphi_G^{\ominus}$ 为玻璃电极的标准电极电位(V);R 为气体常数;T 为绝对温度(K);F 为法拉第常数。

饱和甘汞电极(SCE)(图 1-32)由汞、甘汞糊、饱和 KCl 溶液构成。一定温度下饱和 KCl 溶液的浓度为一定值,故饱和甘汞电极的电极电位 φ_{SCE} 也为一定值,298 K

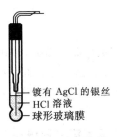

图 1-31 玻璃电极

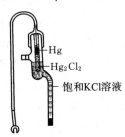

图 1-32 饱和甘汞电极(SCE)

时为 0.241 2 V。

将玻璃电极和饱和甘汞电极插入溶液中组成原电池,电池的电动势为

$$E = \varphi_{SCE} - \varphi_G$$

$$= \varphi_{SCE} - \varphi_G^{\ominus} + \frac{2.303RT}{F}pH$$

由上式可知,E 与 pH 值呈线性关系,只要测得 E 便可求得 pH 值。由于 $\varphi_G^{\ominus}$ 通常是未知的,所以在实际测量中应该用与待测溶液 pH 值相近的标准溶液定位。在原电池中标准溶液的电动势为

$$E_S = \varphi_{SCE} - \varphi_G^{\ominus} + \frac{2.303RT}{F}pH_S$$

待测溶液的电动势为

$$E_x = \varphi_{SCE} - \varphi_G^{\ominus} + \frac{2.303RT}{F}pH_x$$

上两式中的 pH_S 和 pH_x 分别为标准溶液和待测溶液的 pH 值。两式相减,得

$$pH_x = \frac{(E_x - E_S)F}{2.303RT} + pH_S$$

2.PB-10 型酸度计

PB-10 型酸度计的 pH 值测量范围为 0~14.00,精确度为±0.01,具有自动温度补偿功能。该酸度计采用 pH 复合玻璃电极(将玻璃电极和参比电极组装在一起)。酸度计测量出 pH 复合玻璃电极的电压,电压转换成 pH 值,在液晶数字显示屏上显示溶液的 pH 值。PB-10 型酸度计的示意图如图 1-33 所示。

PB-10 型酸度计测量溶液 pH 值的基本操作方法如下。

(1)仪器安装。将 pH 复合玻璃电极与 BNC(电极)和 ATC(温度探头)输入孔连接。将变压器插头与酸度计"Power(电源)"插孔相连,并接好交流电。

(2)校准。

① 按"Mode"键,直至显示屏上出现相应的测量方式(pH),用此键可在 pH 和 mV 模式之间进行切换。

② 按"Setup"键,显示屏显示"Clear",按"Enter"键确认,清除以前的校准数据。

③ 按"Setup"键,直至显示屏显示缓冲溶液组"1.68 4.01 6.86 9.18 12.46"或所要求的其他缓冲溶液组,按"Enter"键确认。

④ 取下复合电极中装有浸泡液的防护帽,将电极用蒸馏水清洗,并用滤纸吸干电极表面液体(注意不要擦拭电极),然后浸入第一种缓冲溶液(6.86)中,等到数值稳定并出现"S"时,按"Standardize"键,仪器将自动校准,校准数值作为第一校准点被存储,显示"6.86"。

⑤ 用蒸馏水清洗电极,滤纸吸干电极表面液体后浸入第二种缓冲溶液(4.01)中,等到数值稳定并出现"S"时,按"Standardize"键,仪器将自动校准,校准数值作为

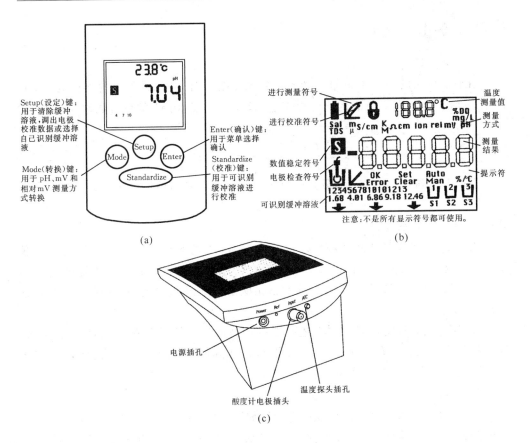

图 1-33 PB-10 型酸度计

(a)仪器正视图；(b)显示内容；(c)仪器后视图

第二校准点被存储,显示"4.01 6.86"。

（3）测量。用蒸馏水清洗电极,滤纸吸干电极表面液体后浸入待测溶液中,等到数值稳定并出现"S",即可读取测量值。

3. 注意事项

（1）校准。为了校准酸度计,至少需用两种缓冲溶液,待测溶液的 pH 值应处于两种缓冲溶液的 pH 值之间。酸度计最多可以使用三种缓冲溶液进行自动校准,若输入第四种缓冲溶液,将替代第一种缓冲溶液的值。

（2）pH 复合玻璃电极下端的玻璃膜易破碎,切忌与硬物接触；电极切忌与油脂类物质接触；用电磁搅拌器搅拌,可使电极的响应速度更快；测量结束后应将电极浸泡在 KCl 溶液中或套上电极的防护帽。

（3）如果使用温度探头,酸度计总是随温度不断调整,由于温度的变化,缓冲溶液的 pH 显示值与其标准值相比可能会有微小的波动。

【723N 分光光度计】

1.基本原理

当某一波长的一束平行单色光照射到某一溶液时,如果入射光的强度为 I_o,透过光的强度为 I_t,则 I_t 与 I_o 的比值称为透光率,用 T 表示。T 的负对数称为吸光度,用 A 表示:

$$T = \frac{I_t}{I_o} \qquad A = -\lg T = \lg \frac{I_o}{I_t}$$

根据 Lambert-Beer 定律,吸光度 A 与溶液浓度 c 和溶液厚度 b 之间的关系为

$$A = abc$$

式中:a 称为吸光系数。

当入射光、吸光系数和溶液液层厚度不变时,透光率或吸光度只随溶液的浓度变化而变化。因此使透过溶液的光经过测光系统中的光电转换器,将光能转变为电能,就可以在测光系统的指示器上显示出相应的吸光度和透光率,从而计算出溶液的浓度。

723N 分光光度计就是根据上述原理设计制造的。其可在紫外-可见光区内,对样品物质做定性、定量分析,可广泛应用于医药卫生、临床检测、生物化学、石油化工、环保检测、食品卫生和质量控制等部门。

2.723N 分光光度计

723N 分光光度计外形结构及按键功能如图 1-34 所示。仪器采用 128×64 位点阵液晶显示器,可直接显示标准曲线和测试数据,主机可存储测试数据(200 组、100条标准曲线),并可选配打印机打印;USB 数据输出接口,可选配 YOKE 3.0 专业软件进行联机操作,实现标准曲线、动力学测试等功能。设计独特的光学系统、高性能1200 条/毫米光栅和进口接收器确保仪器有优良的性能指标;自动波长校准、自动波长设定;操作简单、方便。其技术参数如下:波长范围为 $320 \sim 1\,100$ nm;波长精度为± 0.5 nm;光谱带宽为 2 nm;波长重复性为 0.2 nm;杂散光为 $\leqslant 0.05\%T(360$ nm);光度精度为 $\pm 0.3\%T$;光度重复性为 $0.2\%T$;工作方式为 T、A、C;显示范围为 $0 \sim 200\%T, -0.3A \sim 3A, 0 \sim 9999C$;显示系统为 128×64 位、LCD;调零方式为自动。

723N 分光光度计基本操作方法如下。

(1) 仪器自检。仪器开机后,进入自检状态,自检共有五项,分别为滤色片、检测器、波长校准、系统参数和暗电流。如果任一项自检出错,系统会鸣叫报警,同时显示错误项,通过按任意键继续自检下一项;对错误项如暗电流太大,请检查样品池后,在"系统设定"菜单中重新测定暗电流。

(2) 系统预热。自检结束后仪器进入预热状态,预热时间 20 min。按任意键可以跳过预热过程,进入主菜单:"光度测量""定量测量"和"系统设定"。

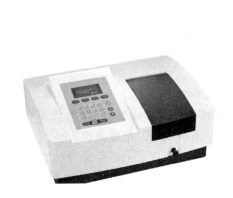
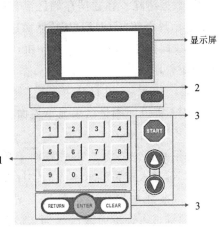

按键面板示意图

图 1-34　723N 分光光度计

1.数字键（"0""1""2""3""4""5""6""7""8""9"·"."""—"—用来输入波长、浓度、日期等数据）；2.功能键（"SET"参数设定，用来设定各个模式下的测量参数；"GOλ"波长设定键；"ZERO"校空白键，用于调0.000Abs和100.0％T；"PRINT"记录打印键）；3.编辑键（"▲"上键，光标向上移动；"▼"下键，光标向下移动；"START/STOP"开始/停止键；"CLEAR"清除/删除键；"RETURN"返回键，用于返回上级菜单；"ENTER"确认键，用于数据和菜单的确认）

（3）光度测量主界面。用"▲""▼"键选择"光度测量"，按"ENTER"键进入光度测量主界面。

（4）设定测量模式。在光度测量主界面下，按"SET"键，进入测量模式选择界面："吸光度""透过率"和"能量"。按"▲""▼"键，选定所需要的测量模式（如吸光度），按"ENTER"键确定。按"RETURN"键返回上一级界面。

（5）设定波长。在光度测量主界面下，按"GOλ"键，进入波长设定界面，通过按数字键"0""1""2""3""4""5""6""7""8""9"和"."输入波长，按"ENTER"键确定并返回上一级界面。

（6）校正空白。将空白溶液和待测溶液分别装入比色皿中（溶液占比色皿体积的3/4），用吸水纸吸干比色皿外壁水珠，打开样品室盖，将比色皿置于比色皿槽中（一般情况下，盛有空白溶液的比色皿放在第一个槽位），盖上样品室盖，此时空白溶液处于光路中，按"ZERO"键校准0.000Abs/100.0％T。

（7）测量样品。将待测溶液拉入光路，从显示器上可以直接读出待测溶液的吸光度。如果需要仪器存储数据，按"START"键进入测量界面，再按"START"键可在当前工作波长下对样品进行测量，每一屏只可显示5行数据，其余数据可以通过按"▲""▼"键翻页显示。在此界面可以重复步骤（5）至（7）测量样品在不同波长下的吸光度。

(8) 数据清除。在数据存储区满(共 200 个数据)或想清除已测数据时,可在测量结果显示界面按"CLEAR"键,然后选择"是",按"ENTER"键,清除已测数据。

(9) 数据打印。连接专用打印机,在测量结果显示界面下,按"PRINT"键,然后选择"确定打印",按"ENTER"键后系统开始打印,打印结束后,系统和屏幕数据将自动清除。如果不想打印,选择"取消打印"后按"ENTER"键退出,也可按"RETURN"键返回测量结果显示界面。

(10) 定量测量。

①定量测量主界面。在主界面菜单下,通过"▲""▼"键选择"定量测量",按"ENTER"键进入定量测量主界面:"标准曲线法""系数法"和"浓度单位"。

②标准曲线法。在定量测量主界面下用"▲""▼"键选择"标准曲线法",按"ENTER"键进入标准曲线法界面,选择"新建曲线",按"ENTER"键进入参数设定界面的第一步,标样数设定界面,用数字键输入想要设定的标样数,按"ENTER"键确定,并设定工作波长、校正空白,按"RETURN"键返回参数设定界面的第二步,在参数设定界面用翻页键选择"标样浓度",按"ENTER"键进入标样浓度设定界面,根据提示放入对应编号的标样,用数字键"0""1""2""3""4""5""6""7""8""9"和"·"输入设定的浓度,按"ENTER"键确定输入,系统将记录当前输入浓度值和测量出的吸光度,并自动进入下一个标样的设定界面,按照同样方法、使用同一比色皿放入对应编号的标样并输入标样浓度值后按"ENTER"键,如此反复直至完成所有标样浓度的设定;此时系统会自动生成工作曲线。

③测量。在工作曲线界面下,按"START"键即进入测量结果数据显示界面,在数据显示界面将待测溶液拉入光路,再次按"START"键即可用刚刚建立的标准曲线进行测量,每按一次"START"键进行一次测量,测量结果顺序编号并依次显示在屏幕上。按"PRINT"键,然后选择"确定打印",按"ENTER"键后系统开始打印,打印结束后,系统将对显示数据进行清空。

(11) 仪器使用完毕,取出比色皿,关闭电源,盖上防尘罩。

3. 注意事项

(1) 改变波长后必须重新将空白溶液放于光路中,按"ZERO"键校准 0.000Abs/100.0%T。

(2) 在比色皿中装入溶液前,必须用该溶液润洗 3~4 次,以保证溶液浓度不发生变化。

(3) 为保护比色皿的透光面,拿取比色皿时,只能用双指捏住毛玻璃面;装入溶液后要用吸水纸吸干外壁水珠方能放进比色皿槽中,使用完毕应洗干净(不能用碱或强氧化剂洗涤)。

(4) 不得将溶液洒落在比色皿槽中,若不慎洒落应擦干净,以免腐蚀仪器。

【鼓风干燥箱】

1.操作方法

烘箱是用来干燥物品、烘焙、熔蜡、灭菌的仪器。下面介绍 DHG-9075A 型电热鼓风干燥箱(图 1-35)的使用方法。

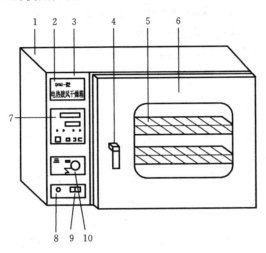

图 1-35　DHG-9075A 型电热鼓风干燥箱
1.箱体;2.铭牌;3.控制面板;4.门拉手;5.搁板;6.箱门;
7.控温仪;8.电源指示灯;9.电源开关;10.风门调节旋钮

(1) 把需干燥处理的物品放入干燥箱内,关好箱门,将风门调节旋钮旋到"∑"处。

(2) 把电源开关拨至"1"处,此时电源指示灯亮,控温仪上有数字显示。

(3) 温度和时间的设置。按"⟳/SET"键,(PV)显示器显示"SP",按"⊡"或"⊡"键,使(SV)显示器显示所需要的设定温度,再按"⟳/SET"键,(PV)显示器显示"ST",按"⊡"或"⊡"键,使(SV)显示器显示所需要的定时时间,再按"⟳/SET"键,仪表回到标准模式。如设定温度为 150 ℃,加热指示灯亮,开始进入加热升温状态,经过一段时间,当显示温度接近设定温度时,指示灯亮灭交替即为恒温点,一般情况下,加热 90 min 后温度控制进入恒温状态。

(4) 鼓风。当被干燥的物品比较潮湿时,可旋转风门调节旋钮至"≡"处,使箱内湿空气排出。

(5) 干燥结束后,如不需要马上取出物品,则应先旋转风门调节旋钮把风门关上,如果仍将风门打开,则需将电源开关拨至"关"处;如马上打开箱门取出物品,则应用干布和手套,防止烫伤。刚取出的玻璃仪器不能碰水,以防炸裂。

2.注意事项

（1）干燥箱外壳必须有效接地，以保证使用安全。

（2）干燥箱应放置在具有良好通风条件的室内，在其周围不可放置易燃、易爆物品。

（3）实验室里的干燥箱是公用的，往干燥箱里放玻璃仪器时应自上而下依次放入，仪器口向上，以免残留的水滴流下使已烘热的玻璃仪器炸裂。箱内物品放置切勿过挤，必须留出空间，以利于热空气循环。

（4）干燥玻璃仪器时一般应先沥干，无水滴下时再放入干燥箱，将温度控制在100～110 ℃。

【数显恒温水浴锅】

恒温水浴锅广泛用于干燥、浓缩、蒸馏及浸渍化学试剂和生物制品，也可用于恒温加热和其他温度实验，是医药、卫生、分析、教育科研的必备工具。其特点是工作室水箱材料为不锈钢，有优越的抗腐蚀性能；自动控温，控温精度高，数字显示；操作简便，使用安全。下面介绍 HH-6 型数显恒温水浴锅(图 1-10(a))。

1.操作方法

（1）向水箱中注入适量的洁净自来水，加热管应低于水面至少5 cm。

（2）将控温旋钮置于最小值(从左向右调节，温度逐渐增大)，接通电源，打开电源开关。

（3）将控制开关置于"设定"端，此时显示屏显示的温度为设定的温度，调节旋钮，设置到工作所需的温度(设定的工作温度应高于环境温度，此时机器开始加热，黄色指示灯亮，否则机器不工作)。

（4）将控制开关置于"测量"端，此时显示屏显示的温度为水箱内水的实际温度，随着水温的变化，显示的数字也会发生相应变化。当加热到所需温度时，加热会自动停止，绿色指示灯亮；当水箱内的水因热量散发，低于所设定的温度时，又会开始加热。

（5）如发现水温不均匀，可打开搅拌功能，慢慢调节搅拌旋钮，让箱内的水自动循环。

（6）工作完毕，将控温旋钮置于最小值，切断电源。

2.注意事项

（1）水浴锅严禁在长时间无人看管的情况下使用，以防水箱内水蒸干后，导致加热管爆裂。水位低于最低限制水位时，应及时加入适量的水。

（2）若水浴锅较长时间不使用，应将水箱中的水排尽，并用软布擦净、晾干。

（3）使用时切记注意防潮，且随时检查水浴锅是否有渗漏现象。

（4）高温使用时，不要直接接触仪器的上部，以免烫伤。

第四节　实验误差和数据处理

【实验误差与误差表示方法】

（一）误差的种类及产生原因

定量分析的任务是准确地测定试样中某组分的含量。由于受分析方法、测量仪器、所用试剂和分析工作者的主观条件等因素影响，所得结果不可能绝对准确，即使对同一试样在同样条件下多次重复测试，也不可能得到完全相同的结果。这说明测量误差是普遍存在的。因此，在测量工作中，不仅要得到测量的结果，而且必须对测量结果进行评价，分析测量结果的准确性（可靠程度）、误差大小及产生误差的原因，采取有效的措施减小误差，以提高测量结果的准确性。

根据误差的性质与产生的原因，可将误差分为系统误差、偶然误差和过失误差三类。

1.系统误差

系统误差（可定误差）是由某些确定的原因引起的，它对测量结果的影响比较固定，在同一条件下，重复测量，它将重复出现，其大小也是相对固定的。根据产生原因，系统误差可分为方法误差（容量分析中计量点和滴定终点不符合）、仪器误差（如天平、砝码和量器刻度不够准确）、试剂误差、操作误差（滴定管读数偏高或偏低，某种颜色的变化辨别不够敏锐）等。常用对照实验、空白实验、仪器校准等办法减小系统误差。

2.偶然误差

偶然误差（随机误差）是由某些难以预料的不确定的因素引起的（如测量时环境温度、湿度、气压、电流、电压的微小波动，仪器性能的微小变化等），它对测量结果的影响不固定。虽然偶然误差的大小、正负具有不确定性，但它具有一定的规律：大小相等的正、负误差出现的概率相等；小误差出现的机会多，大误差出现的机会少。所以，多次测量取平均值是消除偶然误差的最好办法。实践证明偶然误差随测量次数的增加而减小。定量分析中，一般要平行测量 3 次以上。

3.过失误差

过失误差是由分析工作者的粗心大意或不按操作规程操作所造成的误差（如加错试剂，读数、记录和计算错误等）。

为了提高测量结果的准确度，应尽量减小系统误差、偶然误差，消除过失误差。

（二）误差的表示方法

1.准确度与误差

准确度是指测量值与真实值之间的偏离程度，其大小用误差来度量。误差越小,测量结果的准确度越高。其表示方法有以下两种。

(1) 绝对误差(E)。实验测量值(X)与真实值(μ)的差值称为绝对误差(E),即

$$E = X - \mu$$

若测量值(X)大于真实值(μ),E 为正;反之为负。

(2) 相对误差(E_r)。绝对误差(E)与真实值(μ)的百分比称为相对误差,即

$$E_r = \frac{E}{\mu} \times 100\%$$

例如:标定 HCl 溶液时,在分析天平上称取 Na_2CO_3 两份,其质量分别为2.175 0 g 和 0.217 5 g,其真实质量分别为 2.175 1 g 和 0.217 6 g,则它们的绝对误差分别为

$$E_1 = (2.175\ 0 - 2.175\ 1)\ g = -0.000\ 1\ g$$
$$E_2 = (0.217\ 5 - 0.217\ 6)\ g = -0.000\ 1\ g$$

而它们的相对误差分别为

$$E_{r1} = \frac{-0.000\ 1}{2.175\ 1} \times 100\% = -0.005\%$$

$$E_{r2} = \frac{-0.000\ 1}{0.217\ 6} \times 100\% = -0.05\%$$

由此可见,两物体称量的绝对误差虽然相等,但当用相对误差表示时,就可看出第一份称量的准确度比第二份称量的准确度大 10 倍。所以一般用相对误差来表示分析结果的准确度。

但是,真实值往往是未知的。在实际工作中,常用精密度来评价分析的结果。

2. 精密度和偏差

精密度是指多次测量结果之间相吻合的程度,反映了测量结果的重现性。

在实际工作中,被测量组分的真实值并不知道,所以一般用相同条件下多次测量结果的平均值代替真实值。

每次测量结果(X_i)与平均值($\overline{X}$)之差称为偏差(d),它是度量精密度高低的物理量。偏差越小,精密度越高。偏差的表示方法有以下几种。

(1) 绝对偏差(d)。各测量值(X_i)与平均值($\overline{X}$)的差值称为绝对偏差,其有正负之分。

$$d_i = X_i - \overline{X} \qquad (X_i\text{为第 } i \text{ 个测量值})$$

(2) 绝对平均偏差($\overline{d}$)。各个偏差绝对值的平均值称为绝对平均偏差($\overline{d}$),即

$$\overline{d} = \frac{|d_1| + |d_2| + \cdots + |d_n|}{n} \quad (n \text{ 表示测量次数})$$

(3) 相对平均偏差。

$$\overline{d}_r = \frac{\overline{d}}{\overline{X}} \times 100\%$$

（4）标准偏差(s)。

$$s=\sqrt{\frac{d_1^2+d_2^2+\cdots+d_n^2}{n-1}}$$

（5）相对标准偏差(s_r)（也称变异系数（CV））。

$$s_r=\frac{s}{\overline{X}}\times100\%$$

在实际分析工作中,为了更确切地表示测量结果精密度的高低,常用相对平均偏差($\overline{d}_r$)、标准偏差(s)和相对标准偏差(s_r)。其中相对平均偏差比较简单,多用于一般的测量工作中。但为了考虑较大偏差存在的影响,也可用标准偏差(s)和相对标准偏差(s_r)来表示精密度。

滴定分析测量常量组分时,测量结果的相对平均偏差一般应小于0.2%。

【实验数据的处理】

在化学实验,特别是定量分析中,会得到很多实验数据,这些数据有些是直接从仪器上得到的,有些是根据实验数据演算出来的。如何正确地记录、计算这些数据,就是实验数据的处理问题。

掌握分析和处理实验数据的科学方法是十分必要的。

1. 有效数字

记录测量值或在数学运算中,都应真实地反映出误差的大小。实验中所用的仪器上所标出的刻度的精密程度总是有限的,如50 mL量筒上的最小刻度为1 mL,在两刻度间可再估计一位,所以可读至0.1 mL(如35.5 mL)。又如50 mL滴定管,最小刻度为0.1 mL,再估计一位,可读至0.01 mL(如25.41 mL)。也就是说,从仪器上读出的数字中,最后一位是估计数字,是不准确的,它们反映了所用仪器的准确程度。这些从仪器上直接读出的数据(包括最后一位估计数字)称为有效数字。有效数字是指实际测量得到的数据,它包括所有的准确数字和最后一位估计数字。

（1）有效数字的位数确定的几点说明。

① "0"具有双重意义,若作定位用,不是有效数字;若作普通数字用,则是有效数字,即数字前面的"0",不是有效数字,数字中间的"0"和数字末端的"0"是有效数字。另外以"0"结尾的整数,其有效数字的位数不能确定。如500,它可能是两位、三位有效数字等,因为它可表示为5.0×10^2、5.00×10^2等。

② 自然数和在计算中出现的倍数或分数,都不是测量所得到的,所以其有效数字的位数不受限制。

③ 对于pH、pOH、pK、lg$c$等对数值,其有效数字的位数,取决于小数点后面的位数,而小数点前面的整数部分只表明该真数中10的方次数。如pH=10.68,即$c(\mathrm{H^+})=2.1\times10^{-11}$,其有效数字为二位,而不是四位。

（2）有效数字运算法则。

在计算分析数据时，每个测量误差都要传递到结果中去，因此必须按有效数字的运算规则合理取舍，这样既可使计算简单化，又不影响结果的准确度。有效数字的基本运算法则如下。

① 原始记录数值和计算结果只能保留一位估计数字。数据的修约应采用"四舍六入五留双"的原则。

② 加减法。在计算几个数相加或相减时，其和或差的有效数字的位数，应以小数点后位数最少的那个数为准。如求 $50.1+1.46+0.587\ 2$ 的和，应以 50.1 为准，多余数字应按上述规则取舍，因此应为 $50.1+1.5+0.6=52.2$。

③ 乘除法。在计算几个数相乘或相除时，其积或商的有效数字的位数应以有效数字位数最少的那个数为准。如求 $0.043\ 1\times27.84\times1.057\ 8$ 的积，应以 $0.043\ 1$ 为准来保留其他数据的位数，因此应为 $0.043\ 1\times27.8\times1.06=1.27$。

2. 实验数据的表达方式

实验中将得到许多数据，为了准确地表示实验结果、分析其中的规律，就需要将实验数据进行归纳和处理。实验结果的表示方法有列表法、作图法和数学方程法。下面仅就列表法和作图法做简单介绍。

（1）列表法。化学实验中，常用表格来表示实验的测量数据和计算结果，其方法就是将自变量 X 和因变量 Y ——对应排列起来制成表格，以表示两者之间的关系。应用列表法需注意以下几点。

① 注明表格的简明名称；

② 注明表格中各变量的名称和单位；

③ 应注意每一数据的有效数字的位数；

④ 选择较简单的变量作为自变量（如温度、时间、浓度等）。

列表法虽然简单，但不能反映出各数值间连续变化的规律。

（2）作图法。利用实验数据绘出图形，可以直观地显示出实验数据的特点、数据变化的规律。根据图形能简便地找到各函数的中间值、最大值、最小值或转折点的特性以及确定经验方程中的常数等；也可以方便地求出斜率、截距、切线等；同时利用多次测量的数据描绘出的图形，还具有"平均"的意义，从而可以发现和消除一些偶然误差。因此利用实验数据正确地绘出图形，在数据处理上是一种很重要的方法。作图时应注意以下几点。

① 选择适当的坐标纸、坐标轴、比例尺。化学实验中常用的坐标纸有直角坐标纸、对数坐标纸和三角坐标纸，一般用直角坐标纸。用直角坐标纸作图，应以自变量为横轴、因变量（函数值）为纵轴。坐标轴比例尺的选择一般应使坐标刻度表示出全部有效数字。

为了使由图形读出的物理量的准确度与测量的准确度一致，可采取读数的绝对误差在图纸上相当于 0.5~1 小格(坐标纸的最小分度,即 0.5~1 mm);坐标纸上每一格所对应的数值要易读、便于计算;充分利用图纸的全部面积,使图线分布合理,布局匀称,为此,作图时,不必把坐标的原点作为自变量的零点,可从稍低于测量值的数开始;对于直线或近于直线的曲线,应让它与横坐标的夹角为 45°左右(图纸上对角线附近);比例选定后,画出坐标轴,并在轴端或轴旁注明变量的名称和单位,在轴的分度(刻度)边写明该变量的对应值(一般写在逢 5 或 10 的粗刻度线上)。

② 数据的代表点要清楚。根据测得的数值,在坐标纸上清楚地绘出代表点。点的常用符号为○、⊗、△、×、□等(符号的面积近似地表示测量的误差范围)。绘出曲线后这些代表点符号仍保持清晰显现。

③ 绘制出的曲线要平滑。根据代表点可连接成曲线(或直线)。曲线不必通过各个点,但要尽量保证各代表点均匀地分散在曲线两侧(使所有点离曲线的距离的平方和最小)。这样绘出的曲线才能反映出被测物理量之间的变化规律。为了保证曲线所呈现的规律的可靠性,在曲线的极大、极小或转折点处应多测量一些数据。绘制曲线时若发现个别点远离曲线,要分析原因,可以舍弃。总之,绘制的曲线应平滑,不能成折线。

若在同一坐标纸上绘制几条曲线,则每一条曲线上的代表点及对应的曲线要用不同的符号或不同的颜色表示。

④ 图名和说明。曲线绘制好后,应注上图的名称,说明坐标轴所代表的物理量及比例尺,以及主要的测量条件(如温度、压力、浓度等)。

⑤ 在直线上求斜率,必须从线上取点。对于直线 $y = ax + b$,斜率 $a = \dfrac{y_2 - y_1}{x_2 - x_1}$。为了减小误差,所取的两点不能相距太近,所取的点必须在线上(绝对不允许取实验中的两组数据代入计算)。计算时应注意斜率是两点的坐标值差之比,不是纵、横坐标线段长度之比(纵、横坐标的比例尺可能不同)。

第二章　基础化学实验部分

实验一　玻璃仪器认领、清洗、干燥及实验数据的处理方法

【目的要求】

(1) 认识实验室常用的玻璃仪器。

(2) 熟悉玻璃仪器的洗涤方法和干燥方法。

(3) 掌握实验数据的处理方法。

【实验原理】

进行化学实验时,为避免杂质进入反应体系,影响化学反应的进行和实验现象的观察,必须使用干净的玻璃仪器。玻璃仪器的洗涤方法很多,应根据实验的要求、污物的性质、沾污的程度来选用。常用的洗涤方法:刷洗,用去污粉、肥皂或洗涤剂洗,铬酸洗液洗,浓 HCl 溶液洗,$NaOH$ 的 $KMnO_4$ 洗液洗等。用以上方法洗涤后,经自来水冲洗干净的仪器上往往还留有 Ca^{2+}、Mg^{2+}、Cl^- 等离子,如果实验中不允许这些离子存在,应该再用蒸馏水把它们洗去,使用蒸馏水时应符合少量(每次用量少)多次(一般洗 3 次)的原则。

洗净的仪器可被水完全润湿,若把仪器倒过来,水即顺器壁流下,器壁上只留下一层薄而均匀的水膜,且不挂水珠。

玻璃仪器洗净后有时还需要干燥,常用的仪器干燥方法:晾干、烘干、烤干、电吹风吹干、有机溶剂挥发带走水汽等。

该实验通过对常规仪器的认领、洗涤和干燥,达到熟悉本学期实验中使用的仪器的目的;通过学习实验数据的处理方法,为本学期实验数据的正确处理提供保障。

【仪器与试剂】

酸式滴定管(50 mL×1)、碱式滴定管(50 mL×1)、白色试剂瓶(500 mL×2)、棕色试剂瓶(500 mL×1)、碘量瓶(250 mL×3)、三角瓶(250 mL×3,50 mL×2)、容量瓶(100 mL×2,50 mL×5)、烧杯(500 mL×1,300 mL×3,100 mL×2,50 mL×2,10 mL×5)、移液管(25 mL×1,20 mL×1)、吸量管(10 mL×1,5 mL×1,2 mL×1,

1 mL×1)、量筒(100 mL×1)、量杯(25 mL×1,10 mL×1)、滴瓶(2)、洗瓶、洗耳球、瓷坩埚、表面皿、9 cm 长颈漏斗、7 cm 短颈漏斗、酒精灯、200 ℃温度计、蒸发皿、布氏漏斗、吸滤瓶、试管(4)、石棉网、玻棒。

去污粉、肥皂、蒸馏水。

【实验步骤】

(1) 玻璃仪器的认领。根据指导教师的指引逐个认识基础化学实验中常用的玻璃仪器,若发现玻璃仪器破损,应进行登记并更换。

(2) 玻璃仪器的洗涤。洗涤所认领的玻璃仪器,将洗涤干净的两支试管、一个烧杯给指导教师检查。

(3) 玻璃仪器的干燥。对洗涤干净的仪器,用酒精灯烤干一支试管,鼓风干燥箱烘干一支试管。洗涤的其余玻璃仪器存放于实验柜内或抽屉中晾干。

(4) 自主学习基础化学实验须知中的"实验误差和数据处理",并对学习内容进行讨论。

(5) 观看实验录像:实验安排、目的要求、安全事故案例分析、实验室安全、实验预习和实验报告要求、实验数据处理、容量分析仪器操作。

【思考题】

(1) 玻璃仪器洗涤洁净的标志是什么?

(2) 烤干试管时为什么管口要略向下倾斜?

(3) 为什么带有刻度的量器不能用加热的方法进行干燥?

实验二 气体常数 R 的测定

【目的要求】

(1) 了解测定气体常数的方法及其操作。

(2) 掌握理想气体状态方程式和分压定律。

(3) 熟悉称量、量气等操作。

【实验原理】

通过测量金属镁与 HCl 溶液反应产生的 H_2 的体积,可以算出气体常数 R 的数值。反应方程式为

$$Mg + 2HCl \mathrm{=\!=\!=} MgCl_2 + H_2 \uparrow$$

准确称取一定质量的镁与过量的 HCl 溶液反应,在一定温度和压力下,可以测

出反应所放出的 H_2 的体积。实验的温度 T 和压力 p 可以分别由温度计和气压计测得。H_2 的物质的量 n 可以通过反应中镁的质量来求得。由于 H_2 是在水面上收集的,其中混有水汽。在实验温度下水的饱和蒸气压 $p(H_2O)$ 可从表中查出。根据分压定律,H_2 的分压可由下式求得

$$p(H_2) = p - p(H_2O)$$

将以上所得数据代入 $R = \dfrac{pV}{nT}$ 式中,即可算出 R 值。

也可通过铝或锌与 HCl 溶液反应来测定 R 值。测定气体常数 R 的装置如图2-1所示。

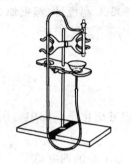

图 2-1 气体常数 R 的测定装置

【仪器与试剂】

电子天平(0.1 mg)、反应管、量气管、乳胶管、铁架台、漏斗。
HCl 溶液(2 mol·L^{-1})、镁条。

【实验步骤】

1.称量

用电子天平称取 3 份镁条,每份质量为 0.03 g 左右(准确称至 0.000 1 g)。

2.安装测定装置

按图 2-1 所示装配好测定装置。向量气管内装水至略低于刻度"0"的位置。上下移动漏斗,以赶尽附着在乳胶管和量气管内壁的气泡,然后把反应管和量气管用乳胶管连接。

3.检漏

把漏斗下移一段距离,并固定在一定位置上。如果量气管中的液面只在开始时(3~5 min)稍有下降,随后便维持恒定,说明装置不漏气。如果液面继续下降,则表明装置漏气,检查各接口处是否密封。经检查与调整后,重复测试,至不漏气为止。

4.测定

(1) 取下反应管,如果需要的话,可以再调整一次漏斗的高度,使量气管内液面保持在略低于刻度"0"的位置。用漏斗将 5 mL 2 mol·L^{-1} HCl 溶液注入反应管中,切勿使酸沾在反应管壁上。用一滴水将镁条沾在反应管内壁上部,使镁条与酸不接触。装好反应管,塞紧磨口塞,再一次检查装置是否漏气。

(2) 将漏斗移至量气管的右侧,使两者的液面保持同一水平,记录量气管中液面的位置。

(3) 将反应管底部抬高,使镁条和 HCl 溶液接触,这时反应产生的 H_2 进入量气管中,将管中的水压入漏斗内。为避免管内压力过大,在管内液面下降时,漏斗也相

应地向下移动,使管内液面和漏斗中的液面大体上保持同一水平。

(4) 镁条反应完后,待反应管冷至室温,使漏斗与量气管的液面处于同一水平,记录液面的位置。1~2 min 后,再记录液面的位置,如两次读数相等,表明管内的气体温度与室温一致。

记下室内的温度和大气压力。用另两份已称量的镁条重复实验。

【结果记录和处理】

实验样号	I	II	III
镁条质量/g			
室温 T/K			
大气压 p/kPa			
$R = pV/(nT)$			
$\bar{R}$			
$\bar{d}_r$			

【思考题】

(1) 计算气体常数 R 时,要用到哪些数据？如何得到？

(2) 检查实验装置是否漏气的原理是什么？

(3) 下列情况对实验结果有何影响？

① 量气管和乳胶管内的气泡没有赶尽;

② 镁条的称量不准;

③ 镁条表面的氧化物没有除尽;

④ 镁条装入时碰到酸;

⑤ 读取液面的位置时,量气管和漏斗中的液面不在同一水平;

⑥ 反应过程中,由量气管压入漏斗的水过多而溢出。

实验三 凝固点降低法测定溶质的相对分子质量

【目的要求】

(1) 掌握溶液的凝固点降低法测定溶质的相对分子质量的原理。

(2) 学会使用 0.1 ℃分度温度计,熟悉移液管的使用方法。

(3) 巩固电子天平的使用方法。

预习内容

【实验原理】

溶液的凝固点(T_f)低于纯溶剂的凝固点(T_f^0),对于非电解质的稀溶液有下列关系:

$$\Delta T_f = T_f^0 - T_f = K_f b_B$$

$$b_B = \frac{m_B / M_B}{m_A} \times 1\,000$$

故

$$M_B = \frac{K_f m_B}{m_A \Delta T_f} \times 1\,000$$

式中:b_B为溶液的质量摩尔浓度(mol·kg^{-1});m_B为溶质的质量(g);M_B为溶质的摩尔质量,当以 g·mol^{-1}为单位时,其数值等于该溶质的相对分子质量;m_A为纯溶剂的质量(g);K_f为溶剂的质量摩尔凝固点降低常数(K·kg·mol^{-1})。

【仪器与试剂】

电子天平(0.01 g)、温度计(0.1 ℃分度)、试管(40 mm×150 mm)、烧杯(500 mL×1)、移液管(50 mL×1)、洗耳球、搅拌器、放大镜、量筒(100 mL×1)、制冰机、玻棒。

葡萄糖(AR,s)、食盐、冰、蒸馏水。

【实验步骤】

1.葡萄糖的称取

精确称取 4.2~5.1 g 葡萄糖放入洁净、干燥的试管中。

2.测定葡萄糖溶液的平均凝固点

用移液管准确吸取 50.00 mL 纯水,放入盛有葡萄糖的试管中,搅拌,使葡萄糖全部溶解。烧杯内加入少量自来水、足量的冰块和食盐(总体积约为 250 mL),搅拌,使冰盐浴的温度在−5 ℃以下。将试管放在烧杯内(图 2-2),一边均匀地搅动试管内

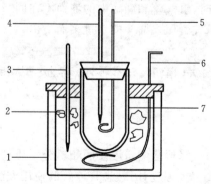

图 2-2 凝固点测定装置图

1.烧杯;2.冰块;3、4.温度计;5、6.搅拌器;7.试管

的溶液,一边搅动冰盐浴,时而补充少量冰和盐,并取出冰盐浴中多余的水。待试管中出现过冷现象,观察到温度迅速回升到某一数值(不再改变),同时溶液出现冰屑时,读取并记录该数值(可借助放大镜观察)。取出试管,流水冲洗管外壁,使管内冰屑完全融化,用此溶液重复操作两次。取三次温度的平均值(任意两次温度值不得相差 0.05 ℃),即为溶液的凝固点 T_f。

3. 测定纯水的凝固点

将洗净的试管用纯水洗涤三次后,用移液管准确吸取 50.00 mL 纯水,放入试管中,测定纯水的凝固点 T_f^0。其方法同步骤 2。

4. 葡萄糖的相对分子质量的计算

从物理化学手册中查得水的 K_f 为 1.86 K·kg·mol^{-1},代入 $M_B = \dfrac{K_f m_B}{m_A \Delta T_f} \times 1\,000$,即可得到葡萄糖的相对分子质量,并按下式计算测定的相对误差。

$$相对误差 = \frac{实验值-理论值}{理论值} \times 100\%$$

葡萄糖的相对分子质量的理论值为 180。

【结果记录和处理】

	I	II	III	平均值
葡萄糖溶液的凝固点 T_f/℃				
纯水的凝固点 T_f^0/℃				
葡萄糖的相对分子质量				
相对误差/(%)				

【思考题】

(1) 冰水中加盐为什么可以作为制冷剂?

(2) 能否用沸点升高法测定葡萄糖的相对分子质量?

(3) 0.256 g 萘($M_r = 128$)溶于 25 g 苯中,试计算所得苯溶液的凝固点(T_f^0(苯) = 5.5 ℃,K_f(苯) = 5.10 K·kg·mol^{-1})。

实验四　酸、碱标准溶液的配制及其浓度的比较

【目的要求】

(1) 熟悉容量分析仪器的使用方法。

(2) 了解酸碱滴定法的基本原理。

预习内容

(3) 练习滴定操作,学会正确地判断滴定终点。

【实验原理】

酸碱滴定法常用的标准溶液是 HCl 溶液和 NaOH 溶液,由于浓 HCl 溶液易挥发出 HCl 气体,NaOH 溶液易吸收空气中的水分和 CO_2,故不宜直接配制成准确浓度的溶液,一般先配制成近似浓度的溶液,然后用一级标准物质(基准物质)进行标定。

酸碱反应的实质是 $H_3O^+ + OH^- \rightleftharpoons 2H_2O$,当 HCl 和 NaOH 反应完全时:

$$n(HCl) = n(NaOH)$$

本实验先配制约 $0.1\ mol \cdot L^{-1}$ 的 HCl 溶液和 NaOH 溶液,再进行酸、碱溶液浓度的比较、滴定,反应达计量点时:

$$c(HCl) \times V(HCl) = c(NaOH) \times V(NaOH)$$

$$\frac{c(HCl)}{c(NaOH)} = \frac{V(NaOH)}{V(HCl)}$$

上式表明,通过酸、碱溶液的体积比较,可准确测出酸、碱溶液的浓度比,如果已知 HCl 溶液的准确浓度,即可由上式计算出 NaOH 溶液的准确浓度。

【仪器与试剂】

酸式滴定管(50 mL×1)、碱式滴定管(50 mL×1)、滴定管架、锥形瓶(250 mL ×3)、烧杯(500 mL×1)、量筒(100 mL×1)、试剂瓶(500 mL×2)、洗瓶。

HCl 溶液($2.0\ mol \cdot L^{-1}$)、NaOH 溶液($2.0\ mol \cdot L^{-1}$)、甲基橙指示剂。

【实验步骤】

1. 标准溶液的配制

(1) $0.1\ mol \cdot L^{-1}$ HCl 溶液。计算配制 500 mL $0.1\ mol \cdot L^{-1}$ HCl 溶液所需 $2.0\ mol \cdot L^{-1}$ HCl 溶液的体积,用 100 mL 量筒量取计算量的 HCl 溶液,倒入洁净的 500 mL 试剂瓶中,加蒸馏水稀释至 500 mL,盖上瓶塞,充分摇匀,贴上标签(注明试剂名称、浓度、班级、姓名、学号及日期),备用。

(2) $0.1\ mol \cdot L^{-1}$ NaOH 溶液。计算配制 500 mL $0.1\ mol \cdot L^{-1}$ NaOH 溶液所需 $2.0\ mol \cdot L^{-1}$ NaOH 溶液的体积,按 $0.1\ mol \cdot L^{-1}$ HCl 溶液的配制方法,配成 500 mL $0.1\ mol \cdot L^{-1}$ NaOH 溶液,贴上标签(注明试剂名称、浓度、班级、姓名、学号及日期),备用。

2. 酸、碱标准溶液浓度的比较

(1) 取酸式滴定管和碱式滴定管各一支,洗净,经检查不漏水后,分别用所配制的 $0.1\ mol \cdot L^{-1}$ HCl 溶液和 NaOH 溶液润洗 2~3 次(每次约用 10 mL),再装入酸、碱标准溶液至"0.00"刻度以上,赶走尖端气泡,调节滴定管内溶液的弯月面至"0.00"刻度或稍低于"0.00"刻度处,静置片刻,准确记录最初读数(准确至小数点后第二位)。

(2) 从碱式滴定管中放出 0.1 mol·L^{-1} NaOH 溶液 20～25 mL 于洁净的250 mL 锥形瓶中,加入1～2滴甲基橙指示剂,摇匀。将 0.1 mol·L^{-1} HCl 溶液滴入锥形瓶中,边滴边旋摇锥形瓶,近终点时,用洗瓶中的蒸馏水淋洗锥形瓶内壁,把滴定过程中附着在内壁上的溶液冲下,继续逐滴滴定(最好控制在半滴半滴加入)至橙色,即为终点。继续滴入几滴 HCl 溶液,溶液由橙色又变为红色(表明过量),再从碱式滴定管中逐滴滴入 NaOH 溶液,使溶液由红色变为橙色,注意观察终点。如此反复练习滴定操作和终点的观察。最后准确读取终点(橙色)时所耗用的 HCl 溶液和NaOH 溶液的体积,并求出 HCl 溶液和 NaOH 溶液的体积比。平行测定 3 次,计算平均结果和相对平均偏差,要求相对平均偏差小于 0.2%。

【结果记录和处理】

编　　号		Ⅰ	Ⅱ	Ⅲ
HCl	终读数/mL			
	初读数/mL			
	V(HCl)/mL			
NaOH	终读数/mL			
	初读数/mL			
	V(NaOH)/mL			
V(NaOH)∶V(HCl)				
平均值				
相对平均偏差 $\bar{d}_r$/(%)				

【思考题】

(1) 滴定管在使用前都要用待装的溶液润洗 2～3 次,锥形瓶要不要润洗?为什么?

(2) 为什么每次滴定前,都要使滴定管内溶液的初读数从"0.00"刻度或稍低于"0.00"刻度处开始?

(3) 下列情况对实验结果有无影响?

① 滴定完毕,滴定管的尖端留有液滴或尖端内部产生了气泡;

② 在滴定过程中,向锥形瓶中淋洗了少量的蒸馏水。

(4) 本实验为什么用甲基橙作指示剂,能否用酚酞作指示剂?

实验五 乙酸解离度与解离常数的测定

预习内容

【目的要求】

(1) 了解测定解离度及解离常数的方法和原理。
(2) 进一步熟悉吸量管、碱式滴定管的使用。
(3) 掌握酸度计的使用。

【实验原理】

乙酸是弱电解质,在水溶液中存在下述解离:

$$HAc + H_2O \rightleftharpoons H_3O^+ + Ac^-$$

一定温度下,解离达平衡时:

$$K_a = \frac{[H_3O^+] \cdot [Ac^-]}{[HAc]}$$

式中:$[H_3O^+]$、$[Ac^-]$、$[HAc]$均为平衡浓度;K_a为解离常数。

根据解离度 α 的定义:$\alpha = [H_3O^+]/c$。c 为乙酸溶液的起始浓度,用标准 NaOH 溶液滴定测出;$[H_3O^+]$通过酸度计测定乙酸溶液的 pH 值获得。由乙酸溶液的 K_a 与 α 之间的关系式 $K_a = \dfrac{c\alpha^2}{1-\alpha}$,即可求出 K_a 值。

【仪器与试剂】

碱式滴定管(50 mL×1)、锥形瓶(250 mL×3)、烧杯(10 mL×4)、容量瓶(50 mL×3)、移液管(25 mL×1,10 mL×1)、吸量管(10 mL×1)、酸度计(PB-10 型)、洗瓶、洗耳球。

乙酸溶液 (约 0.2 mol·L^{-1})、NaOH 标准溶液(约 0.1 mol·L^{-1},已标定)、酚酞指示剂、pH=4.00 和 pH=6.86 的标准缓冲溶液。

【实验步骤】

1. 乙酸溶液浓度的测定(准确至三位有效数字)

用移液管吸取 10.00 mL 乙酸溶液置于 250 mL 锥形瓶中,加 2 滴酚酞指示剂,用 NaOH 标准溶液滴定至溶液呈微红色,30 s 内不褪色,即为终点。记下所消耗的 NaOH 标准溶液的体积。平行测定 3 次,计算乙酸溶液的浓度。

2. 配制不同浓度的乙酸溶液

用吸量管或移液管分别吸取 25.00 mL、5.00 mL 和 2.50 mL 已标定过的乙酸溶液置于 3 个 50 mL 容量瓶中,用蒸馏水稀释至刻度,摇匀,并计算稀释后的浓度。加上步骤 1 所测的乙酸溶液,共得四种浓度的乙酸溶液。

3.测定乙酸溶液的 pH 值

取上述四种不同浓度的乙酸溶液分别置于 4 个干燥的烧杯中,按照由稀到浓的顺序分别在 PB-10 型酸度计上测定它们的 pH 值,并记下温度。酸度计的使用参见基本技能部分。

【结果记录和处理】

1.乙酸溶液浓度的测定

	编　号	I	II	III
NaOH	初读数/mL			
	终读数/mL			
	V(NaOH)/mL			
c(NaOH)/(mol·L^{-1})				
c(HAc)/(mol·L^{-1})				
$\bar{c}$(HAc)/(mol·L^{-1})				
$\bar{d}_r$/(%)				

2.乙酸溶液解离度与解离常数的测定

编　号	I	II	III	IV
c(HAc)/(mol·L^{-1})				
pH 值				
c(H$_3$O$^+$)/(mol·L^{-1})				
α				
K_a				
$\bar{K}_a$				
实验温度/℃				

【思考题】

(1) 如果改变所测乙酸溶液的温度,则解离度和解离常数有无变化?

(2) 使用酸度计时应特别注意哪些事项?

(3) 不同浓度的乙酸溶液的解离度是否相同?其解离常数是否相同?

实验六　化学反应速率与活化能的测定

【目的要求】

(1) 验证浓度、温度、催化剂对化学反应速率的影响。

(2) 了解 $(NH_4)_2S_2O_8$ 氧化 KI 的反应速率的测定原理和方法。

(3) 学会使用图解法确定反应级数和活化能。

【实验原理】

在水溶液中,$(NH_4)_2S_2O_8$ 与 KI 发生如下反应:

$$S_2O_8^{2-}+3I^-=\!=\!=2SO_4^{2-}+I_3^- \tag{1}$$

该反应的反应速率 v 按速率方程可表示为

$$v=k\,[S_2O_8^{2-}]^m\cdot[I^-]^n$$

式中:v 为瞬时速率;k 为反应速率常数;$[S_2O_8^{2-}]$ 与 $[I^-]$ 分别为两种离子的起始浓度;$(m+n)$ 为反应级数。

实验测得的反应速率是在一段时间 (Δt) 内反应的平均速率:$\bar{v}=-\dfrac{\Delta[S_2O_8^{2-}]}{\Delta t}$。由于本实验在 Δt 时间内反应物的浓度变化很小,所以平均速率可以看成是瞬时速率。即

$$v=\bar{v}=-\frac{\Delta[S_2O_8^{2-}]}{\Delta t}=k[S_2O_8^{2-}]^m\cdot[I^-]^n$$

为了能测定出在一定时间 (Δt) 内 $(NH_4)_2S_2O_8$ 的改变量 $\Delta[S_2O_8^{2-}]$,将 $(NH_4)_2S_2O_8$ 溶液与 KI 溶液混合的同时,定量加入 $Na_2S_2O_3$ 溶液和作为指示剂的淀粉溶液。这样在反应(1)进行的同时,还进行如下反应:

$$2S_2O_3^{2-}+I_3^-=\!=\!=S_4O_6^{2-}+3I^- \tag{2}$$

反应(2)比反应(1)快得多,瞬间完成。由于反应(1)生成的 I_3^- 立即与 $S_2O_3^{2-}$ 作用,生成无色的 $S_4O_6^{2-}$ 和 I^-。因此在反应开始的一段时间内看不到碘与淀粉作用所显示的蓝色。但是,一旦 $Na_2S_2O_3$ 耗尽,由反应(1)生成的微量碘就迅速与淀粉作用,使溶液显蓝色。

由于在 Δt 时间内 $S_2O_3^{2-}$ 全部耗尽,浓度为零,所以 $\Delta[S_2O_8^{2-}]$ 实际上就是反应前 $Na_2S_2O_3$ 的浓度。又从反应(1)和(2)可知,$\Delta[S_2O_8^{2-}]:\Delta[S_2O_3^{2-}]=1:2$,所以 $S_2O_8^{2-}$ 在 Δt 时间内的浓度变化量 $\Delta[S_2O_8^{2-}]$ 可从下式求出:

$$\Delta[S_2O_8^{2-}]=\frac{\Delta[S_2O_3^{2-}]}{2}=\frac{c(S_2O_3^{2-})}{2}$$

将速率方程 $v = k[S_2O_8^{2-}]^m \cdot [I^-]^n$ 两边取对数：

$$\lg v = m\lg[S_2O_8^{2-}] + n\lg[I^-] + \lg k$$

由此可知,当 $[I^-]$ 一定时,以 $\lg v$ 对 $\lg[S_2O_8^{2-}]$ 作图得一直线,其斜率为 m;当 $[S_2O_8^{2-}]$ 一定时,以 $\lg v$ 对 $\lg[I^-]$ 作图也得一直线,其斜率为 n,则该反应的反应级数为 $(m+n)$。

利用实验测得的反应速率和反应级数,按速率方程就可以求出反应速率常数 k 的值。

根据 Arrhenius 方程,反应速率常数 k 与反应温度 T 有如下关系:

$$\lg k = -\frac{E_a}{2.303RT} + \lg A$$

式中:E_a 为活化能;R 为气体常数($8.314\ \mathrm{J \cdot mol^{-1} \cdot K^{-1}}$);$T$ 为绝对温度。测出在不同温度下的 k 值,以 $\lg k$ 对 $\frac{1}{T}$ 作图得一直线,其斜率为 $-\frac{E_a}{2.303R}$,从而可以求出反应的活化能 E_a(由文献查得反应 $S_2O_8^{2-} + 3I^- = 2SO_4^{2-} + I_3^-$ 的 E_a 为 $51.58\ \mathrm{kJ \cdot mol^{-1}}$)。

【仪器与试剂】

温度计(2)、秒表、数显恒温水浴锅、烧杯($100\ \mathrm{mL} \times 4$)、量筒($20\ \mathrm{mL} \times 4$,$5\ \mathrm{mL} \times 1$)、吸量管($10\ \mathrm{mL} \times 1$)、玻棒。

$(NH_4)_2S_2O_8$ 溶液($0.2\ \mathrm{mol \cdot L^{-1}}$)、KI 溶液($0.2\ \mathrm{mol \cdot L^{-1}}$)、$Na_2S_2O_3$ 溶液($0.2\ \mathrm{mol \cdot L^{-1}}$)、淀粉溶液($0.2\%$)、$KNO_3$ 溶液($0.2\ \mathrm{mol \cdot L^{-1}}$)、$(NH_4)_2SO_4$ 溶液($0.2\ \mathrm{mol \cdot L^{-1}}$)、$Cu(NO_3)_2$ 溶液($0.2\ \mathrm{mol \cdot L^{-1}}$)。

【实验步骤】

1. 浓度对反应速率的影响

用量筒取 $20.0\ \mathrm{mL}\ 0.2\ \mathrm{mol \cdot L^{-1}}$ KI 溶液置于 $100\ \mathrm{mL}$ 烧杯中,用另一量筒加入 $4.0\ \mathrm{mL}\ 0.2\%$ 淀粉溶液,由吸量管加入 $8.00\ \mathrm{mL}\ 0.2\ \mathrm{mol \cdot L^{-1}}$ $Na_2S_2O_3$ 溶液,混匀。再用第三个量筒量取 $20.0\ \mathrm{mL}\ 0.2\ \mathrm{mol \cdot L^{-1}}$ $(NH_4)_2S_2O_8$ 溶液迅速倒入混合液中,同时启动秒表,并搅匀。注意观察,当溶液刚出现蓝色时,立即停表。记录反应时间 Δt 和室温。

用同样方法按下表中的用量进行另外四组实验,为了使每次实验中溶液的离子强度和总体积不变,不足的量分别用 $0.2\ \mathrm{mol \cdot L^{-1}}$ KNO_3 溶液和 $0.2\ \mathrm{mol \cdot L^{-1}}$ $(NH_4)_2SO_4$ 溶液补充。

编　号		I	II	III	IV	V
试剂用量 /mL	$0.2\ mol \cdot L^{-1}(NH_4)_2S_2O_8$	20.0	10.0	5.0	20.0	20.0
	$0.2\ mol \cdot L^{-1}KI$	20.0	20.0	20.0	10.0	5.0
	$0.2\ mol \cdot L^{-1}Na_2S_2O_3$	8.00	8.00	8.00	8.00	8.00
	0.2%淀粉	4.0	4.0	4.0	4.0	4.0
	$0.2\ mol \cdot L^{-1}KNO_3$	0.0	0.0	0.0	10.0	15.0
	$0.2\ mol \cdot L^{-1}(NH_4)_2SO_4$	0.0	10.0	15.0	0.0	0.0
起始浓度 /(mol · L^{-1})	$c((NH_4)_2S_2O_8)$					
	$c(KI)$					
	$c(Na_2S_2O_3)$					
$\Delta[S_2O_8^{2-}]$						
反应时间 $\Delta t/s$						
反应速率 $v/(mol \cdot L^{-1} \cdot s^{-1})$						

2.温度对反应速率的影响

按上表编号IV中的用量,把 KI、$Na_2S_2O_3$、淀粉、KNO_3溶液加到 100 mL 烧杯中,$(NH_4)_2S_2O_8$溶液加到另一个烧杯中,然后将它们同时置于冰水浴中冷却。当烧杯内溶液与冰水浴温度相同,且低于室温 10 ℃左右时,把$(NH_4)_2S_2O_8$溶液迅速倒入混合溶液中,同时启动秒表,并搅匀。当溶液刚出现蓝色时,立即停表。记录反应时间 Δt 和反应温度。

同理,利用热水浴在高于室温 10 ℃和 20 ℃左右的条件下,重复上述实验。

3.催化剂对反应速率的影响

按上表编号IV的用量,向 KI、$Na_2S_2O_3$、淀粉、KNO_3 混合液中加入 3 滴 0.2 mol · L^{-1} $Cu(NO_3)_2$溶液,混合后,迅速加入 0.2 mol · L^{-1} $(NH_4)_2S_2O_8$溶液,同时启动秒表,并搅匀。当溶液刚出现蓝色时,立即停表。记录反应时间 Δt,并与没加入 $Cu(NO_3)_2$溶液的反应时间进行比较,得出结论。

【结果记录和处理】

1.反应级数的确定及反应速率常数的计算

实验编号	I	II	III	IV	V
lg$v$					
lg$[S_2O_8^{2-}]$					

续表

实验编号	Ⅰ	Ⅱ	Ⅲ	Ⅳ	Ⅴ
$lg[I^-]$					
m					
n					
反应速率常数 k					

当$[I^-]$一定时,以lgv对$lg[S_2O_8^{2-}]$作图得一直线,求斜率m;当$[S_2O_8^{2-}]$一定时,以lgv对$lg[I^-]$作图得一直线,求斜率n。确定该反应的反应级数。

2.反应活化能的计算

实验编号	Ⅰ	Ⅱ	Ⅲ	Ⅳ
反应温度/℃				
反应时间 $\Delta t/s$				
反应速率 $v/(mol \cdot L^{-1} \cdot s^{-1})$				
反应速率常数 k				

以lgk对$\dfrac{1}{T}$作图,求出斜率,计算活化能,并分析误差产生的原因。

【注意事项】

(1) $Na_2S_2O_3$的体积必须取准。$(NH_4)_2S_2O_8$应新鲜配制,其溶液的pH值应大于3,否则说明已分解,不能使用。

(2) 各溶液加入的顺序不可颠倒。

(3) 混合时立即启动秒表。

(4) 测定不同温度下的数据时,温度应以烧杯内溶液的温度为准。

【思考题】

(1) $Na_2S_2O_3$溶液的用量不同,对本实验有无影响?为什么?

(2) 下列情况对实验结果各有何影响?

① 实验中量筒没分开专用;

② 先加$(NH_4)_2S_2O_8$溶液,后加KI溶液;

③ 慢慢加入$(NH_4)_2S_2O_8$溶液。

实验七 有机酸试剂纯度的测定

预习内容

【目的要求】

(1) 学习 NaOH 标准溶液的标定方法。

(2) 进一步训练滴定操作,从严考核滴定结果。

【实验原理】

大部分有机酸是固体弱酸,这类化工产品(试剂级或工业级)纯度的测定很多都采用酸碱滴定法。如果有机酸能溶于水,并且满足 $c_aK_a \geqslant 10^{-8}$,就可用 NaOH 标准溶液进行滴定来确定纯度。本实验测定草酸的纯度,草酸($H_2C_2O_4 \cdot 2H_2O$)是一种白色晶体,可溶于水。草酸是二元弱酸,$K_{a1} = 5.9 \times 10^{-2}$,$K_{a2} = 6.4 \times 10^{-5}$。由于 $K_{a1}/K_{a2} < 10^4$,因此与强碱作用时,草酸可一次被滴定。其反应方程式如下:

$$H_2C_2O_4 + 2NaOH =\!=\!= Na_2C_2O_4 + 2H_2O$$

滴定产物是弱碱(pH 值约为 8.4),滴定突跃范围在弱碱性区域(7.7~10.0),一般选用酚酞为指示剂,滴定至呈现浅红色为终点。根据 NaOH 标准溶液的浓度、消耗的体积及被滴定有机酸的相对分子质量,便可计算试样的纯度:

$$w(H_2C_2O_4 \cdot 2H_2O) = \cfrac{c(NaOH) \times V(NaOH) \times \dfrac{M(H_2C_2O_4 \cdot 2H_2O)}{2 \times 1\,000}}{m(样品) \times \dfrac{25.00}{250.00}} \times 100\%$$

NaOH 易吸收空气中的 H_2O 和 CO_2,如果 NaOH 标准溶液中含有少量的 Na_2CO_3,对观察终点颜色变化和滴定结果都会有影响,所以,必须防止引入 CO_3^{2-}。通常的做法是先配制饱和的 NaOH 溶液,其质量分数约为 50%(在 20 ℃时浓度约为 19 mol·L⁻¹)。这种溶液具有不溶解 Na_2CO_3 的性质,经过离心或放置一段时间后,取一定量的上清液,用刚煮沸过并已冷却的蒸馏水稀释至一定体积后进行标定。

饱和 NaOH 溶液和 NaOH 标准溶液在存放和使用过程中要密封,因此,常安装虹吸管和碱石灰管以防止其吸收空气中的 CO_2,如图 2-3 所示。

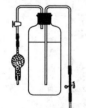

碱溶液浓度标定所用的一级标准物质(基准物质)有多种,本实验选用一种常用的酸性一级标准物质邻苯二甲酸氢钾($KHC_8H_4O_4$)来标定 NaOH 溶液的浓度,标定时的反应方程式为

图 2-3 NaOH 溶液的保存

$$KHC_8H_4O_4 + NaOH =\!=\!= KNaC_8H_4O_4 + H_2O$$

NaOH 溶液的浓度可由下式来计算：

$$c(\text{NaOH}) = \frac{m(\text{KHC}_8\text{H}_4\text{O}_4)}{V(\text{NaOH}) \times M(\text{KHC}_8\text{H}_4\text{O}_4)} \times 1\,000$$

式中：$m(\text{KHC}_8\text{H}_4\text{O}_4)$ 为所称取的邻苯二甲酸氢钾的质量(g)；$M(\text{KHC}_8\text{H}_4\text{O}_4)$ 为邻苯二甲酸氢钾的相对分子质量；$V(\text{NaOH})$ 为所消耗的 NaOH 溶液的体积(mL)。

【仪器与试剂】

电子天平(0.1 mg)、碱式滴定管(50 mL×1)、烧杯(50 mL×1,250 mL×1)、移液管(25 mL×1)、滴定管架、锥形瓶(250 mL×3)、量筒(10 mL×1)、洗瓶、玻棒、容量瓶(250 mL×1)、称量瓶、洗耳球、滴管、试剂瓶(500 mL×1)。

饱和 NaOH 溶液、酚酞指示剂、邻苯二甲酸氢钾(AR,s)、有机酸($H_2C_2O_4 \cdot 2H_2O$,s)、蒸馏水。

【实验步骤】

1. 配制 0.1 mol·L⁻¹NaOH 标准溶液

用干燥的 10 mL 量筒量取一定量饱和 NaOH 溶液,立即倒入刚煮沸并已冷却的蒸馏水中,配制成 500 mL 0.1 mol·L⁻¹NaOH 标准溶液。配制好后随即盖紧,以防吸收空气中的 CO_2,此溶液若只在短时间内使用,不必安装虹吸管和碱石灰管。

2. 标定 NaOH 溶液

用电子天平准确称取邻苯二甲酸氢钾 3 份(每份应消耗 0.1 mol·L⁻¹NaOH 溶液 20～25 mL),分别放入 250 mL 锥形瓶中,加 20～30 mL 水溶解,待完全溶解后,加入 2 滴酚酞指示剂,用 0.1 mol·L⁻¹NaOH 标准溶液滴定至溶液呈粉红色,30 s 内不褪色,即为终点。计算 NaOH 标准溶液的浓度。要求 3 份测定结果的相对平均偏差小于 0.2%,否则重新标定。

3. 有机酸试样纯度的测定

从指导教师处领取一份有机酸试样,准确称取 1.7～1.9 g 有机酸试样,用煮沸并冷却的水溶解后在 250 mL 容量瓶中定容,摇匀。用 25 mL 移液管取出 3 份试液于锥形瓶中,以酚酞为指示剂,分别滴定至终点。由消耗的 NaOH 标准溶液的平均体积及该有机酸的相对分子质量计算试样的纯度,即质量分数 ω。

【结果记录和处理】

1. 标定 NaOH 溶液

编　号	Ⅰ	Ⅱ	Ⅲ
$\text{KHC}_8\text{H}_4\text{O}_4$ 的质量/g			

续表

编　号		I	II	III
NaOH	终读数/mL			
	初读数/mL			
	V(NaOH)/mL			
c(NaOH)/(mol·L^{-1})				
$\bar{c}$(NaOH)/(mol·L^{-1})				
$\bar{d}_r$/(%)				

2. 有机酸试样纯度的测定

编　号		I	II	III
有机酸的质量/g				
NaOH	终读数/mL			
	初读数/mL			
	V(NaOH)/mL			
ω/(%)				
$\bar{\omega}$/(%)				
$\bar{d}_r$/(%)				

【思考题】

（1）已标定好的 NaOH 标准溶液，在存放过程中若吸收了 CO_2，用它来测定 HCl 溶液的浓度，以酚酞为指示剂对测定结果有何影响？如果以甲基橙为指示剂又如何？

（2）NaOH 溶液为什么要储存在塑料瓶中？储存时应注意什么？

（3）具备哪些条件的物质才能成为一级标准物质（基准物质）？

实验八　APC药片中阿司匹林含量的测定

【目的要求】

（1）了解药用 APC 药片中阿司匹林含量测定的原理及方法。

（2）进一步巩固滴定分析操作。

预习内容

【实验原理】

阿司匹林（即乙酰水杨酸）具有解热、镇痛的作用。它的分子结构中含有羧基，

在溶液中可解离出 H^+,是一元弱酸($pK_a=3.5$),可以用碱标准溶液直接滴定,其滴定反应方程式为

$$\underset{OCOCH_3}{\overset{COOH}{\bigcirc}} + NaOH \Longrightarrow \underset{OCOCH_3}{\overset{COONa}{\bigcirc}} + H_2O$$

反应到达计量点时,溶液呈弱碱性,可选用酚酞作指示剂。

阿司匹林的乙酰基很容易水解,使得用 NaOH 溶液滴定时,分析结果偏高,其反应方程式为

$$\underset{OCOCH_3}{\overset{COOH}{\bigcirc}} + 2NaOH \Longrightarrow \underset{OH}{\overset{COONa}{\bigcirc}} + H_2O + CH_3COONa$$

因此,滴定应在中性乙醇溶液中进行,并保持滴定时的温度在 10 ℃ 以下。此外,滴定应在不断振摇下较快地进行,以防止局部碱浓度过高而促使其水解。

【仪器与试剂】

电子天平(0.1 mg)、量筒(50 mL×1)、锥形瓶(250 mL×3)、烧杯(250 mL×1)、碱式滴定管(50 mL×1)、研钵、滴定管架、玻棒、洗瓶。

APC 药片、NaOH 标准溶液(约 0.1 $mol \cdot L^{-1}$,已标定)、酚酞指示剂、中性乙醇溶液(取所需用量的 95% 乙醇溶液,加 2~3 滴酚酞指示剂,用 0.100 0 $mol \cdot L^{-1}$ NaOH 溶液滴定至微红色,加盖,在 10 ℃ 下储存,备用)。

【实验步骤】

1. 标定 NaOH 溶液

见"实验七 有机酸试剂纯度的测定"中实验步骤 2 或按如下方法进行。准确称取 $KHC_8H_4O_4$ 一份于小烧杯中,用蒸馏水溶解后在 250 mL 容量瓶中定容,摇匀。用 25 mL 移液管平行移取 3 份于锥形瓶中,加酚酞指示剂 1~2 滴,用 0.1 $mol \cdot L^{-1}$ NaOH 标准溶液滴至溶液呈粉红色(如果每份应消耗 0.1 $mol \cdot L^{-1}$ NaOH 溶液体积 20~25 mL,则 $KHC_8H_4O_4$ 应称量多少?),30 s 内不褪色,即为终点,计算 NaOH 标准溶液浓度和相对平均偏差。

2. APC 药片中阿司匹林含量的测定

称取研细后的 APC 药粉 0.4~0.5 g(约为 1 片的质量,准确至 0.1 mg)于锥形瓶中,加 20 mL 中性乙醇溶液溶解(由于 APC 药片中除阿司匹林外,还含有其他赋形剂等物质,后者不溶于乙醇,故溶液是白色混浊液,但不影响滴定终点的观察)。溶解后加 2~3 滴酚酞指示剂,在不超过 10 ℃ 的温度下,用 NaOH 标准溶液滴定至粉红色,30 s 不褪色即为终点。平行测定 2~3 次,取其平均值,按下式计算阿司匹林的质量分数。

$$w(C_9H_8O_4) = \frac{c(NaOH) \times V(NaOH) \times M(C_9H_8O_4)}{m(样品) \times 1\,000} \times 100\%$$

【结果记录和处理】

编号		Ⅰ	Ⅱ	Ⅲ
NaOH	终读数/mL			
	初读数/mL			
	$V(\text{NaOH})$/mL			
$c(\text{NaOH})$/(mol·L^{-1})				
样品质量 m/g				
阿司匹林的含量/(%)				
阿司匹林的平均含量/(%)				

【思考题】

为什么测定 APC 药片中阿司匹林的含量要在中性乙醇溶液中进行？

实验九 混合碱的分析

【目的要求】

(1) 掌握多元碱在滴定过程中溶液 pH 值的变化规律。
(2) 熟悉酸碱滴定中指示剂的选择原则。
(3) 进一步熟练掌握滴定管和移液管的正确使用。

【实验原理】

混合碱(工业品烧碱 NaOH 中常含有 Na_2CO_3，纯碱 Na_2CO_3 中常含有 $NaHCO_3$，这两种工业品都称为混合碱)的分析主要涉及对 NaOH、Na_2CO_3 和 $NaHCO_3$ 的测定。常用双指示剂法和 $BaCl_2$ 法。

1. 双指示剂法

以酚酞作指示剂，用 HCl 标准溶液滴定，指示第一化学计量点，消耗的 HCl 溶液的体积为 V_1，试样中 Na_2CO_3 滴至 $NaHCO_3$，NaOH 完全被滴定，若含 $NaHCO_3$，则未被滴定。在同一份溶液中，用甲基橙作指示剂，指示第二化学计量点，消耗的 HCl 溶液(即第一化学计量点到第二化学计量点消耗的)的体积为 V_2，此时 $NaHCO_3$（或是 Na_2CO_3 第一步被中和生成的，或是试样中含有的）滴至 H_2CO_3（H_2O 和 CO_2）。所涉及的化学反应方程式如下：

$$NaOH + HCl \Longrightarrow NaCl + H_2O$$

$$Na_2CO_3 + HCl \Longrightarrow NaCl + NaHCO_3$$

$$NaHCO_3 + HCl \Longrightarrow NaCl + H_2O + CO_2 \uparrow$$

当 $V_1 > V_2$ 时,试样为 Na_2CO_3 与 NaOH 的混合物,中和 Na_2CO_3 所需的 HCl 溶液是分两批加入的,两次用量应该相等。即滴定 Na_2CO_3 所消耗的 HCl 溶液的总体积为 $2V_2$,而中和 NaOH 所消耗的 HCl 溶液的体积为 $(V_1 - V_2)$。故计算 NaOH 和 Na_2CO_3 的含量的公式分别为

$$NaOH 的含量 = \frac{(V_1 - V_2) \times c(HCl) \times M(NaOH)}{V_s}$$

$$Na_2CO_3 的含量 = \frac{V_2 \times c(HCl) \times M(Na_2CO_3)}{V_s}$$

式中: V_s 为混合碱试样溶液的体积(mL)。

当 $V_1 < V_2$ 时,试样为 Na_2CO_3 与 $NaHCO_3$ 的混合物,此时 V_1 为达到第一化学计量点时 Na_2CO_3 所消耗的 HCl 溶液的体积,故 Na_2CO_3 所消耗的 HCl 溶液的体积为 $2V_1$,中和 $NaHCO_3$ 消耗的 HCl 溶液的体积为 $(V_2 - V_1)$。计算 $NaHCO_3$ 和 Na_2CO_3 的含量的公式分别为

$$NaHCO_3 的含量 = \frac{(V_2 - V_1) \times c(HCl) \times M(NaHCO_3)}{V_s}$$

$$Na_2CO_3 的含量 = \frac{V_1 \times c(HCl) \times M(Na_2CO_3)}{V_s}$$

式中: V_s 为混合碱试样溶液的体积(mL)。

2. $BaCl_2$ 法

对烧碱中 NaOH 和 Na_2CO_3 含量的测定:先取一份混合碱试样,加入 $BaCl_2$ 溶液,待 $BaCO_3$ 沉淀析出后,以酚酞作指示剂,用 HCl 标准溶液滴定 NaOH,设用去的 HCl 溶液的体积为 V_1;另取一份试样溶液,以甲基橙作指示剂,用 HCl 标准溶液滴定至橙色,测得的是碱的总量,消耗的 HCl 溶液的体积为 V_2。计算 NaOH 和 Na_2CO_3 含量的公式分别为

$$NaOH 的含量 = \frac{V_1 \times c(HCl) \times M(NaOH)}{V_s}$$

$$Na_2CO_3 的含量 = \frac{(V_2 - V_1) \times c(HCl) \times M(Na_2CO_3)}{2V_s}$$

式中: V_s 为混合碱试样溶液的体积(mL)。

纯碱中 Na_2CO_3 和 $NaHCO_3$ 含量的测定:先取一份混合碱试样,加入 NaOH 标准溶液的体积为 V_1,使 $NaHCO_3$ 转化为 Na_2CO_3,再加入 $BaCl_2$ 溶液使之生成 $BaCO_3$ 沉淀,然后以酚酞作指示剂,用 HCl 标准溶液返滴定过量的 NaOH,所消耗的 HCl 溶液的体积为 V_2;另取一份混合碱试样,以甲基橙为指示剂,用 HCl 标准溶液滴定碱

的总量,消耗的体积为 V_3。计算 $NaHCO_3$ 和 Na_2CO_3 含量的公式分别为

$$NaHCO_3 的含量 = \frac{[c(NaOH) \times V_1 - c(HCl) \times V_2] \times M(NaHCO_3)}{V_s}$$

$$Na_2CO_3 的含量 = \frac{\{c(HCl) \times V_3 - [c(NaOH) \times V_1 - c(HCl) \times V_2]\} \times M(Na_2CO_3)}{2V_s}$$

式中：V_s 为混合碱试样溶液的体积(mL)。

【仪器与试剂】

电子天平(0.1 mg)、酸式滴定管(50 mL×1)、移液管(20 mL×2)、锥形瓶(250 mL×3)、滴定管架、洗瓶、洗耳球。

无水 Na_2CO_3(AR,基准物质)、混合碱试样(l)、酚酞指示剂、甲基橙指示剂、$BaCl_2$ 溶液(1%)、HCl 溶液(约 2 mol·L^{-1})、NaOH 溶液(约 0.1 mol·L^{-1},已标定)。

【实验步骤】

1. 0.1 mol·L^{-1} HCl 溶液的标定

(1) 配制 500 mL 0.1 mol·L^{-1} HCl 溶液。

(2) 准确称取 1.1～1.4 g 基准物质 Na_2CO_3,加入蒸馏水溶解,定量转入 250 mL 容量瓶中,定容,摇匀。准确移取上述 Na_2CO_3 溶液 20.00 mL 于锥形瓶中,加入 1～2 滴甲基橙指示剂,用待标定的 HCl 溶液滴定至溶液由黄色变为橙色,即为终点。计算 HCl 溶液的浓度。

2. 混合碱试样的测定

(1) 双指示剂法。移取 20.00 mL 试样于 250 mL 锥形瓶中,加入 1～3 滴酚酞指示剂,用 HCl 标准溶液滴定至溶液由红色变为无色,消耗 HCl 溶液的体积为 V_1。在同一份溶液中,加入 2～3 滴甲基橙指示剂,继续滴定至溶液由黄色变为橙色,又消耗 HCl 溶液的体积为 V_2。

根据 V_1 与 V_2 的大小,可判断混合碱由何种组分组成,并定量计算其含量。

(2) $BaCl_2$ 法。移取 20.00 mL 试样于 250 mL 锥形瓶中,加入已知浓度的 NaOH 标准溶液的体积为 V_1,若混合溶液为 NaOH 与 Na_2CO_3,则此步可省略(观察 NaOH 的量是否足够,可在沉淀后加酚酞观察,若显红色,表明 NaOH 的量足够,若显无色,则不足)。再加入 1% $BaCl_2$ 溶液至略过量,使 Na_2CO_3 完全沉淀为 $BaCO_3$,加入 2～3 滴酚酞指示剂,用 HCl 标准溶液滴定至溶液由红色变为无色,消耗的 HCl 溶液的体积为 V_2。

另取一份试样 20.00 mL,以甲基橙(1～2 滴)为指示剂,用 HCl 标准溶液滴定至溶液由黄色变为橙色,消耗 HCl 溶液的体积为 V_3,根据 HCl 溶液与 NaOH 溶液的体积与浓度,可判断混合碱的组成,计算各自的含量。

【思考题】

(1) 用 $0.1\ mol\cdot L^{-1}$ HCl 溶液滴定 Na_2CO_3,以甲基橙为指示剂时,有时会出现较大的终点误差,为什么?应注意什么问题?可采取什么措施减小误差?

(2) 比较两种测定混合碱的方法的优缺点。

(3) 用双指示剂法测定混合碱,在同一份溶液中测定,判断在下列五种情况下试样的组成。

①$V_1=0$;②$V_2=0$;③$V_1>V_2$;④$V_1<V_2$;⑤$V_1=V_2$。

实验十　消毒液中 H_2O_2 含量的测定

【目的要求】

(1) 了解 $KMnO_4$ 标准溶液的配制和标定方法。

(2) 掌握用氧化还原滴定法测定消毒液中 H_2O_2 含量的原理和方法。

【实验原理】

双氧水是医药上常用的消毒液,药用双氧水含 H_2O_2 约 3%。本实验用 $KMnO_4$ 法测定其含量。在强酸性介质中 MnO_4^- 氧化 H_2O_2 后产生 O_2 和近乎无色的 Mn^{2+},其反应方程式如下:

$$5H_2O_2+2MnO_4^-+6H^+=\!=\!=2Mn^{2+}+8H_2O+5O_2\uparrow$$

因而,当 $KMnO_4$ 溶液滴加到酸性 H_2O_2 溶液中时,其颜色将褪掉,直至 H_2O_2 反应完全,此时再加入一滴 $KMnO_4$ 溶液将会使溶液显色(即为滴定终点)。根据滴定消耗的 $KMnO_4$ 溶液的体积和浓度,即可计算出 H_2O_2 的含量。

市售的 $KMnO_4$ 试剂不稳定,易被其他还原性物质还原,因此,$KMnO_4$ 标准溶液不宜用直接法配制,而是配成近似浓度的溶液(在中性介质中,其还原产物为难溶的 MnO_2,故标定 $KMnO_4$ 溶液之前,先将 $KMnO_4$ 溶液煮沸让其与杂质反应,并过滤除去难溶的 MnO_2),再用一级标准物质 $Na_2C_2O_4$ 标定 $KMnO_4$ 溶液。其标定反应方程式为

$$5C_2O_4^{2-}+2MnO_4^-+16H^+=\!=\!=2Mn^{2+}+10CO_2\uparrow+8H_2O$$

该标定反应的反应速率较慢,可用多种方法提高其反应速率。较简便的方法之一是,加热溶液至 80~90 ℃,并始终控制滴定时的温度大于 60 ℃。

【仪器与试剂】

电子天平(0.1 mg,0.01 g)、干燥器、称量瓶、酸式滴定管(50 mL×1)、移液管

(10 mL×1,25 mL×2)、容量瓶(250 mL×2)、锥形瓶(250 mL×3)、烧杯(1 000 mL ×1,250 mL×1)、量筒(100 mL×1)、试剂瓶(500 mL×1)、砂芯漏斗、吸滤瓶、滤纸、水流抽气泵、洗瓶、胶头滴管、洗耳球、玻棒。

$KMnO_4$(AR,s)、$Na_2C_2O_4$(AR,s)、H_2SO_4溶液(6 mol·L^{-1})、药用双氧水(约3%)、蒸馏水。

【实验步骤】

1.0.02 mol·L^{-1} $KMnO_4$溶液的配制和标定

(1)用电子天平(0.01 g)称取 $KMnO_4$ 约 1.5 g,置于烧杯中,加蒸馏水溶解,稀释至 500 mL,加热至沸腾并保持微沸状态 1 h,静置过夜,然后用砂芯漏斗过滤。滤液储存于棕色试剂瓶中,在暗处密闭保存。

(2)将 3 g $Na_2C_2O_4$ 放入称量瓶,于 110~120 ℃烘干 1 h,冷却,放置在干燥器中。准确称取 1.6~1.7 g(±0.1 mg)干燥后的 $Na_2C_2O_4$,置于烧杯中,加适量蒸馏水使之溶解,用玻棒转移至 250 mL 容量瓶中,用少量蒸馏水淋洗烧杯 2~3 次,淋洗液一并转入容量瓶中,加蒸馏水稀释至标线附近时改用胶头滴管加至标线,盖好瓶塞,充分摇匀。

(3)用移液管吸取 25.00 mL $Na_2C_2O_4$ 溶液置于 250 mL 锥形瓶中,加 15 mL 6 mol·L^{-1} H_2SO_4溶液。加热溶液至 80~90 ℃,趁热用 $KMnO_4$ 溶液慢慢滴定(滴定过快,$KMnO_4$ 将与产物 Mn^{2+} 反应生成黑色的 MnO_2)。注意控制反应温度大于 60 ℃,边滴加边摇锥形瓶,直至溶液显淡红色且保持 30 s 不褪色(放一张白纸在锥形瓶下方以便于颜色的观察),即达滴定终点。记录数据(由于 $KMnO_4$ 颜色较深,很难观察弯月面,通常读取最高点)。平行标定 3 次。根据滴定所消耗的体积和 $Na_2C_2O_4$ 的质量,按下式计算 $KMnO_4$ 标准溶液的准确浓度:

$$c(KMnO_4) = \frac{2}{5} \times \frac{m(Na_2C_2O_4) \times 1\,000 \times 25.00}{250.0 \times V(KMnO_4) \times M(Na_2C_2O_4)}$$

2.双氧水中 H_2O_2 含量的测定

用移液管吸取 10.00 mL 药用双氧水置于 250 mL 容量瓶中,加蒸馏水稀释至标线,摇匀。然后用移液管吸取 25.00 mL 稀释后的双氧水待测液,置于 250 mL 锥形瓶中,加 15 mL 6 mol·L^{-1} H_2SO_4溶液,摇匀。边摇锥形瓶边用 $KMnO_4$ 标准溶液滴定,至溶液显淡红色且保持 30 s 不褪色为止。平行测定 3 次。根据滴定所消耗的 $KMnO_4$ 标准溶液的体积,按下式计算 H_2O_2 的含量:

$$\rho(H_2O_2) = \frac{5}{2} \times \frac{c(KMnO_4) \times V(KMnO_4) \times M(H_2O_2)}{10.00 \times \frac{25.00}{250.0}}$$

【结果记录和处理】

1. 0.02 mol·L^{-1}KMnO$_4$溶液的标定

编　号		I	II	III
Na$_2$C$_2$O$_4$的质量/g				
KMnO$_4$	初读数/mL			
	终读数/mL			
	V(KMnO$_4$)/mL			
c(KMnO$_4$)/(mol·L^{-1})				
$\bar{c}$(KMnO$_4$)/(mol·L^{-1})				
$\bar{d}_r$/(%)				

2. 双氧水中 H$_2$O$_2$含量的测定

编　号		I	II	III
KMnO$_4$	初读数/mL			
	终读数/mL			
	V(KMnO$_4$)/mL			
ρ(H$_2$O$_2$)/(g·L^{-1})				
$\bar{\rho}$(H$_2$O$_2$)/(g·L^{-1})				
$\bar{d}_r$/(%)				

【思考题】

（1）在本实验中，如果酸度不够，KMnO$_4$会产生 MnO$_2$，而不是 Mn^{2+}，对实验结果会产生什么影响？

（2）在储存过程中，KMnO$_4$标准溶液将会分解为 MnO$_2$，其充当了分解反应继续进行的催化剂。解释一周后用同样的 KMnO$_4$标准溶液重新进行滴定时滴定结果的误差。

（3）下面的反应方程式有什么错误？

$$6H_3O^+ + 2MnO_4^- + 9H_2O_2 \longrightarrow 2Mn^{2+} + 7O_2 + 18H_2O$$

实验十一　注射液中葡萄糖含量的测定

【目的要求】

（1）了解 Na$_2$S$_2$O$_3$标准溶液和 I$_2$标准溶液的配制方法。掌握标定 Na$_2$S$_2$O$_3$标准

溶液和 I_2 标准溶液浓度的原理和方法。

(2)掌握碘量法测定葡萄糖含量的原理和方法。

【实验原理】

碘量法是无机物与有机物分析中应用较为广泛的一种氧化还原滴定法。在本实验中,碘(I_2)与 NaOH 作用可生成次碘酸钠(NaIO),它可将葡萄糖($C_6H_{12}O_6$)定量氧化生成葡萄糖酸($C_6H_{12}O_7$)。反应结束后,在酸性条件下,未与葡萄糖作用的次碘酸钠可转变成单质碘析出,用 $Na_2S_2O_3$ 标准溶液滴定析出的碘,便可计算出样品中葡萄糖的含量。其反应方程式如下:

$$I_2 + C_6H_{12}O_6 + 2NaOH \Longrightarrow C_6H_{12}O_7 + 2NaI + H_2O$$

$$3IO^- \Longrightarrow IO_3^- + 2I^-$$

$$IO_3^- + 5I^- + 6H^+ \Longrightarrow 3I_2 + 3H_2O$$

$$I_2 + 2S_2O_3^{2-} \Longrightarrow S_4O_6^{2-} + 2I^-$$

硫代硫酸钠($Na_2S_2O_3 \cdot 5H_2O$)一般都含有少量杂质,如 S、Na_2SO_3、Na_2SO_4 等,同时还容易风化和潮解,因此不能直接配制准确浓度的溶液。通常用 $K_2Cr_2O_7$ 作为基准物质标定 $Na_2S_2O_3$ 溶液的浓度。$K_2Cr_2O_7$ 先与 KI 反应析出 I_2,再用 $Na_2S_2O_3$ 标准溶液滴定。其反应如下:

$$Cr_2O_7^{2-} + 6I^- + 14H^+ \Longrightarrow 2Cr^{3+} + 3I_2 + 7H_2O$$

$$I_2 + 2S_2O_3^{2-} \Longrightarrow S_4O_6^{2-} + 2I^-$$

【仪器与试剂】

电子天平(0.01 g)、酸式滴定管(50 mL×1)、碱式滴定管(50 mL×1)、移液管(20 mL×3)、碘量瓶(250 mL×3)、试剂瓶(500 mL×2)、洗瓶、洗耳球、烧杯(100 mL×1,250 mL×1)、玻棒、量筒(100 mL×1,10 mL×2)。

HCl 溶液(2 mol·L^{-1},1:1)、NaOH 溶液(0.2 mol·L^{-1})、淀粉溶液(5 g·L^{-1})、$Na_2S_2O_3 \cdot 5H_2O$(AR,s)、KI(AR,s)、I_2(AR,s)、$K_2Cr_2O_7$ 溶液(0.016 67 mol·L^{-1})、葡萄糖注射液(5%)、蒸馏水。

【实验步骤】

1. $Na_2S_2O_3$ 标准溶液的配制与标定

(1)配制 0.05 mol·L^{-1} $Na_2S_2O_3$ 溶液。称取适量 $Na_2S_2O_3 \cdot 5H_2O$ 溶于 500 mL 煮沸并冷却的蒸馏水中,转入细口瓶中,摇匀。

(2)标定。移取 20.00 mL 0.016 67 mol·L^{-1} $K_2Cr_2O_7$ 标准溶液于碘量瓶中,加入 1 g KI,摇动溶解后,加入 3 mL HCl 溶液(1:1),盖上盖子,并置于暗处反应 5 min,然后加入 100 mL 蒸馏水,立即用 $Na_2S_2O_3$ 溶液滴定至溶液由红棕色变为浅黄色,加入 2 mL 淀粉溶液,继续滴定至蓝色刚好消失,即为终点。平行滴定 3 次。按下式计算 $Na_2S_2O_3$ 溶液的浓度。

$$c(Na_2S_2O_3) = \frac{6 \times c(K_2Cr_2O_7) \times V(K_2Cr_2O_7)}{V(Na_2S_2O_3)}$$

2. I_2 溶液的配制与标定

称取 7 g KI 于 100 mL 烧杯中,加入 20 mL 蒸馏水和 2 g I_2,充分搅拌,使 I_2 溶解完全,转移至棕色试剂瓶中,加蒸馏水稀释至 300 mL,摇匀。准确移取 20.00 mL I_2 溶液于 250 mL 锥形瓶中,加 50 mL 蒸馏水稀释,用已标定好的 $Na_2S_2O_3$ 标准溶液滴定至溶液呈黄色,加入 2 mL 淀粉溶液,继续滴定至蓝色刚好消失,即为终点。平行测定 3 份。按下式计算 I_2 溶液的浓度。

$$c(I_2) = \frac{c(Na_2S_2O_3) \times V(Na_2S_2O_3)}{2 \times V(I_2)}$$

3. 葡萄糖含量的测定

将 1.00 mL 5% 葡萄糖注射液准确稀释 100 倍,摇匀后,取 20.00 mL 于碘量瓶中,向其中准确加入 20.00 mL I_2 标准溶液,慢慢滴加 0.2 mol·L^{-1} NaOH 溶液,边加边摇,直到溶液呈淡黄色。将碘量瓶盖好,放置 10~15 min,加入 6 mL 2 mol·L^{-1} HCl 溶液,立即用 $Na_2S_2O_3$ 标准溶液滴定,至溶液呈浅黄色时加入 2 mL 淀粉溶液,继续滴定至蓝色刚好消失,即为终点。平行滴定 2~3 次。按下式计算样品中葡萄糖的含量。

$$葡萄糖的含量 = \frac{[2c(I_2) \times V(I_2) - c(Na_2S_2O_3) \times V(Na_2S_2O_3)] \times M(C_6H_{12}O_6) \times 100}{2\,000 \times 20.00}$$

【思考题】

(1) 配制 I_2 溶液时为什么要加入过量的 KI? 为什么先用少量蒸馏水进行溶解?

(2) 氧化葡萄糖时,加稀 NaOH 溶液的速度能否快? 为什么?

(3) I_2 溶液能否装在碱式滴定管中? 为什么?

实验十二　自来水总硬度的测定

【目的要求】

(1) 掌握 EDTA 法的特性及其在配位滴定中的应用。

(2) 熟悉 EDTA 法测定水的总硬度的原理和方法。

(3) 掌握金属指示剂的作用原理、适宜 pH 值范围及选择方法。

(4) 了解缓冲溶液在配位滴定中的重要性及其配制方法。

【实验原理】

EDTA 能与大多数金属离子形成稳定配合物,因此可用 EDTA 标准溶液对大多数金属离子进行滴定分析。

EDTA 一般不直接配制成标准溶液,而是先配制成浓度大致相近的溶液,再进行标定。标定 EDTA 溶液的基准物质有纯锌、铋、铜、ZnO、$CaCO_3$、$MgSO_4 \cdot 7H_2O$ 等。通常标定条件尽可能与测定条件一致,以免引起系统误差。

水的硬度是一种比较古老的概念,最初是指水沉淀肥皂的能力。使肥皂沉淀的主要原因是水中存在钙、镁离子。总硬度是指水中钙、镁离子的总浓度,其中包括碳酸盐硬度(也叫暂时硬度,即通过加热能以碳酸盐形式沉淀下来的钙、镁离子)和非碳酸盐硬度(亦称永久硬度,即加热后不能沉淀下来的那部分钙、镁离子)。

硬度对工业用水影响很大,尤其是锅炉用水,因此,硬度较高的水都要经过软化处理并经过滴定分析达到一定标准后才能输入锅炉。其他很多工业用水对水的硬度也都有一定的要求。生活饮用水中硬度过高会影响肠胃的消化功能,我国生活饮用水卫生标准中规定水的硬度(以 $CaCO_3$ 计)不得超过 450 mg $\cdot$ L^{-1}。

在国际标准、我国国家标准及有关部门的行业标准中,总硬度的测定方法都是以铬黑 T 为指示剂的配位滴定法。这一方法适用于生活饮用水、工业锅炉用水、冷却水、地下水及没有严重污染的地表水。

在 pH＝10 的 NH_3-NH_4Cl 缓冲溶液中,以铬黑 T 为指示剂,用 EDTA 标准溶液滴定溶液中的 Ca^{2+}、Mg^{2+}。铬黑 T 本身呈蓝色,它与 Mg^{2+} 形成的配合物呈紫红色,用 EDTA 溶液滴定时,EDTA 先与游离的 Ca^{2+} 和 Mg^{2+} 反应形成无色的配合物,达到化学计量点时,EDTA 夺取指示剂配合物中的 Mg^{2+},使指示剂游离出来,溶液由酒红色变成纯蓝色,即为终点(如果水样中没有或有极少量 Mg^{2+},则终点变色不够敏锐,这时应加入少许 $MgNa_2Y$ 溶液,或者改用酸性铬蓝 K 作指示剂)。反应方程式如下:

滴定前 $Mg^{2+} + HIn^{2-}$(纯蓝色) $\Longrightarrow [MgIn]^-$(酒红色)$+ H^+$

化学计量点前 $Ca^{2+} + H_2Y^{2-} \Longrightarrow [CaY]^{2-} + 2H^+$

$Mg^{2+} + H_2Y^{2-} \Longrightarrow [MgY]^{2-} + 2H^+$

化学计量点时 $[MgIn]^-$(酒红色)$+ H_2Y^{2-} \Longrightarrow [MgY]^{2-} + HIn^{2-}$(纯蓝色)$+ H^+$

根据消耗的 EDTA 标准溶液的体积计算水的总硬度(以 $CaCO_3$ 计,mg $\cdot$ L^{-1})。

$$水的总硬度 = \frac{c(\text{EDTA}) \times V(\text{EDTA}) \times M(\text{CaCO}_3)}{V(水样)} \times 1\ 000$$

根据滴定第一份水样所消耗的 EDTA 标准溶液的体积,在滴定第二份和第三份水样时,应在水样中先加入所需总体积 95% 左右的 EDTA 标准溶液,然后再加入缓冲溶液(升高 pH 值)进行滴定,这样可以降低水或试剂中的 CO_3^{2-} 对 Ca^{2+} 的干扰,使终点变色比较敏锐。

【仪器与试剂】

电子天平(0.1 mg,0.01 g)、称量瓶(2)、酸式滴定管(50 mL×1)、移液管(20 mL×1,100 mL×1)、吸量管(20 mL×1,10 mL×1)、容量瓶(250 mL×1)、锥形瓶(250 mL×3)、烧杯(100 mL×1,250 mL×1)、量筒(100 mL×1,50 mL×1,10 mL×2)、试剂瓶(500 mL×1)、洗瓶、胶头滴管、洗耳球、玻棒、表面皿、电炉。

乙二胺四乙酸二钠(简写为 $Na_2H_2Y \cdot 2H_2O$ 或 EDTA,AR,s)、$CaCO_3$(GR,s)、HCl 溶液(1:1)、三乙醇胺溶液(1:3)、铬黑 T 指示剂、NH_3-NH_4Cl 缓冲溶液(pH=10,将 67 g NH_4Cl 溶于 300 mL 重蒸水中,加入 570 mL 氨水,稀释至 1 L,混匀)、Mg-EDTA 溶液(称取 5.0 g $MgNa_2Y \cdot 4H_2O$ 或 $MgK_2Y \cdot 2H_2O$,溶解于 1 L 水中;还可将 2.44 g $MgCl_2 \cdot 6H_2O$ 及 4.44 g $Na_2H_2Y \cdot 2H_2O$ 溶于 200 mL 水中,加入 20 mL NH_3-NH_4Cl 缓冲溶液及适量铬黑 T 指示剂,显紫红色,如是蓝色,应再加入少量 $MgCl_2 \cdot 6H_2O$ 至显紫红色,在搅拌下滴加 0.02 mol·L^{-1} EDTA 溶液至刚刚变为蓝色,然后加水稀释到 1 L)。

【实验步骤】

(1) 配制 500 mL 0.01 mol·L^{-1} EDTA 标准溶液。

(2) 0.01 mol·L^{-1} 钙标准溶液的配制。准确称取约 0.25 g $CaCO_3$ 置于 100 mL 烧杯中,加几滴水润湿,盖上表面皿,从烧杯嘴处缓慢滴加 1:1 HCl 溶液(约 5 mL)使 $CaCO_3$ 完全溶解,再加 20 mL 水,小火煮沸 2 min 以除去 CO_2,冷却后定量转移至 250 mL 容量瓶中,加水稀释至刻度,摇匀。计算钙标准溶液的浓度。

(3) EDTA 标准溶液的标定。移取 20.00 mL 钙标准溶液于锥形瓶中,加 25 mL 水及 2 mL Mg-EDTA 溶液,预加 15.00 mL EDTA 标准溶液,再加 5 mL NH_3-NH_4Cl 缓冲溶液及适量的铬黑 T 指示剂,立即用 EDTA 标准溶液滴定至溶液由酒红色变成纯蓝色,即为终点。平行滴定 3 次(从滴定第二份开始,应将预加 EDTA 标准溶液的量调整为所需总体积的 95%),以其平均体积计算 EDTA 标准溶液的浓度。

(4) 自来水总硬度的测定。用 100 mL 移液管量取 100.00 mL 自来水样置于锥形瓶中,加 5 mL NH_3-NH_4Cl 缓冲溶液及少量铬黑 T 指示剂,立即用 EDTA 标准溶液滴定。滴定时要用力摇动,近终点时应慢滴多摇,溶液由紫红色变成纯蓝色为终点。平行滴定 3 份,所消耗的 EDTA 标准溶液的体积差应不大于 0.10 mL。计算水的总硬度,以 $CaCO_3$(mg·L^{-1})表示。

从滴定第二份开始,应先加所需总体积 95% 的 EDTA 标准溶液,然后再加其他试剂。

【注意事项】

(1) 如果水样中 HCO_3^-、H_2CO_3 含量较高,滴定终点变色不敏锐,可经酸化并煮沸后再滴定,或采用返滴定法。

(2) 水样中若含有 Fe^{3+}、Al^{3+}、Cu^{2+}、Pb^{2+} 等离子,会干扰 Ca^{2+}、Mg^{2+} 的测定,可加入三乙醇胺、KCN、Na_2S 等进行掩蔽,本实验只提供三乙醇胺溶液。所测水样是否需要加三乙醇胺及 Mg-EDTA 溶液,应根据实验中的具体情况来确定。

【思考题】

(1) 在 pH=10,以铬黑 T 为指示剂时,为什么滴定的是 Ca^{2+}、Mg^{2+} 的总量?

(2) 用钙标准溶液标定 EDTA 溶液时,为什么在加入 NH_3-NH_4Cl 缓冲溶液前,先预加一部分 EDTA 溶液?

(3) 配制 Mg-EDTA 溶液时,为什么两者的比例一定要恰好为 1:1? 否则,对实验结果有何影响?

实验十三　同离子效应与沉淀平衡

【目的要求】

(1) 掌握并验证同离子效应对弱电解质解离平衡的影响,加深理解同离子效应。

预习内容

(2) 根据溶度积规则判断沉淀的生成和溶解、沉淀的转化和分步沉淀。

(3) 掌握离心机的使用和离心分离技术。

【实验原理】

在弱电解质溶液中加入含有相同离子的易溶强电解质时,弱电解质的解离度将减小,这种现象称为"同离子效应"。这种效应可借助酸碱指示剂产生的颜色变化来观察。

在难溶强电解质 A_mB_n 的饱和溶液中,当温度一定时,存在如下平衡:

$$A_mB_n \rightleftharpoons mA^{n+} + nB^{m-}$$

此时,离子浓度幂的乘积为一常数,称为溶度积常数 K_{sp},即 $K_{sp} = [A^{n+}]^m[B^{m-}]^n$。

根据溶度积常数可以判断沉淀的生成与溶解,对于一个给定的难溶强电解质,其离子积用 IP 表示,则

① 当 IP=K_{sp}时,达到平衡(饱和溶液);

② 当 IP>K_{sp}时,沉淀生成;

③ 当 IP $<K_{sp}$ 时,沉淀溶解。

此即溶度积规则。

如果在溶液中有两种或两种以上的离子都可以与同一种沉淀剂反应生成难溶电解质,沉淀的先后顺序根据所需沉淀剂离子浓度的大小而定。所需沉淀剂离子浓度小的优先沉淀出来,所需沉淀剂离子浓度大的后沉淀出来,这种先后沉淀的现象,称为"分步沉淀"。使一种难溶电解质转化为另一种难溶电解质的过程称为"沉淀的转化"。一般来说,溶解度大的难溶电解质容易转化为溶解度小的难溶电解质。

【仪器与试剂】

离心机、烧杯(100 mL×4)、离心试管(2)、试管(10)、量筒(50 mL×3,10 mL×1)。

NaAc(AR,s),NaAc 溶液(0.1 mol · L^{-1})、NH_4Cl(s)、HAc 溶液(0.1 mol · L^{-1})、HNO_3 溶液(6 mol · L^{-1})、NaOH 溶液(0.2 mol · L^{-1},0.002 mol · L^{-1})、氨水(0.1 mol · L^{-1},2 mol · L^{-1})、HCl 溶液(0.1 mol · L^{-1},6 mol · L^{-1})、$Pb(NO_3)_2$ 溶液(0.1 mol · L^{-1},0.001 mol · L^{-1})、KI 溶液(0.1 mol · L^{-1},0.001 mol · L^{-1})、NH_4Cl 溶液(1 mol · L^{-1})、$CdCl_2$ 溶液(0.1 mol · L^{-1})、$FeCl_3$ 溶液(0.1 mol · L^{-1})、K_2CrO_4 溶液(0.1 mol · L^{-1})、Na_2S 溶液(0.1 mol · L^{-1})、Na_2CO_3 溶液(0.1 mol · L^{-1})、NaCl 溶液(1 mol · L^{-1},0.1 mol · L^{-1})、$MgCl_2$ 溶液(0.2 mol · L^{-1})、$(NH_4)_2C_2O_4$ 饱和溶液、$AgNO_3$ 溶液(0.1 mol · L^{-1})、$CuSO_4$ 溶液(0.1 mol · L^{-1})、$CaCl_2$ 溶液(0.1 mol · L^{-1})、$BaCl_2$ 溶液(0.3 mol · L^{-1})、pH 试纸(5.5～9.0)、甲基橙指示剂、酚酞指示剂。

【实验步骤】

1.同离子效应

(1) 在试管中加入 5 mL 0.1 mol · L^{-1} HAc 溶液,再加入 1～2 滴甲基橙指示剂,摇匀,观察溶液的颜色。然后分盛两支试管,在其中一支试管中加入少量 NaAc 晶体,摇动试管以促使 NaAc 晶体溶解,观察溶液颜色的变化,并加以解释。

(2) 试以 0.1 mol · L^{-1} 氨水为例,设计一个实验,证明同离子效应使氨水的解离度降低(应选用哪种指示剂)。

(3) 在烧杯中加入 15 mL 0.1 mol · L^{-1} HAc 溶液和 15 mL 0.1 mol · L^{-1} NaAc 溶液,搅匀,用 pH 试纸测其 pH 值;然后将溶液分成三份,第一份加入 10 滴 0.1 mol · L^{-1} HCl 溶液,第二份加入 10 滴 0.1 mol · L^{-1} NaOH 溶液,第三份加入 10 滴去离子水,分别测其 pH 值。解释缓冲溶液的作用。

2.溶度积规则的应用

(1) 沉淀的生成。

① 在试管中加 1 mL 0.1 mol · L^{-1} $Pb(NO_3)_2$ 溶液,然后加入 1 mL 0.1 mol · L^{-1}

KI 溶液,观察有无沉淀生成;在另一支试管中加 1 mL 0.001 mol·L^{-1}Pb$(NO_3)_2$ 溶液,然后加入 1 mL 0.001 mol·L^{-1}KI 溶液,观察有无沉淀生成。试以溶度积规则解释之。

② 取 1 支离心试管,加入 2 滴 0.1 mol·L^{-1}CuSO$_4$ 溶液和 6 滴 0.1 mol·L^{-1}CdCl$_2$ 溶液,稀释至 2 mL,摇匀后加入 3 滴 0.1 mol·L^{-1}Na$_2$S 溶液,边滴加边观察先生成的沉淀是黄色还是黑色的。离心沉降,往清液中滴加数滴 0.1 mol·L^{-1}Na$_2$S 溶液,观察出现什么颜色的沉淀。试根据有关溶度积数据给予解释。

（2）沉淀的溶解。

① 取 5 滴 0.3 mol·L^{-1}BaCl$_2$ 溶液,加 3 滴饱和草酸铵溶液,此时有白色沉淀生成,在沉淀上滴加数滴 6 mol·L^{-1}HCl 溶液,观察有何现象发生,写出反应方程式。

② 取 10 滴 0.1 mol·L^{-1}AgNO$_3$ 溶液,加 10 滴 0.1 mol·L^{-1}NaCl 溶液,此时有白色沉淀生成,在沉淀上滴加数滴 2 mol·L^{-1}氨水,观察有何现象发生,写出反应方程式。

③ 取 5 滴 0.1 mol·L^{-1}FeCl$_3$ 溶液,加 5 滴 0.2 mol·L^{-1}NaOH 溶液,生成 Fe$(OH)_3$ 沉淀;另取 5 滴 0.1 mol·L^{-1}CaCl$_2$ 溶液,加 5 滴 0.1 mol·L^{-1}Na$_2$CO$_3$ 溶液,得 CaCO$_3$ 沉淀。分别在上述沉淀中滴加数滴 6 mol·L^{-1}HCl 溶液,观察有何现象发生,写出反应方程式。

④ 在试管中加入 10 滴 0.2 mol·L^{-1}MgCl$_2$ 溶液,再滴加 2 滴 2 mol·L^{-1}氨水,观察有何现象发生。然后再滴加 10 滴 1 mol·L^{-1}NH$_4$Cl 溶液,观察又有何现象发生,写出反应方程式。

⑤ 在试管中加入 5 滴 0.1 mol·L^{-1}CuSO$_4$ 溶液,再滴加 5 滴 0.1 mol·L^{-1}Na$_2$S 溶液,观察有何现象发生。然后向该试管中滴加 10 滴 6 mol·L^{-1}HNO$_3$ 溶液,并微热之,观察有何现象发生,写出反应方程式。

（3）沉淀的转化。

① 在盛有 10 滴 0.1 mol·L^{-1}AgNO$_3$ 溶液的试管中,加 5 滴 0.1 mol·L^{-1}K$_2$CrO$_4$ 溶液,然后滴加 0.1 mol·L^{-1}NaCl 溶液,观察有何现象发生,写出反应方程式。

② 取 1 支离心试管,分别加入 10 滴 0.1 mol·L^{-1}Pb$(NO_3)_2$ 溶液和 1 mol·L^{-1}NaCl 溶液。离心分离,弃去清液,向沉淀中滴加 0.1 mol·L^{-1}KI 溶液并剧烈搅拌,观察沉淀颜色的变化。说明原因并写出有关反应方程式。

3. Mg$(OH)_2$ 溶度积的预测

取 50 mL 烧杯 1 只,加 25 mL 0.2 mol·L^{-1}MgCl$_2$ 溶液,烧杯底部衬一黑纸。在 MgCl$_2$ 溶液中逐滴滴入 0.002 mol·L^{-1}NaOH 溶液,并不断搅拌,直到开始有沉淀产生(在强光下观察,NaOH 溶液不能过量),放置,用 pH 试纸测定溶液的 pH 值,计算$[OH^-]$和K_{sp}。

【思考题】

（1）同离子效应对弱电解质的解离度及难溶电解质的溶解度各有什么影响？

（2）如何进行沉淀和溶液的分离？在离心分离操作中有哪些应注意之处？

（3）同离子效应与缓冲溶液的原理有何异同？

实验十四　缓冲溶液的配制与性质

【目的要求】

（1）加深对缓冲溶液缓冲作用及原理的理解。

预习内容

（2）掌握缓冲溶液的性质、缓冲容量与缓冲溶液总浓度及缓冲比的关系。

（3）学习缓冲溶液的配制方法，进一步熟练掌握吸量管的使用，学会用缓冲比色法测定溶液的 pH 值。

【实验原理】

缓冲溶液具有在少量强酸、强碱或稍加稀释的作用下仍保持其 pH 值基本不变的性质。缓冲溶液一般由弱酸（HB）及其共轭碱（B^-）组成，其 pH 值可用下式计算：

$$pH = pK_a + \lg \frac{c(B^-)}{c(HB)}$$

K_a 为共轭酸的酸解离常数。

上式表明，缓冲溶液的 pH 值取决于共轭酸的解离常数以及平衡时溶液中所含共轭碱和共轭酸的浓度比值。配制缓冲溶液时，若使用相同浓度的共轭酸和共轭碱，则可用其体积比代替浓度比，即

$$pH = pK_a + \lg \frac{V(B^-)}{V(HB)}$$

缓冲比色法测定溶液 pH 值的步骤：选择适当的指示剂与一系列已知 pH 值的缓冲溶液配成标准比色系列，然后在待测溶液中加入同类同量的指示剂，并将待测溶液所呈的颜色与标准比色系列进行比较，确定待测溶液的 pH 值。标准比色系列每管间隔约为 0.2pH 单位，故此法一般可准确到 0.1pH 单位。

缓冲溶液缓冲能力的大小可用缓冲容量 β 表示。β 值取决于缓冲溶液的总浓度及缓冲比。

【仪器与试剂】

比色管(10 mL×10)、吸量管(10.00 mL×4,5.00 mL×1)、烧杯(100 mL×4)、试管(6)、洗耳球、洗瓶。

K_2HPO_4 溶液(0.2 mol · L^{-1})、KH_2PO_4 溶液(0.2 mol · L^{-1})、NaOH 溶液(0.2 mol · L^{-1})、HCl 溶液(0.2 mol · L^{-1})、溴百里酚蓝指示剂、甲基橙指示剂、广泛 pH 指示剂。

【实验步骤】

1.配制比色系列

取 9 支比色管,按表中数据分别加入相应的 0.2 mol · L^{-1} KH_2PO_4 溶液和 0.2 mol · L^{-1} K_2HPO_4 溶液,再各加 4 滴溴百里酚蓝指示剂,摇匀后,观察比色系列的颜色变化,并计算各自的 pH 值。(H_3PO_4 $pK_{a1}=2.12$;$pK_{a2}=7.21$;$pK_{a3}=12.67$)

比色管编号	I	II	III	IV	V	VI	VII	VIII	IX
0.2 mol · L^{-1} KH_2PO_4/mL	1.00	2.00	3.00	4.00	5.00	6.00	7.00	8.00	9.00
0.2 mol · L^{-1} K_2HPO_4/mL	9.00	8.00	7.00	6.00	5.00	4.00	3.00	2.00	1.00
溴百里酚蓝指示剂/滴	4	4	4	4	4	4	4	4	4
pH 值理论值									
自制缓冲溶液的 pH 值测定值									

2.配制缓冲溶液

在浓度均为 0.2 mol · L^{-1} 的三种溶液(KH_2PO_4、NaOH、HCl)中选择两种溶液配制出 30.00 mL pH=7.40 的缓冲溶液。移取 10.00 mL 自制缓冲溶液于比色管中,滴入 4 滴溴百里酚蓝指示剂,摇匀后,与比色系列比较颜色,测定其 pH 值。

3.缓冲溶液的性质

分别取 2 mL 自制缓冲溶液于 3 支试管中,各加 4 滴广泛 pH 指示剂,摇匀后观察并记录其颜色。再在这 3 支试管中分别加入 2 滴水、0.2 mol · L^{-1} HCl 溶液、0.2 mol · L^{-1} NaOH 溶液,观察现象,说明原因。另取 2 支试管,分别加入 2 mL 纯水和 4 滴广泛 pH 指示剂,观察颜色;再分别加 2 滴 0.2 mol · L^{-1} HCl 溶液、0.2 mol · L^{-1} NaOH 溶液,观察现象,说明原因。

编号	试 剂	广泛 pH 指示剂	现象	加入液体	现象	原因
I	自制缓冲溶液,2 mL	4 滴		2 滴 H_2O		
II	自制缓冲溶液,2 mL	4 滴		2 滴 HCl 溶液		

续表

编号	试　　　剂	广泛 pH 指示剂	现象	加入液体	现象	原因
Ⅲ	自制缓冲溶液,2 mL	4 滴		2 滴 NaOH 溶液		
Ⅳ	H_2O,2 mL	4 滴		2 滴 HCl 溶液		
Ⅴ	H_2O,2 mL	4 滴		2 滴 NaOH 溶液		

4.影响缓冲容量的因素

(1) β 与缓冲比的关系。

取 2 支比色管,一支加入 2.00 mL 浓度均为 0.2 mol·L^{-1} 的 KH_2PO_4 溶液和 K_2HPO_4 溶液,另一支加入 3.00 mL 0.2 mol·L^{-1} KH_2PO_4 溶液和 1.00 mL 0.2 mol·L^{-1} K_2HPO_4 溶液,再在 2 支比色管中各加入 1 滴甲基橙指示剂,摇匀,观察颜色。向 2 支比色管中分别滴加 0.2 mol·L^{-1} HCl 溶液,记下整个溶液刚好变色时所用 HCl 溶液的滴数。

编号	0.2 mol·L^{-1} KH_2PO_4/mL	0.2 mol·L^{-1} K_2HPO_4/mL	甲基橙	颜色	使其刚好变色的 HCl 溶液滴数	结论
Ⅰ	2.00	2.00	1 滴			
Ⅱ	3.00	1.00	1 滴			

(2) β 与缓冲溶液总浓度 $c_{总}$ 的关系。

取 2 支比色管,一支加入 2.00 mL 浓度均为 0.2 mol·L^{-1} 的 KH_2PO_4 溶液和 K_2HPO_4 溶液,另一支加入 0.50 mL 浓度均为 0.2 mol·L^{-1} 的 KH_2PO_4 溶液和 K_2HPO_4 溶液、3.00 mL 纯水。再在 2 支比色管中各加入 1 滴甲基橙指示剂,摇匀,观察颜色。向 2 支比色管中分别滴加 0.2 mol·L^{-1} HCl 溶液,记下使整个溶液刚好变色时所用 HCl 溶液的滴数。

编号	0.2 mol·L^{-1} KH_2PO_4/mL	0.2 mol·L^{-1} K_2HPO_4/mL	H_2O /mL	甲基橙	颜色	使其刚好变色的 HCl 溶液滴数	结论
Ⅰ	2.00	2.00	0.00	1 滴			
Ⅱ	0.50	0.50	3.00	1 滴			

【思考题】

(1) $NaHCO_3$ 溶液是否具有缓冲能力？为什么？

(2) 试证明在什么情况下缓冲溶液的缓冲容量有最大值。

实验十五　氧化还原反应和电极电位

预习内容

【目的要求】

(1) 了解氧化还原反应和电极电位的关系,定性比较氧化还原电对的电极电位高低。

(2) 了解浓度、酸度变化对氧化还原反应的影响。

【实验原理】

氧化还原反应是氧化剂和还原剂之间发生电子转移的过程。氧化剂和还原剂得失电子能力可由其氧化还原电对的电极电位确定。对于半反应:

$$p\text{Ox} + ne^- \Longleftrightarrow q\text{Red}$$

$$\varphi(\text{Ox/Red}) = \varphi^{\ominus}(\text{Ox/Red}) + \frac{RT}{nF}\ln\frac{(c_{\text{Ox}})^p}{(c_{\text{Red}})^q}$$

这就是著名的电极电位的 Nernst 方程。式中:R 为气体常数($8.314 \text{ J} \cdot \text{mol}^{-1} \cdot \text{K}^{-1}$);$F$ 为法拉第常数($96\,485 \text{ C} \cdot \text{mol}^{-1}$);$T$ 为绝对温度;n 表示电极反应中的电子转移数;c_{Ox} 和 c_{Red} 分别代表电对中氧化型和还原型物质的浓度;p、q 分别代表一个已配平的氧化还原半反应中各氧化型和还原型物质前的系数。

电极电位高的氧化还原电对的氧化型物质得电子能力强,是强氧化剂;电极电位低的氧化还原电对的还原型物质失电子能力强,是强还原剂。

根据电极电位的大小还可判断氧化还原反应进行的方向,只有电极电位高的电对中的氧化型物质与电极电位低的电对中的还原型物质作用时,氧化还原反应才能自发进行。相反,根据氧化还原反应能否发生,也可判断和比较电极电位的相对高低。

浓度、介质酸度、温度等均影响电极电位的相对高低,从而影响氧化还原反应的方向和反应产物。

氧化剂和还原剂的强弱是相对的,如 H_2O_2 遇到强氧化剂(如 $KMnO_4$)呈现还原性,遇到强还原剂(如 I^-)则呈现氧化性。

【仪器与试剂】

试管(10)、试管架、滴瓶、盐桥(称取 1 g 琼脂,放在 100 mL 饱和 KCl 溶液中浸泡一会,加热煮成糊状,趁热倒入 U 形玻璃管(里面不能有气泡)中,冷却后即成)、烧杯(50 mL×10)、数字式电子电位差计,离心机(2),离心试管(6)。

$ZnSO_4$ 溶液($1 \text{ mol} \cdot \text{L}^{-1}$,$0.1 \text{ mol} \cdot \text{L}^{-1}$)、$CuSO_4$ 溶液($1 \text{ mol} \cdot \text{L}^{-1}$,$0.1 \text{ mol} \cdot \text{L}^{-1}$)、

$KMnO_4$ 溶液(0.01 mol $\cdot$ L^{-1})、KI 溶液(0.1 mol $\cdot$ L^{-1})、KBr 溶液(0.1 mol $\cdot$ L^{-1})、$FeCl_3$ 溶液(0.1 mol $\cdot$ L^{-1})、$FeSO_4$ 溶液(0.1 mol $\cdot$ L^{-1})、KSCN 溶液(0.1 mol $\cdot$ L^{-1})、H_2O_2 溶液(0.1 mol $\cdot$ L^{-1})、Br_2 水(饱和)、I_2 水(饱和)、H_2SO_4 溶液(1.0 mol $\cdot$ L^{-1})、HAc 溶液(6 mol $\cdot$ L^{-1})、NaOH 溶液(6 mol $\cdot$ L^{-1},1 mol $\cdot$ L^{-1})、KIO_3 溶液(0.1 mol $\cdot$ L^{-1})、Na_2SO_3(s)、浓氨水、蒸馏水、MnO_2(s)、HCl 溶液(2 mol $\cdot$ L^{-1},浓)、CCl_4、锌片、铜片。

【实验步骤】

1. 电池电动势的测量

在两只 50 mL 的烧杯中,分别注入 20 mL 1 mol $\cdot$ L^{-1} $ZnSO_4$ 溶液和 20 mL 1 mol $\cdot$ L^{-1} $CuSO_4$ 溶液,在 $ZnSO_4$ 溶液中插入锌片,$CuSO_4$ 溶液中插入铜片,组成两电极。中间以盐桥相通。用导线将锌片和铜片分别连接电位差计,近似测量原电池的电动势。取出盐桥,将其中的 1 mol $\cdot$ L^{-1} 的 $CuSO_4$ 溶液,换成 0.1 mol $\cdot$ L^{-1} $CuSO_4$ 溶液,重新测定电池的电动势,与前者的实验数据进行比较,并解释之。

另取两只 50 mL 的烧杯,分别注入 20 mL 0.1 mol $\cdot$ L^{-1} $ZnSO_4$ 溶液和 20 mL 0.1 mol $\cdot$ L^{-1} $CuSO_4$ 溶液,在 $ZnSO_4$ 溶液中插入锌片,$CuSO_4$ 溶液中插入铜片,组成两电极。中间以盐桥相通。用导线将锌片和铜片分别连接电位差计,近似测量电池的电动势。取出盐桥,在不断搅拌的条件下滴加浓氨水至 $CuSO_4$ 溶液中生成沉淀,离心分离,将滤液与 0.1 mol $\cdot$ L^{-1} $ZnSO_4$|Zn 电极组成原电池,测量电池的电动势。并对比前者结果,解释之。

另取两只 50 mL 的烧杯,首先测量电池的电动势:Zn | Zn^{2+}(0.1 mol $\cdot$ L^{-1}) ‖ Cu^{2+}(0.1 mol $\cdot$ L^{-1})|Cu。取出盐桥,在 $CuSO_4$ 溶液中注入浓氨水至生成的沉淀溶解为止,形成深蓝色溶液,再放入盐桥,观察电池的电动势有何变化。再在 $ZnSO_4$ 溶液中加浓氨水至生成的沉淀完全溶解为止,观察电动势又有何变化。利用 Nernst 方程解释实验现象。

测定浓差电池的电动势:Cu | Cu^{2+}(0.1 mol $\cdot$ L^{-1}) ‖ Cu^{2+}(1 mol $\cdot$ L^{-1})|Cu

2. 氧化还原反应与电极电位的关系

在两支试管中分别加入 10 滴 0.1 mol $\cdot$ L^{-1} KBr 溶液和 0.1 mol $\cdot$ L^{-1} KI 溶液,然后均加入 10 滴 0.1 mol $\cdot$ L^{-1} $FeCl_3$ 溶液和 20 滴 CCl_4,充分振荡。观察 CCl_4 层中颜色的变化(I_2 在 CCl_4 层中显紫红色),解释现象并写出反应方程式。

在两支试管中分别加入 10 滴 Br_2 和 I_2 的饱和水溶液,然后各加入 10 滴 0.1 mol $\cdot$ L^{-1} $FeSO_4$ 溶液,振荡后,分别加入 5 滴 0.1 mol $\cdot$ L^{-1} KSCN 溶液(KSCN 遇 Fe^{3+} 呈血红色)。观察颜色变化,解释现象并写出反应方程式。

根据以上实验结果,定性比较电对 I_2/I^-、Br_2/Br^- 和 Fe^{3+}/Fe^{2+} 的电极电位的相对高低,指出其中最强的氧化剂和最强的还原剂,并由此推出电极电位与氧化还原反应方向的关系。

3.氧化还原的相对性

(1) H_2O_2 的氧化性。在试管中加入 10 滴 0.1 mol·L^{-1} KI 溶液,再加入 3 滴 1.0 mol·L^{-1} H_2SO_4 溶液,然后边摇边加入 2 滴 0.1 mol·L^{-1} 双氧水及 20 滴 CCl_4。观察 CCl_4 层的颜色变化,解释原因并写出反应方程式。

(2) H_2O_2 的还原性。在试管中加入 5 滴 0.01 mol·L^{-1} $KMnO_4$ 溶液及 3 滴 1.0 mol·L^{-1} H_2SO_4 溶液,再逐滴加入 0.1 mol·L^{-1} 双氧水,边加边摇。观察现象,解释原因并写出反应方程式。

总结上述实验,应用电极电位说明 H_2O_2 在什么条件下为氧化剂,什么条件下为还原剂,并通过半反应式写出 H_2O_2 为氧化剂或还原剂时,其分别对应的产物各为什么。

4.介质酸度对氧化还原反应的影响

(1) 在两支各盛有 10 滴 0.1 mol·L^{-1} KBr 溶液的试管中,分别加入 5 滴 1.0 mol·L^{-1} H_2SO_4 溶液和 5 滴 6.0 mol·L^{-1} HAc 溶液,然后各加入 1 滴 0.01 mol·L^{-1} $KMnO_4$ 溶液。观察两支试管中溶液褪色的快慢,解释原因。

(2) 取少量 Na_2SO_3 固体,用蒸馏水溶解。取三支试管,各加入 10 滴上述 Na_2SO_3 溶液,分别加入 10 滴 1.0 mol·L^{-1} H_2SO_4 溶液、10 滴蒸馏水和 10 滴 6.0 mol·L^{-1} NaOH 溶液,混匀后,再各加入 5 滴 0.01 mol·L^{-1} $KMnO_4$ 溶液,振荡。观察颜色变化,解释现象并写出反应方程式。

(3) 在试管中加入 10 滴 0.1 mol·L^{-1} KI 溶液和 2~3 滴 0.1 mol·L^{-1} KIO_3 溶液,振荡混合后,观察有无变化;再加入几滴 1 mol·L^{-1} H_2SO_4 溶液,观察现象。再逐滴加入 1 mol·L^{-1} NaOH 溶液,使溶液呈碱性,观察反应现象。试解释反应现象,并写出化学反应方程式,指出介质对上述氧化还原反应的影响。

(4) 取两支干燥的试管加入 MnO_2 固体,在通风橱中分别加入 1 mL 2 mol·L^{-1} HCl 溶液和浓盐酸,用湿润的淀粉碘化钾试纸,检验有无气体产生,写出反应方程式,并加以解释。

【思考题】

(1) 为什么 $KMnO_4$ 能氧化浓 HCl 溶液中的 Cl^-,而不能氧化 NaCl 中的 Cl^-?

(2) 氧化还原反应进行的程度和反应速度是否必然一致?为什么?

(3) 介质中的 H^+ 或 OH^- 本身并不得失电子,为什么仍会影响氧化还原反应?

实验十六　配合物的生成和性质

【目的要求】

预习内容

（1）了解配离子与简单离子的区别。

（2）比较配离子的稳定性，了解配位平衡的移动与溶液酸碱性、沉淀及氧化还原平衡的关系。

（3）了解螯合物的形成及特点。

【实验原理】

由中心原子和一定数目的配体通过配位键结合并按一定的组成和空间构型形成的复杂离子称为配离子。含配离子的化合物属于配合物。

配离子在溶液中存在着配位平衡，例如：

$$Cu^{2+} + 4NH_3 \rightleftharpoons [Cu(NH_3)_4]^{2+}$$

$$K_s = \frac{[[Cu(NH_3)_4]^{2+}]}{[Cu^{2+}][NH_3]^4}$$

K_s 值越大，配离子越稳定。

配位平衡属化学平衡，服从化学平衡移动原理，若平衡体系的某一条件（如浓度、酸碱性等）发生改变，平衡将发生移动。增加配位剂（如 NH_3）的浓度，上述平衡向生成配离子的方向移动，反之，平衡向相反的方向移动；若配离子的配体是弱碱（如 NH_3），则加入强酸会促使配离子解离。在一个配合物的溶液中，加入一种可以与中心原子结合生成难溶物的沉淀剂，就会导致溶液中未配位的金属离子的浓度降低，促进配离子的解离；反之，一种配位剂若能与金属离子结合生成稳定的配合物，并且此配合物是易溶性的，则加入足量的配位剂可以使该金属离子的难溶盐溶解。沉淀剂与配位剂对金属离子的竞争结果，取决于相应的难溶物的 K_{sp} 和相应的配离子的 K_s 的相对大小。在配离子中，配体能够改变中心原子原来的电子结构，因而改变其氧化还原性质。如 $[Co(CN)_6]^{4-}$ 的还原性要比 Co^{2+} 的还原性强得多。

中心原子与多齿配体形成的环状结构的配合物，则称螯合物。很多金属螯合物具有特征颜色，并且难溶于水而易溶于有机溶剂。如丁二酮肟在碱性条件下与 Ni^{2+} 生成鲜红色且难溶于水的螯合物：

$$Ni^{2+} + 2\begin{array}{c} H_3C-C=NOH \\ H_3C-C=NOH \end{array} + 2NH_3 \cdot H_2O \longrightarrow \begin{array}{c} H_3C-C=N \quad N=C-CH_3 \\ Ni \\ H_3C-C=N \quad N=C-CH_3 \end{array} + 2NH_4^+ + 2H_2O$$

【仪器与试剂】

电子天平(0.01 g)、小烧杯(50 mL×2)、玻棒、试管(10)、滴管、水流抽气泵、布氏漏斗、滤纸、吸滤瓶。

$CuSO_4 \cdot 5H_2O$(AR,s)、HCl 溶液(1 mol·L^{-1},6 mol·L^{-1})、氨水(2 mol·L^{-1},浓)、NaOH 溶液(1 mol·L^{-1})、Na_2CO_3 溶液(0.1 mol·L^{-1})、Na_2S 溶液(0.1 mol·L^{-1})、$BaCl_2$溶液(0.1 mol·L^{-1})、$(NH_4)_2S$溶液(0.1 mol·L^{-1})、$(NH_4)_2C_2O_4$溶液(0.1 mol·L^{-1})、$FeCl_3$溶液(0.1 mol·L^{-1})、KSCN 溶液(1 mol·L^{-1})、NaBr 溶液(0.1 mol·L^{-1})、Na_2H_2Y 溶液(EDTA,0.1 mol·L^{-1})、$Na_2S_2O_3$溶液(0.1 mol·L^{-1})、$AgNO_3$溶液(0.1 mol·L^{-1})、$CuSO_4$溶液(0.1 mol·L^{-1})、$CoCl_2$溶液(0.5 mol·L^{-1})、$NiCl_2$溶液(0.1 mol·L^{-1})、乙醇溶液(95%)、H_2O_2溶液(30%)、丁二酮肟溶液(1%)、pH 试纸或红色石蕊试纸。

【实验步骤】

1. 配合物的形成——硫酸四氨合铜的制备、组成和性质

(1)制备。在小烧杯中放入 2.5 g $CuSO_4 \cdot 5H_2O$,加入 10 mL 水,搅拌至全部溶解。然后加入 5 mL 浓氨水,混匀,加等体积乙醇溶液(15 mL),混匀,放置 2~3 min,析出晶体后减压过滤,得结晶状[$Cu(NH_3)_4$]$SO_4 \cdot H_2O$,用少量乙醇溶液洗 1~2 次。记录产品的性状。

(2)组成和性质。

① 取少量硫酸四氨合铜晶体,溶于几滴水中,观察并记录溶液的颜色,逐滴加入 1 mol·L^{-1}HCl 溶液至过量,观察并记录溶液颜色的变化。再加入过量浓氨水,观察溶液颜色的变化。根据以上现象,讨论该配合物在溶液中的形成和解离。

② 取三支试管,各加少量硫酸四氨合铜晶体,溶于几滴水中。然后在第一支试管中加入 0.1 mol·$L^{-1}$$Na_2CO_3$溶液,观察有无碱式碳酸铜沉淀生成;在第二支试管中加入 0.1 mol·$L^{-1}$$Na_2S$溶液,观察有无硫化铜沉淀生成;在第三支试管中加入 0.1 mol·$L^{-1}$$BaCl_2$溶液,观察有无硫酸钡沉淀生成。

③ 取少量硫酸四氨合铜晶体(已干燥),闻一闻有无氨臭味,然后放在一支干试管内,管口挂一条湿润的 pH 试纸或红色石蕊试纸,微火加热。观察并记录试纸的颜色变化、残余固体的颜色、有无氨臭味。写出反应方程式。

根据实验结果,讨论配合物的组成,并说明 NH_3 分子是否参与组成配合物,其结合是否牢固。

2. 配位平衡与沉淀-溶解平衡的关系

(1)在两支试管中分别加入 5 滴 0.1 mol·$L^{-1}$$(NH_4)_2S$ 溶液和 5 滴 0.1

$mol \cdot L^{-1}(NH_4)_2C_2O_4$ 溶液,再各加入 5 滴 $0.1\ mol \cdot L^{-1}CuSO_4$ 溶液,观察有无沉淀生成。然后,分别在两种沉淀中加入 10 滴 $6\ mol \cdot L^{-1}$ 氨水,观察有何现象发生。

根据实验结果,试判断 CuS 和 CuC_2O_4 两种难溶电解质溶度积的大小,并查出它们的溶度积来验证你的判断。写出有关反应方程式。

（2）在两支试管中各加入 10 滴 $0.1\ mol \cdot L^{-1}AgNO_3$ 溶液,向第一支试管中逐滴加入 $0.1\ mol \cdot L^{-1}Na_2S_2O_3$ 溶液,待生成的沉淀溶解后,再多加几滴 $Na_2S_2O_3$ 溶液;向第二支试管中逐滴加入 $2\ mol \cdot L^{-1}$ 氨水,待生成的沉淀溶解后,再多加几滴氨水。然后分别向两支试管中加入 $0.1\ mol \cdot L^{-1}NaBr$ 溶液,观察有何现象发生。

根据实验结果,判断 $[Ag(NH_3)_2]^+$ 和 $[Ag(S_2O_3)_2]^{3-}$ 的稳定性大小,并查出它们的稳定常数来验证你的判断。写出有关反应方程式。

3. 配位平衡与溶液 pH 值

在试管中加 4～5 滴 $0.1\ mol \cdot L^{-1}FeCl_3$ 溶液,再加 $1\ mL\ 1\ mol \cdot L^{-1}KSCN$ 溶液,分成两份。一份中加数滴 $1\ mol \cdot L^{-1}HCl$ 溶液,另一份中加数滴 $1\ mol \cdot L^{-1}$ NaOH 溶液,观察并记录溶液颜色变化。讨论 $[Fe(SCN)_6]^{3-}$ 在酸性和碱性溶液中的稳定性。

4. 配体对中心原子氧化还原能力的影响

（1）取 4～5 滴 $CoCl_2$ 溶液,加 4～5 滴 30% H_2O_2 溶液,观察并记录现象。H_2O_2 能否把 Co^{2+} 氧化成 Co^{3+}（Co^{3+} 为棕色）?

（2）取 4～5 滴 $CoCl_2$ 溶液,加过量浓氨水至沉淀溶解,观察溶液颜色的变化。再加 H_2O_2 溶液,观察有无颜色变化。在该溶液中加 $6\ mol \cdot L^{-1}HCl$ 溶液酸化,记录并观察溶液颜色的变化。此时钴的氧化值是多少?形成氨配合物对 Co^{2+} 的还原性有什么影响?

5. 其他配位平衡的影响

分别在 10 滴 $[Fe(SCN)_6]^{3-}$ 溶液(步骤 3)和 $[Cu(NH_3)_4]^{2+}$ 溶液(步骤 1)中滴加足量的 $0.1\ mol \cdot L^{-1}$ EDTA 溶液,各有何现象产生?试解释之,并写出有关反应方程式。

6. 螯合物的生成

在试管中加入 2 滴 $0.1\ mol \cdot L^{-1}NiCl_2$ 溶液和 1 滴 $2\ mol \cdot L^{-1}$ 氨水溶液,然后加入 2 滴 1% 丁二酮肟(多齿配体)溶液,观察现象并解释之。

【思考题】

（1）怎样用实验证明在溶液中形成了 $[Cu(NH_3)_4]^{2+}$?

（2）配合物与复盐有何区别?怎样证明?

（3）怎样判断配合物的相对稳定性?影响配合物稳定性的主要因素有哪些?

（4）螯合剂与配位剂有何区别和联系?

实验十七　过渡金属化合物的性质与应用

【目的要求】

(1) 掌握过渡金属(Cr、Mn、Fe、Co、Ni、Cu、Ag、Zn、Cd、Hg)化合物的酸碱性和氧化还原性。

(2) 掌握过渡金属常见配合物的生成和性质。

【实验原理】

1. Cr 的重要化合物性质

$Cr(OH)_3$ 是灰蓝色的典型两性氢氧化物,能与过量的 NaOH 反应生成绿色 $[Cr(OH)_4]^-$。$Cr(Ⅲ)$ 在酸性溶液中很稳定,但在碱性溶液中具有较强的还原性,易被 H_2O_2 氧化成 CrO_4^{2-}。

铬酸盐与重铬酸盐可以互相转化,溶液中存在下列平衡:

$$2CrO_4^{2-} + 2H^+ \rightleftharpoons Cr_2O_7^{2-} + H_2O$$

因重铬酸盐的溶解度较铬酸盐的溶解度大,因此,向重铬酸盐溶液中加入 Ag^+、Pb^{2+}、Ba^{2+} 等离子时,通常生成铬酸盐沉淀。例如:

$$Cr_2O_7^{2-} + 2Ba^{2+} + H_2O \Longrightarrow 2BaCrO_4(黄色) + 2H^+$$

在酸性条件下,$Cr_2O_7^{2-}$ 具有强氧化性,可氧化乙醇,其反应方程式如下:

$$2Cr_2O_7^{2-} + 3C_2H_5OH + 16H^+ \Longrightarrow 4Cr^{3+}(绿色) + 3CH_3COOH + 11H_2O$$

通过此实验,可判断是否酒后驾车或酒精中毒。

2. Mn 的重要化合物的性质

$Mn(Ⅱ)$ 在碱性条件下具有还原性,易被空气中的氧气所氧化。其反应式如下:

$$Mn^{2+} + 2OH^- \Longrightarrow Mn(OH)_2(白色)$$

$$2Mn(OH)_2 + O_2 \Longrightarrow 2MnO(OH)_2(红棕色)$$

在酸性溶液中,Mn^{2+} 很稳定,只有强氧化剂如 $NaBiO_3$、PbO_2、$S_2O_8^{2-}$ 等,才能将它氧化成 MnO_4^-。其反应式如下:

$$2Mn^{2+} + 5NaBiO_3(s) + 14H^+ \Longrightarrow 2MnO_4^- + 5Bi^{3+} + 5Na^+ + 7H_2O$$

此反应可用来鉴定 Mn^{2+}。

MnO_4^{2-} 能稳定存在于强碱性溶液中,而在酸性或弱碱性溶液中会发生歧化反应:

$$3MnO_4^{2-} + 2H_2O \Longrightarrow 2MnO_4^- + MnO_2 + 4OH^-$$

MnO_4^- 是强氧化剂。介质的酸碱性不仅影响它的氧化能力,也影响它的还原产物。在酸性介质中,其还原产物是 Mn^{2+};在弱碱性(或中性)介质中,其还原产物是

MnO_2；在强碱性介质中，其还原产物是 MnO_4^{2-}。

3. Fe、Co、Ni 的重要化合物的性质

Fe(Ⅱ)、Co(Ⅱ)、Ni(Ⅱ)的氢氧化物依次为白色、粉红色和绿色。

Fe(OH)$_2$具有很强的还原性，易被空气中的氧气所氧化，生成红棕色的Fe(OH)$_3$。Fe(OH)$_2$主要呈碱性，酸性很弱，但能溶于浓碱溶液而形成[Fe(OH)$_6$]$^{4-}$。

CoCl$_2$溶液与 OH$^-$ 反应，先生成蓝色 Co(OH)Cl 沉淀，稍放置后生成粉红色 Co(OH)$_2$沉淀。Co(OH)$_2$也能被空气中的氧气所氧化，生成褐色的 CoO(OH)沉淀。Co(OH)$_2$显两性，不仅能溶于酸，而且能溶于过量的浓碱而形成[Co(OH)$_4$]$^{2-}$。

Ni(OH)$_2$在空气中是稳定的，只有在碱性溶液中用强氧化剂(如 Br$_2$、NaClO、Cl$_2$ 等)才能将其氧化成黑色 NiO(OH)。Ni(OH)$_2$显碱性。

Fe(Ⅲ)、Co(Ⅲ)、Ni(Ⅲ)的氢氧化物都显碱性，颜色依次为红棕色、褐色、黑色。将 Fe(Ⅲ)、Co(Ⅲ)、Ni(Ⅲ)的氢氧化物溶于酸后，则分别得到三价的 Fe^{3+} 和二价的 Co^{2+}、Ni^{2+}。这是因为在酸性溶液中，Co^{3+}、Ni^{3+}是强氧化剂，它们能将 H$_2$O 氧化为 O$_2$，将 Cl$^-$ 氧化为 Cl$_2$。其反应式如下：

$$4M^{3+} + 2H_2O \Longrightarrow 4M^{2+} + 4H^+ + O_2$$
$$2M^{3+} + 2Cl^- \Longrightarrow 2M^{2+} + Cl_2 \text{(M 为 Co、Ni)}$$

Co(Ⅲ)、Ni(Ⅲ)氢氧化物的获得，通常是由 Co(Ⅱ)、Ni(Ⅱ)盐在碱性条件下被强氧化剂(Br$_2$、NaClO、Cl$_2$)氧化而得到。例如：

$$2Ni^{2+} + 6OH^- + Br_2 \Longrightarrow 2Ni(OH)_3 + 2Br^-$$

Fe、Co、Ni 均能生成多种配合物。Fe^{2+}、Fe^{3+}与氨水反应只生成氢氧化物沉淀，而不生成氨配合物。Co^{2+}、Ni^{2+}与氨水反应先生成碱式盐沉淀，而后溶于过量氨水中，形成 Co(Ⅱ)、Ni(Ⅱ)的氨配合物。但是，[Co(NH$_3$)$_6$]$^{2+}$(土黄色)不稳定，易被空气中的氧气氧化为[Co(NH$_3$)$_6$]$^{3+}$(棕红色)，而[Ni(NH$_3$)$_6$]$^{2+}$(蓝紫色)能在空气中稳定存在。[Co(NH$_3$)$_6$]$^{2+}$被空气中氧气氧化的反应方程式如下：

$$4[Co(NH_3)_6]^{2+} + O_2 + 2H_2O \Longrightarrow 4[Co(NH_3)_6]^{3+} + 4OH^-$$

4. Cu、Ag、Zn、Cd、Hg 的重要化合物的性质

Cu^{2+}、Ag$^+$、Zn^{2+}、Cd^{2+}与过量氨水反应，分别生成氨配合物，但是 Hg^{2+}与过量氨水反应时，在没有大量 NH$_4^+$ 存在的情况下，并不生成氨配离子。其反应方程式如下：

$$HgCl_2 + 2NH_3 \Longrightarrow HgNH_2Cl \downarrow \text{(白色)} + NH_4Cl$$
$$2Hg(NO_3)_2 + 4NH_3 \cdot H_2O \Longrightarrow HgO \cdot HgNH_2NO_3 \downarrow \text{(白色)} + 3NH_4NO_3 + 3H_2O$$

Hg^{2+}与 I$^-$ 作用生成红色 HgI$_2$沉淀。HgI$_2$溶于过量 KI 中，生成无色[HgI$_4$]$^{2-}$配离子，[HgI$_4$]$^{2-}$配离子的强碱性溶液称为"奈氏试剂"，用来鉴定 NH$_4^+$。其反应方程式如下：

$$HgI_2 + 2KI \Longrightarrow K_2[HgI_4]$$

Cu^{2+} 与 I^- 反应生成白色 CuI 沉淀,CuI 能溶于过量 KI,生成 $[CuI_2]^-$ 配离子,该配离子不稳定,将溶液加水稀释时,又可得到 CuI 白色沉淀。其反应方程式如下:

$$2Cu^{2+} + 4I^- \Longrightarrow 2CuI\downarrow + I_2$$

$$CuI + I^- \Longrightarrow [CuI_2]^-$$

$$[CuI_2]^- \underset{}{\overset{稀释}{\Longleftrightarrow}} CuI\downarrow + I^-$$

【仪器与试剂】

点滴板、离心机(4)、离心试管(10)、试管、酒精灯、试管夹。

$(NH_4)_2Fe(SO_4)_2 \cdot 6H_2O(CP,s)$、$NaBiO_3(CP,s)$、$MnO_2(CP,s)$、$NH_4Cl(AR,s)$、HCl 溶液（2 mol·$L^{-1}$,浓）、$HNO_3$ 溶液（6 mol·L^{-1}）、H_2SO_4 溶液（3 mol·L^{-1}）、HAc 溶液（2 mol·L^{-1}）、NaOH 溶液（2 mol·L^{-1},6 mol·L^{-1},40%）、氨水（2 mol·L^{-1},浓）、$CoCl_2$ 溶液（0.1 mol·L^{-1}）、$NiSO_4$ 溶液（0.1 mol·L^{-1},0.5 mol·L^{-1}）、$MnSO_4$ 溶液（0.1 mol·L^{-1}）、$CrCl_3$ 溶液（0.1 mol·L^{-1}）、$FeCl_3$ 溶液（0.1 mol·L^{-1}）、$K_2Cr_2O_7$ 溶液（0.1 mol·L^{-1}）、$KMnO_4$ 溶液（0.01 mol·L^{-1}）、Na_2SO_3 溶液（0.1 mol·L^{-1}）、$CoCl_2$ 溶液（0.5 mol·L^{-1}）、NH_4Cl 溶液（1 mol·L^{-1}）、H_2O_2 溶液（3%）、$CuSO_4$ 溶液（0.1 mol·L^{-1}）、$AgNO_3$ 溶液（0.1 mol·L^{-1}）、$ZnSO_4$ 溶液（0.1 mol·L^{-1}）、$CdSO_4$ 溶液（0.1 mol·L^{-1}）、$Hg(NO_3)_2$ 溶液（0.1 mol·L^{-1}）、KI 溶液（0.1 mol·L^{-1},2 mol·L^{-1}）、Br_2、乙醇溶液（95%）、淀粉-碘化钾试纸。

【实验步骤】

1.低价氢氧化物的生成和性质

（1）氢氧化铁(Ⅱ)。在一支试管中加入 1 mL 蒸馏水和 2 滴 3 mol·L^{-1} H_2SO_4 溶液,加热至沸腾以赶尽溶于其中的氧气,冷却后向试管中加入少量固体 $(NH_4)_2Fe(SO_4)_2 \cdot 6H_2O$。在另一支试管中加入 1 mL 6 mol·$L^{-1}$ NaOH 溶液,加热至沸腾以赶尽氧气,冷却后,用滴管吸取 NaOH 溶液,插入亚铁溶液底部,慢慢挤出,观察沉淀的颜色和状态。把沉淀分成三份,一份放置在空气中,观察沉淀颜色是否变化;另两份分别滴入 2 mol·L^{-1} HCl 溶液和 40% NaOH 溶液,观察沉淀是否溶解。写出反应方程式。

（2）氢氧化钴(Ⅱ)。用 0.1 mol·L^{-1} $CoCl_2$ 溶液和 2 mol·L^{-1} NaOH 溶液制取 $Co(OH)_2$ 沉淀,观察沉淀的颜色和状态。把沉淀分成三份,一份放置在空气中,观察沉淀颜色是否变化;另两份分别滴入 2 mol·L^{-1} HCl 溶液和 40% NaOH 溶液,观察沉淀是否溶解。写出反应方程式。

（3）氢氧化镍（Ⅱ）。用 $0.1\ mol \cdot L^{-1} NiSO_4$ 溶液和 $2\ mol \cdot L^{-1} NaOH$ 溶液制取 $Ni(OH)_2$ 沉淀，观察沉淀的颜色和状态。把沉淀分成三份，一份放置在空气中，观察沉淀颜色是否变化；另两份分别滴入 $2\ mol \cdot L^{-1} HCl$ 溶液和 $40\% NaOH$ 溶液，观察沉淀是否溶解。写出反应方程式。

（4）氢氧化锰（Ⅱ）。用 $0.1\ mol \cdot L^{-1} MnSO_4$ 溶液和 $2\ mol \cdot L^{-1} NaOH$ 溶液制取 $Mn(OH)_2$ 沉淀，观察沉淀的颜色和状态。把沉淀分成三份，一份放置在空气中，观察沉淀颜色是否变化；另两份分别滴入 $2\ mol \cdot L^{-1} HCl$ 溶液和 $40\% NaOH$ 溶液，观察沉淀是否溶解。写出反应方程式。

（5）氢氧化铬（Ⅲ）。用 $0.1\ mol \cdot L^{-1} CrCl_3$ 溶液和 $2\ mol \cdot L^{-1} NaOH$ 溶液制取 $Cr(OH)_3$ 沉淀，观察沉淀的颜色和状态。把沉淀分成三份，一份放置在空气中，观察沉淀颜色是否变化；另两份分别滴入 $2\ mol \cdot L^{-1} HCl$ 溶液和 $6\ mol \cdot L^{-1} NaOH$ 溶液，观察沉淀是否溶解。写出反应方程式。

通过以上实验，总结低价氢氧化物的性质。

2.高价氢氧化物的生成和性质

（1）氢氧化铁（Ⅲ）。用 $0.1\ mol \cdot L^{-1} FeCl_3$ 溶液和 $2\ mol \cdot L^{-1} NaOH$ 溶液制取 $Fe(OH)_3$ 沉淀，观察沉淀的颜色和状态。把沉淀分成三份，一份加浓 HCl 溶液，检查是否有 Cl_2 产生；另两份分别滴入 $2\ mol \cdot L^{-1} HCl$ 溶液和 $40\% NaOH$ 溶液，观察沉淀是否溶解。写出反应方程式。

（2）氢氧化钴（Ⅲ）、氢氧化镍（Ⅲ）。用 $0.1\ mol \cdot L^{-1} CoCl_2$、$NiSO_4$ 溶液，$6\ mol \cdot L^{-1}$ NaOH 溶液和溴水分别制备 $Co(OH)_3$、$Ni(OH)_3$ 沉淀，观察沉淀的颜色，然后向所制取的 $Co(OH)_3$、$Ni(OH)_3$ 沉淀中分别滴加浓 HCl 溶液，检查是否有 Cl_2 产生。写出反应方程式。

3.低价盐的还原性

（1）碱性介质中 Cr（Ⅲ）的还原性。取少量 $0.1\ mol \cdot L^{-1} CrCl_3$ 溶液，滴加 $2\ mol \cdot L^{-1} NaOH$ 溶液，观察沉淀的颜色，继续滴加 NaOH 溶液至沉淀溶解，再加入适量 $3\% H_2O_2$ 溶液，加热，观察溶液颜色的变化。写出反应方程式。

（2）酸性介质中 Mn（Ⅱ）的还原性。取少量 $0.1\ mol \cdot L^{-1} MnSO_4$ 溶液，加入少量 $NaBiO_3$ 固体，然后滴加 $6\ mol \cdot L^{-1} HNO_3$ 溶液，观察溶液颜色的变化。写出反应方程式。

4.高价盐的氧化性

（1）Cr（Ⅵ）的氧化性。取数滴 $0.1\ mol \cdot L^{-1} K_2Cr_2O_7$ 溶液，用 $3\ mol \cdot L^{-1}$ H_2SO_4 溶液酸化，再滴加少量 95% 乙醇溶液，微热，观察溶液颜色的变化。写出反应方程式。

（2）Mn(Ⅶ)的氧化性。

① 取三支试管,各加入少量 $0.01\ mol \cdot L^{-1}KMnO_4$ 溶液,然后在第一支试管中加入几滴 $3\ mol \cdot L^{-1}H_2SO_4$ 溶液,第二支试管中加入几滴蒸馏水,第三支试管中加入几滴 $6\ mol \cdot L^{-1}NaOH$ 溶液,最后向各试管中分别滴加几滴 $0.1\ mol \cdot L^{-1}Na_2SO_3$ 溶液,振荡溶液,观察紫红色溶液颜色的变化。写出反应方程式。

② 另取三支试管,各加入少量 $0.01\ mol \cdot L^{-1}KMnO_4$ 溶液,然后将滴加介质及还原剂的次序颠倒,观察实验结果有何不同。为什么?

5. $Cr_2O_7^{2-}$ 与 CrO_4^{2-} 的转化

（1）取 5 滴 $0.1\ mol \cdot L^{-1}K_2Cr_2O_7$ 溶液于试管中,加入 2 滴 $2\ mol \cdot L^{-1}NaOH$ 溶液,观察溶液颜色的变化,在此溶液中加入 2 滴 $0.5\ mol \cdot L^{-1}BaCl_2$ 溶液,观察沉淀的生成。写出反应方程式。

（2）取 5 滴 $0.1\ mol \cdot L^{-1}K_2Cr_2O_7$ 溶液于试管中,加入 2 滴 $2\ mol \cdot L^{-1}HAc$ 溶液,观察溶液颜色的变化,在此溶液中加入 2 滴 $0.5\ mol \cdot L^{-1}BaCl_2$ 溶液,观察沉淀的生成。写出反应方程式。

6. 锰酸盐的生成及不稳定性

（1）取适量 $0.01\ mol \cdot L^{-1}KMnO_4$ 溶液,加入过量 40% NaOH 溶液,再加入少量 MnO_2 固体,微热,搅拌,静置片刻,离心,绿色清液即 K_2MnO_4 溶液。

（2）取少量绿色清液,滴加 $3\ mol \cdot L^{-1}H_2SO_4$ 溶液,观察现象,写出反应方程式。

（3）取少量绿色清液,加入少许 NH_4Cl 固体,振荡试管,使 NH_4Cl 溶解,微热,观察现象,写出反应方程式。

7. Co、Ni、Cu、Ag、Zn、Cd、Hg 的氨配合物

（1）钴氨配合物。取少量 $0.5\ mol \cdot L^{-1}CoCl_2$ 溶液,滴加少量 $1\ mol \cdot L^{-1}NH_4Cl$ 溶液,然后逐滴加入 $2\ mol \cdot L^{-1}$ 氨水,振荡试管,观察沉淀的颜色。再继续加入过量的浓氨水至沉淀溶解为止,观察反应产物的颜色。最后将溶液放置一段时间,观察溶液的颜色变化。说明钴氨配合物的性质,写出反应方程式。

（2）镍氨配合物。取适量 $0.5\ mol \cdot L^{-1}NiSO_4$ 溶液,滴加少量 $1\ mol \cdot L^{-1}NH_4Cl$ 溶液,然后逐滴加入 $2\ mol \cdot L^{-1}$ 氨水,振荡试管,观察沉淀的颜色。再继续加入过量的浓氨水至沉淀溶解为止,观察反应产物的颜色。把溶液分成四份,第一份溶液中加入几滴 $2\ mol \cdot L^{-1}NaOH$ 溶液,第二份溶液中加入几滴 $3\ mol \cdot L^{-1}H_2SO_4$ 溶液,有何现象?将第三份溶液用水稀释,是否有沉淀产生?将第四份溶液煮沸,有何变化?综合实验结果,说明镍氨配合物的稳定性。

（3）Cu、Ag、Zn、Cd、Hg 的氨配合物。取少量浓度均为 $0.1\ mol \cdot L^{-1}$ 的 $CuSO_4$、$AgNO_3$、$ZnSO_4$、$CdSO_4$、$Hg(NO_3)_2$ 溶液,分别加入几滴 $2\ mol \cdot L^{-1}$ 氨水,观察沉淀的生成,然后加入过量的浓氨水,观察沉淀是否溶解。

8. Cu、Hg 的碘配合物

（1）在少量 $0.1\ mol \cdot L^{-1} CuSO_4$ 溶液中滴加数滴 $0.1\ mol \cdot L^{-1} KI$ 溶液，观察溶液的变化。分离和洗涤沉淀后，在沉淀中加入 $2\ mol \cdot L^{-1} KI$ 溶液，观察其溶解的情况，写出反应方程式。

（2）取 $1 \sim 2$ 滴 $0.1\ mol \cdot L^{-1} Hg(NO_3)_2$ 溶液，滴加 $0.1\ mol \cdot L^{-1} KI$ 溶液，观察沉淀的颜色，然后加入过量的 $2\ mol \cdot L^{-1} KI$ 溶液，观察现象，写出反应方程式。

【思考题】

（1）比较 $Fe(OH)_3$、$Al(OH)_3$、$Cr(OH)_3$ 的性质。

（2）设计实验，分离并鉴定含 Fe^{3+}、Al^{3+}、Cr^{3+} 的混合液。

（3）$FeCl_3$ 的水溶液呈黄色，当它与什么试剂作用时，可以呈现下列现象：①血红色；②红棕色沉淀；③先呈血红色，后变为无色溶液；④深蓝色沉淀。

（4）有三个同学分别采用了下列三种方法分离 Zn^{2+}、Cd^{2+}、Hg^{2+}。

甲：用过量 NaOH 溶液将 Zn^{2+} 分离，然后在沉淀中加入过量氨水，将 Cd^{2+} 与 Hg^{2+} 分离。

乙：用过量氨水将 Hg^{2+} 分离，然后在溶液中加入过量 NaOH 溶液，将 Zn^{2+} 与 Cd^{2+} 分离。

丙：通 H_2S 于酸化的混合液中，将 Zn^{2+} 分离，然后在沉淀中加入 HNO_3 溶液，将 Cd^{2+}、Hg^{2+} 分离。

这三种方法是否都合理？为什么？你将采用什么方法？

实验十八　蛋白质的分光光度法测定

【目的要求】

（1）掌握分光光度法测定蛋白质含量的原理和方法。

（2）进一步熟悉 723N 型分光光度计的使用方法。

【实验原理】

偶氮胂 M 是一种良好的光度分析显色剂，在 $pH = 2.2 \sim 2.8$ 的条件下，蛋白质与偶氮胂 M 生成稳定的蓝色复合物，此复合物的最大吸收波长为 605 nm，通过测定该复合物的吸光度可求出蛋白质的含量。生物体内存在的金属离子和阴离子如 K^+、Na^+、Ca^{2+}、Mg^{2+}、Cu^{2+}、Zn^{2+}、Cl^- 以及维生素、肌苷、尿酸、葡萄糖等对蛋白质的测定均无影响，因此可以将样品粉碎、提取、过滤后直接进行分光光度法测定。

【仪器与试剂】

723N 型分光光度计、比色皿(2.0 cm×4)、电子天平(0.01 g)、PB-10 型酸度计、高速匀浆器、高速离心机、比色管(10 mL×7)、烧杯(250 mL×1,500 mL×1)、移液管(2 mL×1,1 mL×1)、吸量管(1 mL×3)、量筒(100 mL×1)、容量瓶(100 mL×1)、纱布。

蛋白质标准溶液(约 1 g·L^{-1})、偶氮胂 M 溶液(5.0×10^{-4} mol·L^{-1})、KH_2PO_4 溶液(5.0×10^{-3} mol·L^{-1})、乳化剂 OP 水溶液(0.050%)、NaCl 溶液(1.0%)、乳酸-乳酸钠缓冲溶液(pH=2.5)、含蛋白质的样品(干花生)、去离子水。

【实验步骤】

1.含蛋白质的样品的预处理

称取 25 g 干花生,用含 5.0×10^{-3} mol·L^{-1} KH_2PO_4 和 1.0% NaCl 的溶液(pH=7.2)在室温下浸泡 4~8 h(溶液加至刚好淹没全部花生后再过量 20 mL 左右)。然后用匀浆器匀浆,浆液于 4 ℃下静置过夜。用三层纱布过滤,并用30 mL pH=7.2 的缓冲溶液分多次洗涤滤渣,用水稀释滤液至 100 mL。取滤液适量,在 12 000 r·min^{-1} 转速下离心 20 min,清液在 4 ℃下保存。

2.样品中蛋白质含量的测定

取七支 10 mL 比色管,依次编号,按下表中数据加入各种溶液,七支比色管最后均用去离子水稀释至刻度,摇匀,放置 15 min。以Ⅰ号为参比溶液测定 605 nm 波长处吸光度。以Ⅴ、Ⅵ、Ⅶ号溶液的吸光度对标准溶液的浓度作图,将得一直线,延长此直线与横轴相交,交点的绝对值即为样品清液中蛋白质的含量。

编　　　号	Ⅰ	Ⅱ	Ⅲ	Ⅳ	Ⅴ	Ⅵ	Ⅶ
乳酸-乳酸钠缓冲溶液/mL	2.00	2.00	2.00	2.00	2.00	2.00	2.00
乳化剂 OP 溶液/mL	1.00	1.00	1.00	1.00	1.00	1.00	1.00
偶氮胂 M 溶液/mL	0.80	0.80	0.80	0.80	0.80	0.80	0.80
样品清液/mL	0	0.50	0.50	0.50	0.50	0.50	0.50
蛋白质标准溶液/mL	0	0	0	0	0.20	0.40	0.60
吸光度 A							

【思考题】

(1) 蛋白质样品处理后所得清液为什么不需提纯就可以进行分光光度法测定?

(2) 蛋白质含量的测定还有哪些方法?

实验十九　磺基水杨酸合铁(Ⅲ)配合物的组成和稳定常数的测定

预习内容

【目的要求】

(1) 学习用浓比递变法测定配合物的组成和稳定常数。

(2) 进一步熟悉 723N 型分光光度计的使用。

【实验原理】

当一束波长一定的单色光通过有色溶液时,吸光度 A 与有色溶液的浓度 c 和液层厚度 b 的乘积成正比,这就是 Lambert-Beer 定律,其数学表达式为

$$A = \varepsilon bc$$

式中:ε 是摩尔吸光系数,它是吸光物质在一定波长下的特征常数。在分光光度法中,当条件一定时,ε、b 均为常数,此时,吸光度 A 与有色物质的浓度 c 成正比。

运用该定律可以测定配合物的组成和稳定常数。浓比递变法是一种十分有效的方法。该方法适用于仅有一种配合物生成时,测定其组成和稳定常数。所谓浓比递变法就是在保持溶液中金属离子的浓度(c_m)与配体的浓度(c_x)之和 c_t 不变的前提下(即 $c_x + c_m = c_t$),改变 c_m 与 c_x 的相对量。在一定波长下,溶液中的配合物对光产生强烈吸收而金属离子与配体几乎没有吸收。配体的摩尔分数 $x = \dfrac{c_x}{c_t}$,由于 $\dfrac{c_x}{c_t} + \dfrac{c_m}{c_t} = \dfrac{c_t}{c_t}$,则 $1 - x = \dfrac{c_m}{c_t}$。以吸光度 A 对配体的摩尔分数 x 作图(图 2-4),得一曲线。将曲线两边的切线延长相交于 P' 点,交点所对应的摩尔分数即为配合物的组成比。当金属离子和配体恰好完全生成配合物时,ML_n 的浓度最大,对应的吸光度也最大。其反应式为

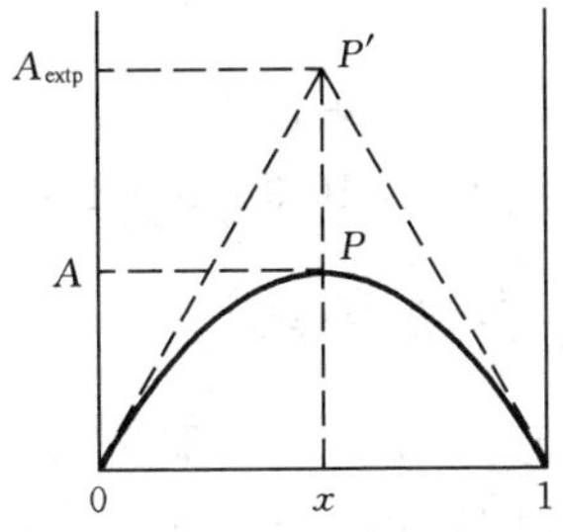

$$M + nL = ML_n$$

其中

$$n = \frac{c_x}{c_m} = \frac{x}{1-x}$$

图 2-4　浓比递变法图

实际的吸光度 A 与 P' 处的 A_{extp} 有偏差,此差值可以用来确定配合物的稳定常数。其中 A_{extp} 代表完全生成配合物时的吸光度,由于配合物部分解离,其浓度要稍小一些,实验测得的最大吸光度 A 在 P 点,也稍小一些,则配合物的解离度为

$$\alpha = \frac{A_{extp} - A}{A_{extp}}$$

1∶1 型配合物的稳定常数可由下列平衡关系导出:

$$ML \rightleftharpoons M+L$$

开始浓度 $\qquad c \qquad 0 \quad 0$

平衡浓度 $\qquad c-c\alpha \quad c\alpha \; c\alpha$

$$K_s = \frac{[ML]}{[M][L]} = \frac{1-\alpha}{c\alpha^2}$$

式中:c 为配合物的浓度。

本实验测定磺基水杨酸合铁(Ⅲ)配合物的组成和稳定常数。配合物的组成随溶液 pH 值的不同而改变。当 pH=2~3 时,生成配合比为 1∶1 的紫红色配合物,反应方程式表示如下:

当 pH=4~9 时,生成配合比为 1∶2 的红色配合物;当 pH >10 时,生成配合比为 1∶3 的黄色配合物。本实验是测定 pH=2~3 时形成的紫红色的磺基水杨酸合铁(Ⅲ)配合物的组成及其稳定常数。

【仪器与试剂】

723N 型分光光度计、比色皿(1.0 cm×4)、容量瓶(100 mL×2)、吸量管(10 mL×2)、干燥烧杯(50 mL×11)、洗耳球、胶头滴管。

$NH_4Fe(SO_4)_2$ 溶液(0.010 0 mol·L^{-1},用 0.010 0 mol·L^{-1} $HClO_4$ 溶液配制)、磺基水杨酸溶液(0.010 0 mol·L^{-1},用 0.010 0 mol·L^{-1} $HClO_4$ 溶液配制)、$HClO_4$ 溶液(0.010 0 mol·L^{-1})。

【实验步骤】

(1) 配制浓度为 0.001 00 mol·L^{-1} 的磺基水杨酸溶液。用吸量管吸取 10.00 mL 0.010 0 mol·L^{-1} 磺基水杨酸溶液于 100 mL 容量瓶中,用 0.010 0 mol·L^{-1} $HClO_4$ 溶液定容。

配制浓度为 0.001 00 mol·L^{-1} 的 Fe^{3+} 溶液。用吸量管吸取 10.00 mL 0.010 0 mol·L^{-1} $NH_4Fe(SO_4)_2$ 溶液于 100 mL 容量瓶中,用 0.010 0 mol·L^{-1} $HClO_4$ 溶液定容。

(2) 配制系列溶液。依下表所示溶液体积,用吸量管依次向 11 个 50 mL 干燥烧杯中移取 0.001 00 mol·L^{-1} 磺基水杨酸溶液(溶液 A)和 0.001 00 mol·L^{-1} $NH_4Fe(SO_4)_2$ 溶液(溶液 B),混合均匀。

混合溶液编号	I	II	III	IV	V	VI	VII	VIII	IX	X	XI
V(溶液 A)/mL	10.00	9.00	8.00	7.00	6.00	5.00	4.00	3.00	2.00	1.00	0.00
V(溶液 B)/mL	0.00	1.00	2.00	3.00	4.00	5.00	6.00	7.00	8.00	9.00	10.00
磺基水杨酸的摩尔分数											
吸光度 A											

注意:11 个烧杯中金属离子与配体的总的物质的量相等。

(3) 用表中Ⅵ号溶液,以蒸馏水为空白,在 $400\sim620$ nm 波长范围内制作吸收曲线,找出最大吸收波长。然后,在最大吸收波长下,以蒸馏水为空白,分别测定上述 11 种系列溶液的吸光度。以吸光度对摩尔分数作图,确定磺基水杨酸合铁(Ⅲ)配合物的组成,并计算其稳定常数。

【思考题】

阐述用浓比递变法如何确定配合物的稳定常数。用该方法确定配合物的稳定常数时有什么条件?

实验二十　分光光度法测定$[\mathrm{Ti}(\mathrm{H_2O})_6]^{3+}$ 的晶体场分裂能

【目的要求】

(1) 学习应用分光光度法测定配合物的分裂能。
(2) 进一步熟练掌握 723N 型分光光度计的使用方法。

【实验原理】

过渡金属离子的 d 轨道在晶体场的影响下会发生能级分裂(图 2-5)。金属离子的 d 轨道没有被电子充满时,处于低能量 d 轨道上的电子吸收了一定波长的可见光后,就跃迁到高能量的 d 轨道,这种 d-d 跃迁的能量差可以通过实验测定。

仅有一个 3d 电子的配离子$[\mathrm{Ti}(\mathrm{H_2O})_6]^{3+}$,在八面体场的影响下,$\mathrm{Ti}^{3+}$ 的 5 个简并的 d 轨道分裂为二重简并的 $\mathrm{d_\gamma}(\mathrm{e_g})$ 轨道和三重简并的 $\mathrm{d_\varepsilon}(\mathrm{t_{2g}})$ 轨道,$\mathrm{d_\gamma}$ 轨道和 $\mathrm{d_\varepsilon}$ 轨道的能量差等于分裂能 Δ_o(10 Dq)。

根据

$$E_光 = E_{\mathrm{d_\gamma}} - E_{\mathrm{d_\varepsilon}} = \Delta_\mathrm{o}$$

得

$$\Delta_\mathrm{o} = E_光 = h\nu = \frac{hc}{\lambda}$$

式中:h 是普朗克常数(6.626×10^{-34} J・s);c 是光速(2.998×10^8 m・s^{-1});$E_光$ 是可

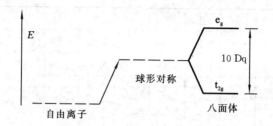

图 2-5 Ti^{3+} 中 d 轨道在八面体场中的能级分裂

见光光能(J);ν 是频率(s^{-1});λ 是波长(nm)。

当 Δ_{o} 用波数(1/λ)的单位 cm^{-1} 表示时,则有

$$\Delta_{o} = \frac{1}{\lambda} \times 10^{7}$$

【仪器与试剂】

7200 型分光光度计、容量瓶(50 mL×1)、烧杯(50 mL×1)、移液管(5 mL×1)、洗耳球、洗瓶、胶头滴管。

TiCl$_3$ 溶液(15%)、HCl 溶液(2 mol·L^{-1})。

【实验步骤】

1. [Ti(H$_2$O)$_6$]$^{3+}$ 溶液的配制

用移液管吸取 5.00 mL 15% TiCl$_3$ 水溶液于 50 mL 容量瓶中,用蒸馏水稀释至刻度,摇匀。

2. 测定吸光度

在 420~600 nm 波长范围内,以蒸馏水作参比,每隔 10 nm 波长测定上述溶液的吸光度(在吸收峰附近时,波长间隔可适当减少,一般为 2 nm)。

【结果记录和处理】

(1) [Ti(H$_2$O)$_6$]$^{3+}$ 的吸收曲线。

λ/nm	
A	

(2) 计算 [Ti(H$_2$O)$_6$]$^{3+}$ 配离子的 Δ_{o} 值。

【思考题】

(1) 配合物的分裂能 Δ_{o}(10 Dq)受哪些因素的影响?

(2) 本实验测定吸收曲线时,溶液浓度的高低对测定 10 Dq 值是否有影响?

实验二十一 生理盐水中氯离子含量的测定

【目的要求】

(1) 掌握 $AgNO_3$ 标准溶液配制与标定的方法。

(2) 熟悉莫尔(Mohr)法以 K_2CrO_4 为指示剂测定氯离子含量的方法和原理。

【实验原理】

莫尔法是以 K_2CrO_4 为指示剂，$AgNO_3$ 标准溶液为滴定剂，在中性或弱碱性溶液中滴定 Cl^- 等的方法。由于 AgCl 沉淀的溶解度比 Ag_2CrO_4 的溶解度小，因此溶液中首先析出 AgCl 沉淀，滴定终点时，稍微过量的 Ag^+ 与 K_2CrO_4 生成砖红色的 Ag_2CrO_4 沉淀，指示终点的到达。主要反应方程式如下：

$$Ag^+ + Cl^- \longrightarrow AgCl \downarrow （白色）$$
$$2Ag^+ + CrO_4^{2-} \longrightarrow Ag_2CrO_4 \downarrow （砖红色）$$

滴定的适宜 pH 范围为 $6.5 \sim 10.5$。溶液中若存在铵盐，则 pH 范围应控制在 $6.5 \sim 7.2$。溶液中若存在较多的 Cu^{2+}、Co^{2+}、Cr^{3+} 等有色离子，将影响终点的观察。凡是能与 Ag^+ 或 CrO_4^{2-} 发生化学反应的阴、阳离子都干扰测定。

【仪器与试剂】

分析天平(0.1 mg)、酸式滴定管(棕色,50 mL×1)、移液管(25 mL×1)、锥形瓶(250 mL×3)、容量瓶(250 mL×2)、小烧杯等。

$AgNO_3$(CP)、NaCl(基准试剂,500～600 ℃灼烧至恒重)、K_2CrO_4 溶液(5%)、生理盐水。

【实验步骤】

1. $0.02\ mol \cdot L^{-1}\ AgNO_3$ 标准溶液的配制

称取约 0.85 g $AgNO_3$ 于烧杯中，加入 250 mL 纯水中，摇匀，将溶液转入棕色试剂瓶中，置于暗处保存，避免见光分解。

2. $AgNO_3$ 溶液的标定

准确称取 0.25～0.3 g 基准 NaCl 于小烧杯中，用少量蒸馏水溶解后，转入 250 mL 的容量瓶中，定容，摇匀。

用移液管移取 25.00 mL NaCl 溶液于锥形瓶中，加入 25 mL 蒸馏水、1.00 mL 5% 的 K_2CrO_4 溶液，用 $AgNO_3$ 溶液滴定至砖红色，即为终点。平行标定三份。根据

所消耗的 $AgNO_3$ 溶液的体积和 $NaCl$ 的质量,计算 $AgNO_3$ 溶液的浓度。

3.试样分析

用移液管移取 25.00 mL 生理盐水样品至 250 mL 的容量瓶中,稀释至刻度,摇匀。

用移液管移取 25.00 mL 稀释后的生理盐水于锥形瓶中,加入 25 mL 蒸馏水及 1 mL 5‰的 K_2CrO_4 溶液,用 $AgNO_3$ 溶液滴定至砖红色,即为终点。平行测定三份。根据所消耗的 $AgNO_3$ 溶液的体积,计算 $NaCl$ 的含量,测定结果以 g/100 mL 表示。

实验完毕后,将装 $AgNO_3$ 溶液的滴定管先用蒸馏水冲洗 2～3 次,再用自来水洗净,以免 $AgCl$ 残留于管内。

【结果记录与处理】

$$c(AgNO_3) = \frac{m(NaCl) \times 1\,000}{M(NaCl) \times V} \times \frac{25.00}{250.00}$$

根据以下公式计算生理盐水中 $NaCl$ 的含量:

$$\rho(NaCl)(g/100\ mL) = \frac{c(AgNO_3) \times V \times M(NaCl)}{25.00} \times \frac{250.00}{25.00} \times 100$$

【思考题】

(1) 莫尔法测定氯离子,为什么溶液的 pH 须控制在 6.5～10.5?

(2) 莫尔法可以用 $NaCl$ 标准溶液直接滴定 Ag^+ 吗?

实验二十二　食品中亚硝酸盐含量的测定

【目的要求】

(1) 熟悉分光光度计的基本原理和使用方法。

(2) 了解食品中亚硝酸盐含量的测定方法。

【实验原理】

亚硝酸盐被广泛地用作肉制品的发色剂和防腐剂,但亚硝酸盐可以与胺反应产生致癌物质亚硝胺。因此必须对食品中亚硝酸盐的含量进行严格监测。食品样品经沉淀蛋白质、去除脂肪后,亚硝酸盐与对氨基苯磺酸发生重氮化反应生成重氮盐,然后重氮盐与盐酸萘乙二胺偶合,生成紫红色偶氮化合物。其化学反应方程式如下:

重氮化:$H_2N\!-\!\!\left\langle\;\right\rangle\!-\!SO_3H\ +\ NO_2^-\ \xrightarrow{HCl}\ ClN_2^+\!-\!\!\left\langle\;\right\rangle\!-\!SO_3H$

偶合：

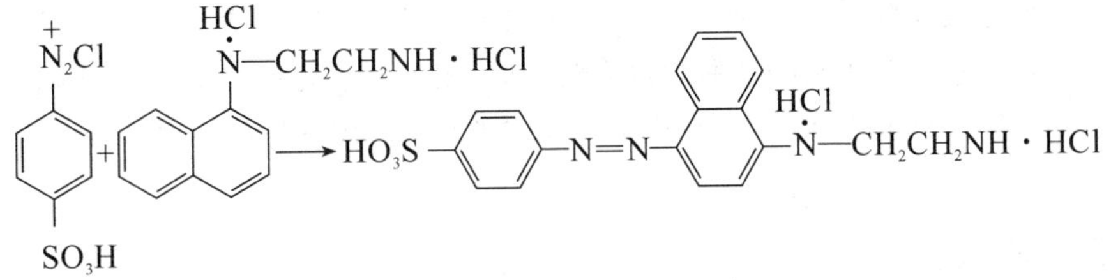

$$\text{(偶合反应式)}$$

生成的紫红色产物的吸光度 A 与亚硝酸盐含量成正比。因此,以吸光度对标准溶液浓度作图,即可绘制标准曲线。通过标准曲线可获得对应的被测溶液浓度。

【仪器与试剂】

紫外-可见分光光度计、比色皿(1 cm×4)、电子天平(0.01 g)、移液管(25 mL×1)、吸量管(2.00 mL×4)、容量瓶(50 mL×7)、烧杯(50 mL×1)等。

亚硝酸钠标准储备液(400 μg · mL^{-1})、亚硝酸钠标准应用液(10.00 μg · mL^{-1})、盐酸萘乙二胺溶液(0.3%)、对氨基苯磺酸溶液(1.0%)。

【实验步骤】

1. 处理食品样品,制备待测溶液

实验步骤自行设计。

2. 标准曲线的绘制

分别准确吸取亚硝酸钠标准应用液(10.00 μg · mL^{-1})0.00 mL、0.30 mL、0.60 mL、0.90 mL、1.20 mL、1.50 mL 于六只 50 mL 容量瓶中,加入蒸馏水 30 mL,分别加入 1.0%对氨基苯磺酸溶液 2.00 mL,摇匀,放置 3 min,再加入 0.3%盐酸萘乙二胺溶液 2 mL 并加蒸馏水稀释至刻度,摇匀,放置 15 min,用 1 cm 比色皿,以试剂空白为参比溶液,在 538 nm 波长处测定上述各溶液的吸光度,绘制标准曲线。

3. 样品中亚硝酸盐含量的测定

准确移取 25.00 mL 待测溶液于 50 mL 容量瓶中,同上加入显色剂并用蒸馏水定容,摇匀。放置 15 min 后测定其吸光度。根据吸光度在标准曲线上查得相应浓度,并以 mg · kg^{-1} 表示食品中亚硝酸盐的含量。

【数据记录与处理】

1. 标准曲线与样品中亚硝酸盐含量的测定

$V(NaNO_2)/mL$	0.00	0.30	0.60	0.90	1.20	1.50	待测溶液(25 mL)
$c(NaNO_2)/(\mu g \cdot mL^{-1})$							
吸光度 A							

2.结果处理

以标准溶液亚硝酸钠的含量为横坐标,相应的吸光度为纵坐标,绘制标准曲线。根据待测溶液的吸光度,在标准曲线上查得其亚硝酸盐含量,并计算原食品中亚硝酸盐的含量($mg \cdot kg^{-1}$)。

【思考题】

(1) 如果溶液为红色,表明该溶液对红色的光是吸收还是透过?

(2) 为什么要及时测定试样中亚硝酸盐的含量?

实验二十三　双波长分光光度法测定水样中硝酸盐的含量

【目的要求】

(1) 掌握双波长分光光度法测定硝酸盐含量的基本原理。

(2) 熟悉紫外-可见分光光度计的基本结构和使用方法。

【实验原理】

当某一组分的吸收光谱对待测组分的吸收光谱产生干扰或者测定背景吸收较大的溶液时,可采用双波长分光光度法进行测定。在干扰组分亚硝酸盐存在时,双波长等吸收测定法测定硝酸盐的原理如下(图 2-6)。

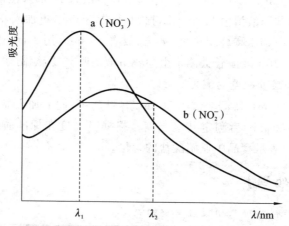

图 2-6　双波长等吸收测定法测定硝酸盐的原理

依据吸光度的加和性原则:

$$A_1 = A_1^a + A_1^b \quad A_2 = A_2^a + A_2^b$$

$$\Delta A = A_1 - A_2 = A_1^a - A_2^a = (\varepsilon_1^a - \varepsilon_2^a)bc$$

上式表明,硝酸盐在 λ_1 和 λ_2 处的吸光度差值 ΔA 与硝酸盐的浓度 c 成正比,而与干扰组分亚硝酸盐的量无关,从而可以消除亚硝酸盐的干扰。

【仪器与试剂】

紫外-可见分光光度计、比色皿(1 cm×2)、容量瓶(50 mL×7)、吸量管(5 mL×2)、小烧杯等。

硝酸钠标准储备液(1.000 mg·mL^{-1})、硝酸钠标准应用液(50.00 μg·mL^{-1},5.00 μg·mL^{-1})、亚硝酸钠标准储备液(250.0 μg·mL^{-1})、亚硝酸钠标准应用液(5.00 μg·mL^{-1}),硝酸钠、亚硝酸钠均为分析纯。

【实验步骤】

1. 绘制吸收光谱曲线

以蒸馏水为参比溶液,在 190～230 nm 波长范围内,分别测定 5.00 μg·mL^{-1} 硝酸钠标准溶液和 5.00 μg·mL^{-1} 亚硝酸钠标准溶液的吸光度(波长间隔为 1 nm),绘制硝酸钠和亚硝酸钠的吸收光谱曲线。

2. 选择测定波长 λ_1 和 λ_2

根据绘制的吸收光谱曲线,选择测定波长 λ_1 和 λ_2。

3. 配制标准系列溶液

分别移取 50.00 μg·mL^{-1} 硝酸钠标准溶液 0.00 mL、1.00 mL、2.00 mL、3.00 mL、4.00 mL 和 5.00 mL 于六只 50 mL 容量瓶中,用蒸馏水稀释定容后摇匀。

4. 吸光度测定

用蒸馏水为参比溶液,在波长 λ_1 和 λ_2 处测定标准系列溶液和待测溶液的吸光度。以标准系列溶液在两波长处吸光度的差值 ΔA 为纵坐标,硝酸钠的浓度为横坐标,绘制标准曲线,将待测溶液吸光度差值代入回归方程,计算待测试样中硝酸盐的浓度。

【结果记录和处理】

(1) 绘制吸收光谱曲线,并确定测定波长 λ_1 和 λ_2。

(2) 绘制标准曲线,确定待测溶液浓度,数据记录如下:

$V(NaNO_3)$/mL	1.00	2.00	3.00	4.00	5.00	待测溶液
$c(NaNO_3)$/(μg·mL^{-1})						
$A_1(\lambda_1)$						
$A_2(\lambda_2)$						
$\Delta A = A_1 - A_2$						

【思考题】

(1) 双波长分光光度法选择波长的原则是什么？

(2) 双波长分光光度法测定的优点是什么？

实验二十四　火焰原子吸收光谱法测定人头发中的锌

【目的要求】

(1) 掌握原子吸收光谱法的基本原理。

(2) 熟悉发样的湿法消化技术。

(3) 熟悉原子吸收分光光度计的基本结构和使用方法。

【实验原理】

发样经湿法消化,采用火焰原子化器进行原子化,当锐线光源(空心阴极灯)辐射出的待测元素的特征谱线通过火焰的原子化区时,待测元素的气态基态原子对谱线产生吸收,在一定实验条件下,吸光度与溶液中被测组分浓度成正比,$A=Kc$,可采用标准曲线法进行定量分析。

【仪器与试剂】

原子吸收分光光度计、锌空心阴极灯、空气压缩机、乙炔钢瓶、电子天平(0.01 g)、电热板、吸量管(2 mL×2)、容量瓶(50 mL×7,25 mL×1)、锥形瓶(50 mL×1)、烧杯等。

锌标准储备液(1.000 mg·mL^{-1})、锌标准应用液(50.00 μg·mL^{-1})、硝酸溶液(1%)、混合酸(硝酸:高氯酸为 4:1)、金属锌(GR)、硝酸(GR)、高氯酸(GR)。

【实验步骤】

1. 样品处理

取受检者枕部距头皮 2 cm 左右的头发约 0.5 g,剪碎至 1 cm 左右,置于烧杯中,用中性洗涤剂浸洗 30 min,并不断搅拌,用自来水洗至无泡沫,再用蒸馏水冲洗多次,滤干后,用无水乙醇浸泡 2 min,捞出,待乙醇挥发干后,置于 80 ℃干燥箱中干燥 30 min。准确称取 0.1~0.15 g 发样于锥形瓶中,加入 2.0 mL 混合酸,置于电热板上,逐步升温消化至溶液澄清透明。冷却,将消化液完全转移至 25 mL 容量瓶中,定容,摇匀备用,试剂空白溶液用同样的方法处理。

2. 配制标准系列溶液

在六只 50 mL 容量瓶中，分别加入 0.00 mL（空白）、0.30 mL、0.60 mL、0.90 mL、1.20 mL 和 1.50 mL 的 50.00 $\mu g \cdot mL^{-1}$ 锌标准应用液，用 1％硝酸溶液稀释定容后摇匀。

3. 仪器调试和操作条件

检测波长 213.9 nm、光谱通带 0.5 nm、灯电流 3.0 mA、乙炔流量 1.2 $L \cdot min^{-1}$、空气流量 6.0 $L \cdot min^{-1}$。仪器预热 30 min。

4. 样品测定

用空白溶液调节仪器吸光度为 0，按由稀到浓的顺序测定标准系列溶液的吸光度，在同样条件下测定试剂空白溶液和试样溶液的吸光度。用标准曲线法定量。

【结果记录和处理】

以吸光度对标准系列溶液浓度绘制标准曲线，并按下式计算分析结果：

$$\omega = \frac{(c-c_0)KV}{m_s} \times 10^{-6}$$

式中：ω 为发样中锌含量（$\mu g \cdot g^{-1}$）；V 为试样溶液体积；K 为试样稀释倍数；c 为试样溶液中锌的浓度（$\mu g \cdot mL^{-1}$）；c_0 为试剂空白溶液中锌的浓度（$\mu g \cdot mL^{-1}$）；m_s 为发样质量（g）。

【思考题】

(1) 测定头发中的锌有何实际意义？

(2) 狭缝宽度对测定有何影响？如何选择狭缝宽度？

实验二十五　荧光分光光度法测定牛奶中的核黄素

【目的要求】

(1) 掌握荧光分光光度法的基本原理和测量方法。

(2) 了解牛奶中核黄素测定的实验方法。

【实验原理】

核黄素（维生素 B_2）在中性和弱酸性溶液中可以发出荧光，通过测定溶液的荧光强度，就能确定物质中核黄素的含量。采用 pH＝4.6 的醋酸盐缓冲溶液沉淀蛋白质，连二亚硫酸钠作为熄灭剂，测定样品在加入熄灭剂前后的荧光强度的差值，求出样品中核黄素的含量，从而消除杂散光对测定的干扰。

【仪器与试剂】

荧光分光光度计、比色皿(1 cm×1)、容量瓶(50 mL×1)、吸量管(5 mL×3)、比色管(10 mL×7)、漏斗、玻棒、小烧杯(50 mL)等。

维生素 B_2 标准储备液(100.0 $\mu g \cdot mL^{-1}$)、维生素 B_2 标准应用液(2.00 $\mu g \cdot mL^{-1}$)、HAc-NaAc 缓冲溶液(pH=4.6)、HCl 溶液(0.1 mol · L^{-1})、HAc 溶液(1%)、连二亚硫酸钠($Na_2S_2O_4$),所有试剂均为分析纯。

【实验步骤】

1. 样品处理

准确移取牛奶 5.00 mL 于 50 mL 小烧杯中,加入 0.1 mol · L^{-1} HCl 溶液 10 mL,搅匀,放暗处静置 10 min。将溶液完全转移至 50 mL 容量瓶中,加入 20 mL HAc-NaAc 缓冲溶液,用蒸馏水定容,重复振摇,静置数分钟后,用快速定性滤纸过滤,弃去前 10 mL 滤液,收集后面的滤液测定。

2. 标准曲线法

(1) 标准曲线的制作。分别移取 2.00 $\mu g \cdot mL^{-1}$ 维生素 B_2 标准应用液 0.00 mL、0.50 mL、1.00 mL、1.50 mL、2.00 mL、2.50 mL 于六支 10 mL 比色管中,用 1% HAc 溶液稀释至刻度,摇匀。选择激发波长 425 nm,荧光发射波长 525 nm,测定标准系列溶液的荧光强度。以 $F-F_0$ 为纵坐标,维生素 B_2 的浓度为横坐标,绘制标准曲线。

(2) 样品测定。吸取待测样品滤液 5.00 mL 于 10 mL 比色管中,用 1% HAc 溶液稀释至刻线,摇匀。与标准系列溶液在相同条件下测定 F_x,将待测溶液荧光强度差值 F_x-F_0 代入回归方程,计算待测试样中维生素 B_2 的浓度。

3. 直接比较法

(1) 配制 0.25 $\mu g \cdot mL^{-1}$ 的维生素 B_2 标准溶液。准确吸取 2.00 $\mu g \cdot mL^{-1}$ 维生素 B_2 标准溶液 1.25 mL 于 10 mL 比色管中,用 1% HAc 溶液定容至刻度,摇匀。

(2) 测定。测定 0.25 $\mu g \cdot mL^{-1}$ 的维生素 B_2 标准溶液的荧光强度,加入 $Na_2S_2O_4$ 约 10 mg 于比色皿中,迅速摇匀,立即测定荧光强度。然后用相同方法测定样品滤液在加入 $Na_2S_2O_4$ 前后的荧光强度。平行测定三份。

【结果记录和处理】

1. 标准曲线法

绘制标准曲线,确定待测溶液浓度,数据记录如下:

V(维生素 B_2 标准应用液)/mL	0.00	0.50	1.00	1.50	2.00	2.50	待测溶液
c(维生素 B_2)/($\mu g \cdot mL^{-1}$)							
F							

2. 直接比较法

根据下列公式计算样品中的维生素 B_2 含量：

$$\omega(\mu g \cdot mL^{-1}) = \frac{(F_x - F_0{'}) \times 0.25}{F_s - F_0} \times \frac{50.00}{5.00}$$

式中：F_x、F_s 分别为样品、标准品在加 $Na_2S_2O_4$ 前测得的荧光强度；$F_0{'}$、F_0 分别为样品、标准品在加 $Na_2S_2O_4$ 后测得的荧光强度。

【思考题】

(1) 试述本方法的测定原理。

(2) 能否用荧光分光光度计测定核黄素的荧光光谱和激发光谱？

实验二十六　pH 玻璃电极性能检查及饮料 pH 值的测定

【目的要求】

(1) 掌握测定溶液 pH 值的原理。

(2) 熟悉 pH 计测定溶液 pH 值的方法。

(3) 了解电极性能的评价方法。

【实验原理】

电位法测定溶液 pH 值，以玻璃电极为指示电极，饱和甘汞电极为参比电极，组成原电池：

$(-)$Ag,AgCl(s) | 0.1 mol $\cdot$ L^{-1} HCl | 玻璃膜 | H^+(x mol $\cdot$ L^{-1}) ‖ KCl(饱和) | Hg_2Cl_2(s),Hg$(+)$

电池电动势为

$$E = \varphi_+ - \varphi_- = K + \frac{2.303RT}{F} pH$$

目前，实验室多采用将 pH 电极与参比电极组合在一起制成的复合 pH 玻璃电极，不使用时，应将其浸泡于含 KCl 的 pH=4 的缓冲溶液中。

用 pH 计测定 pH 值时，可采用两次测量法，即先用标准缓冲溶液校准 pH 计，然后测定待测溶液的电动势，得到待测溶液的 pH 值。

$$E_s = K + \frac{2.303RT}{F}\text{pH}_s$$

$$E_x = K + \frac{2.303RT}{F}\text{pH}_x$$

两式相减,可得

$$E_s = E_x + \frac{2.303RT}{F}(\text{pH}_s - \text{pH}_x)$$

pH 值变化一个单位,电池的电动势变化 $\frac{2.303RT}{F}$ 伏,此值随温度变化而不同,因此 pH 计上有温度补偿装置来调节温度改变引起的变化。一只性能良好的 pH 玻璃电极,应该具有理论上的能斯特响应,但在实际工作中,电极的实际响应斜率 S 与理论响应斜率有一定的偏差。

【仪器与试剂】

pH 计、电极(玻璃电极和饱和甘汞电极,或复合电极一个)、分析天平(0.01 g)、小烧杯(10 mL×5)。

pH=4.00 的邻苯二甲酸氢钾标准缓冲溶液(0.05 mol·L^{-1})、pH=6.86 的混合磷酸盐标准缓冲溶液(KH$_2$PO$_4$ 0.025 mol·L^{-1},Na$_2$HPO$_4$ 0.025 mol·L^{-1})、pH=9.18 的硼砂标准缓冲溶液(0.05 mol·L^{-1})。所有试剂均为分析纯。

【实验步骤】

1. pH 计的校正

依次采用 pH=6.86、pH=4.00 和 pH=9.18 的缓冲溶液进行校正。

2. 饮料 pH 值的测定

以玻璃电极为指示电极,饱和甘汞电极为参比电极,与待测溶液组成原电池,测定其 pH 值。

3. pH 玻璃电极性能检查

测定三种不同标准缓冲溶液的电动势。在 10 mL 小烧杯中倒入 pH=4.00 的标准缓冲溶液,将电极浸入其中,测定电池电动势,记录读数,清洗电极。依次测定 pH=6.86 和 pH=9.18 标准缓冲溶液的电动势。

【结果记录和处理】

(1) 记录饮料的 pH 值。

(2) 以缓冲溶液的 pH 值为横坐标,以电动势为纵坐标作图,检验玻璃电极对 H$^+$ 响应的线性关系,求得玻璃电极的实际响应斜率,与理论响应斜率进行比较。

【思考题】

(1) 用 pH 计测定溶液 pH 值时,为什么用标准缓冲溶液进行校正?

(2) pH 玻璃电极为什么不能测定过酸或过碱的溶液?

实验二十七　电导法测定水质纯度

【目的要求】

(1) 掌握电导法测定水质纯度的基本原理和实验方法。

(2) 熟悉电导池常数的测定方法。

(3) 了解电导率仪的结构。

【实验原理】

电导率 $\kappa(S \cdot cm^{-1})$ 与溶液中离子的浓度、迁移速度、价态和温度等因素有关,可作为水中电解质含量的参考指标,是评价水质的综合指标之一。电导 $G(S)$、电导率与电导池常数 θ 的关系式如下:

$$G = \kappa \frac{A}{l} = \frac{\kappa}{\theta}$$

式中:A 为电极面积(cm^2);l 为电极间的距离(cm);$\theta = \dfrac{l}{A}$,为电导池常数(cm^{-1})。25 ℃时,纯水的理论电导率为 $5.48 \times 10^{-2}\ \mu S \cdot cm^{-1}$,一般实验室使用的蒸馏水或去离子水的电导率要求小于 $1\ \mu S \cdot cm^{-1}$。

【仪器与试剂】

电导率仪、电极(铂黑电极和铂光亮电极各一个)、恒温水槽、容量瓶(1 000 mL× 1)、小烧杯(50 mL×7)等。

KCl 标准溶液(0.01 mol · L^{-1},准确称取 120 ℃干燥 4 h 的 KCl 0.745 6 g,溶于纯水(电导率<1 $\mu S \cdot cm^{-1}$)中,转移至 1 000 mL 容量瓶中,定容,储存于塑料瓶备用)。

【实验步骤】

1.电导池常数 θ 的测定

清洗电极,取 0.01 mol · L^{-1} 的 KCl 标准溶液约 30 mL 倒入 50 mL 小烧杯中,25 ℃恒温水浴约 15 min,插入电导电极,调节仪器温度为 25 ℃,测定其电导 $G(KCl)$。

2.去离子水、蒸馏水、市售纯净水电导率的测定

调节常数补偿按钮,使仪器显示值与所用电极电导池常数一致;调节温度补偿按钮,使仪器显示温度与溶液温度一致。分别用去离子水、蒸馏水、市售纯净水润洗3个小烧杯3次,然后分别倒入约30 mL,选用铂光亮电极,插入试液中,选择合适量程,读数即为被测溶液电导率。每种试液测定3次,取平均值。

3.自来水、湖水的电导率测定

用待测水样润洗小烧杯3次,倒入约30 mL,选用铂黑电极,插入试液中,按照与步骤2相同的操作测定水样电导率。

【结果记录和处理】

(1)电导池常数 θ:记录 KCl 溶液的电导值,查出 25 ℃下 0.01 mol·L^{-1} KCl 溶液的电导率,计算电导池常数。

(2)记录各水样电导率值,并进行比较。

【思考题】

(1)电导率仪使用直流电还是交流电? 为什么?

(2)为什么要测定电极的电导池常数? 如何测定?

实验二十八　氟离子选择电极法测定
水样中氟离子的浓度

【目的要求】

(1)掌握氟离子选择电极法测定氟离子浓度的原理和方法。

(2)熟悉用标准曲线法和标准加入法测定水样中氟离子浓度的方法。

【实验原理】

氟离子选择电极是一种晶体膜电极,其敏感膜为氟化镧(LaF$_3$)单晶膜,它对氟离子有选择性响应,膜电位大小与氟离子活度的关系遵守 Nernst 方程。测定溶液中的氟离子浓度时,将氟离子选择电极作为指示电极,饱和甘汞电极作为参比电极,组成工作电池,电池电动势与氟离子活度的对数呈线性关系:

$$E = \varphi_{F^-} - \varphi_{ref} = K - 0.059 \lg a_{F^-}$$

当保持溶液离子强度一定时,有

$$E = K - 0.059 \lg c_{F^-}$$

【仪器与试剂】

酸度计、氟离子选择电极和饱和甘汞电极(或复合电极一个)、电磁搅拌器、容量瓶(25 mL×6)、吸量管(2 mL×2,10 mL×3)、小烧杯(50 mL×7)等。

氟离子标准储备液(1.000 mg·mL^{-1})、氟离子标准应用液(10.00 μg·mL^{-1})、总离子强度调节缓冲溶液(称取 58 g 氯化钠、57 mL 冰乙酸、3.4 g 五水合柠檬酸三钠,溶于蒸馏水,用 10 mol·L^{-1}氢氧化钠溶液调节至 pH=5.0～5.5,最后用蒸馏水稀释至 1 000 mL),以上试剂均为分析纯。

【实验步骤】

1.标准曲线法测定水样中氟化物的浓度

分别移取 10.00 μg·mL^{-1}的氟离子标准应用液 0.40 mL、0.60 mL、1.00 mL、1.50 mL、2.00 mL 于 25 mL 容量瓶中,加入 10.00 mL 总离子强度调节缓冲溶液,去离子水定容至 25 mL,摇匀。将配制的标准系列溶液按浓度从低到高,依次倒入洁净小烧杯中,插入电极,磁力搅拌,读取电动势 E 值,以氟离子浓度的对数为横坐标,电动势 E 为纵坐标,绘制标准曲线。

移取 10.00 mL 水样于 25 mL 容量瓶中,加入 10.00 mL 总离子强度调节缓冲溶液,去离子水定容,摇匀,倒入洁净小烧杯中,插入电极,磁力搅拌,读取电动势 E_x值。

2.标准加入法测定水样中氟化物的浓度

移取 10.00 mL 水样于小烧杯中,加入 10.00 mL 总离子强度调节缓冲溶液,插入电极,持续搅拌下读取电动势 E_1 值,然后加入 0.20 mL 1.000 mg·mL^{-1}的氟离子标准储备液,持续搅拌下读取电动势 E_2 值。

【结果记录和处理】

(1) 在标准曲线上查得氟离子浓度,并计算水样中氟离子的浓度。

(2) 标准加入法,由 E_1 和 E_2 计算水样中氟离子的浓度。

(3) 对两种测定方法的结果进行比较。

【思考题】

(1) 总离子强度调节缓冲溶液的作用是什么?

(2) 用上述方法测得的结果是活度还是浓度? 为什么?

实验二十九　气相色谱法测定废水中的苯系物

【目的要求】

(1) 了解气相色谱仪的基本结构和使用方法。

(2) 掌握气相色谱法测定苯系物的原理及实验方法。

(3) 熟悉内标标准曲线法的定量方法。

【实验原理】

苯及苯系物在弱极性或中等极性固定相上的分配系数不同,因而在气相色谱中的保留时间不同,通过保留时间对样品中的苯系物进行定性分析,通过峰面积进行定量分析。

【仪器与试剂】

气相色谱仪(FID)、毛细管柱(HP-1、DB-5 或 OV1701 等,规格为 30 m×0.25 mm×0.25 μm)、微量注射器(10 μL×1)、容量瓶(10 mL×7)、移液枪、分液漏斗(125 mL)等。

苯标准储备液(100 μg·mL^{-1})(移取适量苯,溶于二硫化碳中,定容至 10 mL,摇匀)、甲苯标准储备液(100 μg·mL^{-1})(移取适量甲苯,溶于二硫化碳中,定容至 10 mL,摇匀)、乙苯标准储备液(100 μg·mL^{-1})(移取适量乙苯,溶于二硫化碳中,定容至 10 mL,摇匀),以上试剂均为色谱纯。

【实验步骤】

1.色谱条件

气化室温度:230 ℃。柱温:80 ℃。检测器温度:230 ℃。载气:N$_2$。载气流速:2.0 mL·min^{-1}。氢气流速:30 mL·min^{-1}。空气流速:300 mL·min^{-1}。尾吹气流速:25 mL·min^{-1}。分流比为 10∶1。

2.标准系列的配制

分别准确吸取苯、甲苯标准储备液 0.10 mL、0.20 mL、0.50 mL、1.00 mL、2.00 mL 于 5 只 10 mL 容量瓶中,各瓶中均加入乙苯标准储备液 0.50 mL,加二硫化碳至刻度,摇匀。配制成苯和甲苯的混合标准系列溶液,苯和甲苯的浓度分别为 1.00 μg·mL^{-1}、2.00 μg·mL^{-1}、5.00 μg·mL^{-1}、10.0 μg·mL^{-1}、20.0 μg·mL^{-1},乙苯的浓度均为 5.00 μg·mL^{-1}。

3. 样品溶液的制备

准确移取 25 mL 待测水样于 125 mL 分液漏斗中,加入 5.0 mL 二硫化碳,振摇,静置分层,分出下层二硫化碳,取萃取液 1.0 mL 于 10 mL 容量瓶中,加入乙苯标准储备液 0.50 mL,加二硫化碳至刻度,摇匀。

4. 标准品保留时间的测定

分别配制 5.00 $\mu g \cdot mL^{-1}$ 苯标准溶液、5.00 $\mu g \cdot mL^{-1}$ 甲苯标准溶液和 5.00 $\mu g \cdot mL^{-1}$ 乙苯标准溶液,各取 0.2 μL 分别进样到气相色谱仪,测定苯、甲苯和乙苯的保留时间。

5. 内标标准曲线绘制

将配制好的混合标准系列溶液,按照浓度从低到高依次进样 0.2 μL,计算苯、甲苯与内标物乙苯的峰面积之比,以峰面积之比为纵坐标,浓度为横坐标,分别绘制苯和甲苯的内标标准曲线。

6. 样品测定

在相同的色谱条件下测定样品溶液,进样 0.2 μL,计算苯、甲苯与内标物乙苯的峰面积之比。

【数据记录与处理】

1. 定性分析

将样品溶液中各组分的保留时间与标准溶液中各组分的保留时间进行比较,对样品中各组分进行定性分析。

2. 定量结果处理

根据样品溶液中,苯、甲苯与内标物乙苯的峰面积之比,分别在苯和甲苯的内标标准曲线上查得苯和甲苯的浓度,并计算原水样中苯和甲苯的浓度($\mu g \cdot mL^{-1}$)。

【思考题】

(1) 内标标准曲线法的优点是什么?

(2) 试解释苯、甲苯和乙苯的出峰顺序。

实验三十　高效液相色谱法测定食品中的色素

【目的要求】

(1) 了解高效液相色谱仪的基本结构和使用方法。

(2) 掌握高效液相色谱法测定食品中色素的原理及实验方法。

【实验原理】

柠檬黄和日落黄是我国食品中允许使用的合成色素,可以用于果味水、果味粉、果子露、汽水、配制酒、红绿丝、罐头,以及糕点表面上彩等,但用量有严格限制。柠檬黄和日落黄的结构式如下:

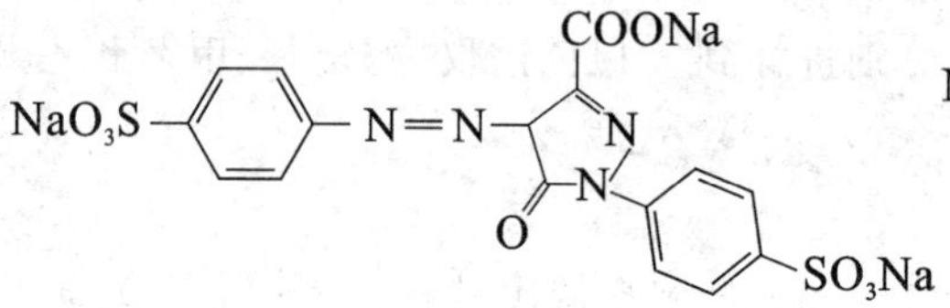

柠檬黄 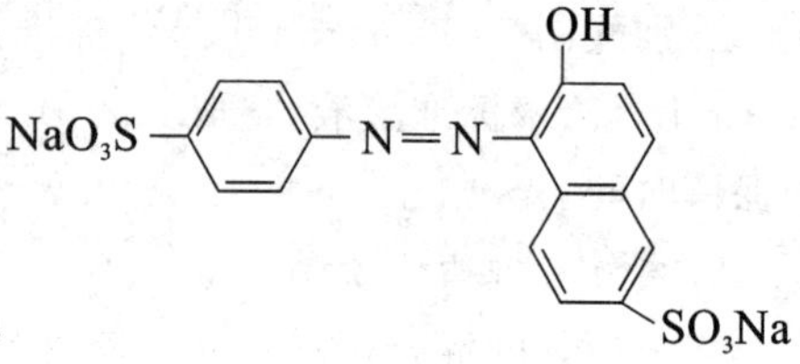　　　　　　　　　　　日落黄

柠檬黄和日落黄在紫外-可见光区有吸收,因此可以采用高效液相色谱法对二者进行分离,然后采用紫外检测器对饮料中的柠檬黄和日落黄进行定量分析。

【仪器与试剂】

高效液相色谱仪(紫外检测器)、色谱柱(C18 柱,规格为 150 mm×4.6 mm×5 μm)、微量注射器(100 μL×1)、分析天平(0.01 g)、超声振荡器、移液枪等。

柠檬酸溶液(称取 20 g 柠檬酸($C_6H_8O_7 \cdot H_2O$),加双蒸水至 100 mL,溶解混匀),pH=6 的水(双蒸水加柠檬酸溶液,调 pH 值到 6),柠檬黄、日落黄标准储备液(1 mg·mL^{-1},准确称取按其纯度折算为 100%质量的柠檬黄、日落黄各 0.1 g(精确至 0.000 1 g),置于 100 mL 容量瓶中,各自加 pH=6 的水到刻度,配成水溶液),柠檬黄、日落黄标准应用液(50 μg·mL^{-1},临用时,将标准储备液加双蒸水稀释 20 倍,经 0.45 μm 微孔滤膜过滤),乙酸铵溶液(0.02 mol·L^{-1},称取 1.54 g 乙酸铵,加双蒸水至 1 000 mL,溶解,经 0.45 μm 微孔滤膜过滤)。

【实验步骤】

1.色谱条件

色谱柱:C18 柱,150 mm×4.6 mm×5 μm。进样量:20 μL。柱温:35 ℃。紫外检测波长:254 nm。流动相:甲醇-0.02 mol·L^{-1}乙酸铵溶液(体积比为 35∶65)。流动相流速:1 mL·min^{-1}。

2.试样制备

果汁饮料及果汁、果味碳酸饮料等:准确称取 20~40 g 样品,放入 100 mL 烧杯中,超声去除二氧化碳。

配制酒类:准确称取 20~40 g 样品,放入 100 mL 烧杯中,加小碎瓷片数片,加热去除乙醇。

硬糖、蜜饯、淀粉软糖等:准确称取 5～10 g 粉碎样品,放入 100 mL 烧杯中,加水 30 mL,温热溶剂,若样品溶液 pH 值较高,用柠檬酸溶液调 pH 值到 6 左右。

巧克力豆及着色糖衣制品:准确称取 5～10 g 样品,放入 100 mL 烧杯中,用水反复洗涤色素,到巧克力都无色素为止,合并色素漂洗液为样品溶液。

3.色素提取

样品溶液加柠檬酸溶液调节 pH 值到 6,加热至 60 ℃,取 1 g 聚酰胺粉加少许水调成糊状,加入样品溶液中,搅拌片刻,以 G3 垂熔漏斗抽滤,用 60 ℃ pH＝4 的水洗涤 3～5 次,然后用甲醇-甲酸混合溶液洗涤 3～5 次,再用水洗至中性,用乙醇-氨水-水混合溶液解吸 3～5 次,直至色素完全解吸,收集解吸液,加乙酸中和,蒸发至近干,加水溶液,定容至 5 mL,经 0.45 μm 微孔滤膜过滤。

4.测定

将样品提取液和柠檬黄、日落黄标准应用液分别注入高效液相色谱仪分析。

【数据记录与处理】

1.定性分析

将样品溶液中各组分的保留时间与标准溶液中各组分的保留时间进行比较,对样品中各组分进行定性分析。

2.定量结果处理

根据样品溶液中柠檬黄、日落黄的峰面积,采用外标峰面积法定量。

【思考题】

(1) 样品在进样前为何要过滤?

(2) 应如何选择流动相和色谱柱?

实验三十一　　粗食盐的提纯

【目的要求】

(1) 熟悉称量、过滤、结晶和干燥等基本操作。

(2) 了解 Mg^{2+}、Ca^{2+}、Ba^{2+} 的鉴定和去除方法。

【实验原理】

许多无机盐均含有杂质,杂质的种类及含量的高低与无机盐的来源及制备方法、条件有关。纯化无机盐的方法有多种,最常用的是重结晶法。

食盐是能溶于水的固态物质。其中所含杂质的去除方法如下。

(1) 机械杂质如泥沙可采取过滤法去除。

(2) 一些能溶解的杂质可根据其性质借助化学方法去除。如加入 $BaCl_2$ 溶液可使 SO_4^{2-} 生成 $BaSO_4$ 沉淀,加入 Na_2CO_3 溶液可使 Mg^{2+}、Ca^{2+}、Ba^{2+} 等离子生成难溶物,再滤去。

(3) 少量可溶性杂质如 Br^-、I^-、K^+ 等离子,可根据溶解度不同,在重结晶时,使其残留在母液中弃去。

【仪器与试剂】

电子天平(0.01 g)、烧杯(100 mL×1)、酒精灯、滤纸、吸滤瓶、布氏漏斗、干燥器、离心机、石棉网、电炉、蒸发皿、试管(6)、离心试管(4)、水流抽气泵。

粗食盐(s)、HCl 溶液(6 mol·L^{-1})、H_2SO_4 溶液(3 mol·L^{-1})、$BaCl_2$ 溶液(1 mol·L^{-1})、Na_2CO_3 溶液(饱和)。

【实验步骤】

(1) 粗食盐的溶解。称取 5 g 粗食盐,加 20 mL 水,加热搅拌使其溶解。

(2) 除 SO_4^{2-}。溶液加热至接近沸腾,一边搅拌,一边逐滴加入 0.8～1.3 mL 1 mol·L^{-1} $BaCl_2$ 溶液,继续加热 5 min,使沉淀颗粒长大而易于沉降。

(3) 检查 SO_4^{2-} 是否除尽。将烧杯从石棉网上取下,待沉淀沉降后取少量上层溶液,离心分离,在离心中加入几滴 6 mol·L^{-1} HCl 溶液,再加入几滴 $BaCl_2$ 溶液,如果有混浊,表示 SO_4^{2-} 尚未除尽,需要再加入 $BaCl_2$ 溶液。如果不混浊,表示 SO_4^{2-} 已除尽,过滤,弃去沉淀。

(4) 除 Mg^{2+}、Ca^{2+}、Ba^{2+} 等阳离子。将上述滤液加热至接近沸腾,一边搅拌,一边滴加饱和 Na_2CO_3 溶液,至不生成沉淀为止,再多加入 0.2 mL Na_2CO_3 溶液,静置。

(5) 检查 Ba^{2+} 是否除尽。取少量上层溶液,离心分离,在离心液中加入几滴 3 mol·L^{-1} H_2SO_4 溶液,如果有混浊,表示 Ba^{2+} 未除尽,需继续加 Na_2CO_3 溶液,至除尽为止(检查液用后弃去),过滤,弃去沉淀。

(6) 用 HCl 溶液调整酸度除去剩余的 CO_3^{2-}。在滤液中滴加 6 mol·L^{-1} HCl 溶液,加热搅拌,直到溶液的 pH 为 2～3。

(7) 浓缩、结晶。把溶液蒸发浓缩到原体积的 1/3,冷却结晶,过滤,用少量蒸馏水洗涤晶体,抽干。把 NaCl 晶体放在蒸发皿内,用小火边搅拌边烘干,以防止溅出与结块,再用大火灼烧 1～2 min,冷后称量。

(8) 产品质量鉴定。取原料、产品各 0.5 g,分别溶于 1.5 mL 蒸馏水中,定性鉴定溶液中有无 SO_4^{2-}、Ca^{2+}、Mg^{2+}、Ba^{2+},比较实验结果。

【结果记录和处理】

1.产率计算

粗食盐的质量 m_1/g	
纯食盐的质量 m_2/g	
产率/(%)	

2.质量鉴定

项　目	粗　食　盐	纯　食　盐
SO_4^{2-}		
Ca^{2+}		
Mg^{2+}		
Ba^{2+}		

【思考题】

（1）粗食盐中不溶性、可溶性杂质如何除去？

（2）$BaCl_2$毒性很大,切勿入口。能否用其他无毒盐如 $CaCl_2$ 等来除去 SO_4^{2-}？

（3）能否用其他酸来除去多余的 CO_3^{2-}？

（4）除去可溶性杂质离子的先后顺序是否合理？可否任意变换顺序？

（5）加沉淀剂除去杂质时,为了得到较大晶粒的沉淀,沉淀的条件是什么？

实验三十二　硫酸亚铁铵的制备(含微型实验)

【目的要求】

（1）学习复盐的制备及性质。

（2）进一步熟练掌握水浴加热、蒸发、结晶、常压过滤和减压过滤等基本操作。

预习内容

（3）进一步熟悉比色管和吸量管的使用,了解微型实验方法与操作。

【实验原理】

硫酸亚铁铵($FeSO_4 \cdot (NH_4)_2SO_4 \cdot 6H_2O$)俗称莫尔盐,为浅蓝绿色单斜晶体,易溶于水,难溶于乙醇,在空气中比亚铁盐稳定,不易被氧化,可作为氧化还原滴定法中的一级标准物质。

常用的制备方法是用过量的 Fe 与稀 H_2SO_4 作用制得 $FeSO_4$,再用等物质的量的 $FeSO_4$ 与 $(NH_4)_2SO_4$ 在水溶液中相互作用。由于复盐的溶解度比组成它的简单盐小,因此经冷却后复盐在水溶液中首先结晶,形成 $FeSO_4 \cdot (NH_4)_2SO_4 \cdot 6H_2O$ 复盐。反应如下:

$$Fe + H_2SO_4 \!=\!=\!= FeSO_4 + H_2\uparrow$$

$$FeSO_4 + (NH_4)_2SO_4 + 6H_2O \!=\!=\!= FeSO_4 \cdot (NH_4)_2SO_4 \cdot 6H_2O$$

【仪器与试剂】

电子天平(0.01 g)、锥形瓶(50 mL×1,15 mL×1)、容量瓶(1 L×1)、水浴锅、量筒(50 mL×1,10 mL×1)、玻璃漏斗、酒精灯、滤纸、水流抽气泵、烧杯(250 mL×1,15 mL×1)、比色管(25 mL×4)、吸量管(1 mL×1,2 mL×1,5 mL×1)、吸滤瓶(口径 19 mm,容积20 mL)、布氏漏斗(20 mm,19 mm)、蒸发皿(10 mL)、玻棒。

Na_2CO_3溶液(10%)、H_2SO_4 溶液(3 mol·L^{-1})、HCl 溶液(3 mol·L^{-1})、$(NH_4)_2SO_4$(AR,s)、KSCN 溶液(1 mol·L^{-1})、乙醇溶液(95%)、去氧蒸馏水(取一定量蒸馏水,在石棉网上小火加热煮沸 10~20 min,冷却后即可使用)、铁片或铁屑、pH 试纸、标准 Fe^{3+} 溶液(0.1 g·L^{-1}:准确称取 0.863 4 g $NH_4Fe(SO_4)_2 \cdot 12H_2O$ 溶于水中,加入浓 H_2SO_4溶液 2.5 mL,定量转移到 1 L 容量瓶中,用水稀释至刻度,充分摇匀)。

【实验步骤】

1.铁片或铁屑的净化(去油污)

用电子天平称取 2.0 g 铁片或铁屑,放入 50 mL 锥形瓶中,加入 10 mL 10% Na_2CO_3溶液,放在石棉网上加热煮沸,用倾析法倾出碱液,然后用蒸馏水把碎铁片或铁屑洗至中性。

2.$FeSO_4$ 的制备

在盛有处理过的碎铁片或铁屑的锥形瓶中,加入 10 mL 3 mol·L^{-1} H_2SO_4溶液,在水浴中加热,使 Fe 与 H_2SO_4充分反应,在加热过程中注意补充蒸发掉的水分,防止 $FeSO_4$结晶。待反应速度明显减慢(无气泡冒出,大约需 30 min),趁热过滤,滤液承接于蒸发皿中,分别用 1 mL 3 mol·L^{-1} H_2SO_4溶液和少量去离子水洗涤未反应完的 Fe 和残渣,洗涤液合并至滤液中。未反应完的铁片用滤纸吸干后称量,计算已参加反应的 Fe 的质量。

3.$FeSO_4 \cdot (NH_4)_2SO_4 \cdot 6H_2O$ 的制备

根据反应中消耗的 Fe 的质量或生成 $FeSO_4$ 的理论产量,计算制备 $FeSO_4 \cdot (NH_4)_2SO_4 \cdot 6H_2O$ 所需 $(NH_4)_2SO_4$ 的理论量(考虑到 $FeSO_4$ 在过滤等操作中的损失,$(NH_4)_2SO_4$ 的用量可按生成 $FeSO_4$ 的理论产量的 80% 计算,约 4.75 g),将其加

到 $FeSO_4$ 溶液中,混合均匀,并用 3 mol·L^{-1} H_2SO_4 溶液调节混合溶液的 pH 值为 1.0~2.0,将该溶液置于水浴中或小火加热溶解,继续蒸发浓缩至表面出现晶膜为止 (蒸发、浓缩过程中不宜搅拌),静置使其自然冷却至室温,得到浅蓝绿色的 $FeSO_4$·$(NH_4)_2SO_4$·$6H_2O$ 晶体。减压过滤,用少量 95% 乙醇溶液洗涤晶体两次,取出晶体用滤纸吸干,再转移到表面皿上,称量,计算产率。

4. 微型实验

称取 0.5 g 铁屑于 15 mL 锥形瓶中,加入 3 mL 10% Na_2CO_3 溶液,加热去油,然后用去离子水洗净,加入 2.5 mL 3 mol·L^{-1} H_2SO_4 溶液,在水浴中加热 5 min,使反应完全。用微型布氏漏斗、吸滤瓶抽滤,依次用 0.3 mL 3 mol·L^{-1} H_2SO_4 溶液、几滴去离子水洗涤,滤液转移至微型蒸发皿中,加入 1.2 g $(NH_4)_2SO_4$,加热溶解并蒸发至出现晶膜,冷却结晶,抽滤,称量,计算产率。

5. 产品检验——Fe^{3+} 的限量分析

产品的主要杂质是 Fe^{3+},根据 Fe^{3+} 与 KSCN 所形成的血红色配离子 $[Fe(SCN)]^{2+}$ 的颜色深浅,用目视比色法可确定其含 Fe^{3+} 的级别。

(1) 标准溶液的配制。依次取 0.1 g·L^{-1} Fe^{3+} 溶液 0.50 mL、1.00 mL、2.00 mL,分别置于 3 支 25 mL 比色管中,各加 1.00 mL 3 mol·L^{-1} H_2SO_4 溶液和 1.00 mL 1 mol·L^{-1} KSCN 溶液,最后用去氧蒸馏水稀释至刻度,摇匀。3 支比色管中分别含 Fe^{3+} 0.05 mg(符合Ⅰ级试剂)、0.10 mg(符合Ⅱ级试剂)、0.20 mg(符合Ⅲ级试剂)。注意:此标准溶液的配制应与产品同时、同样处理。

(2) 产品分析。称 1.00 g 产品,放入 25 mL 比色管中,加 15.00 mL 去氧蒸馏水溶解。加入 1.00 mL 3 mol·L^{-1} H_2SO_4 溶液和 1.00 mL 1 mol·L^{-1} KSCN 溶液,加入去氧蒸馏水至刻度,摇匀。再将该溶液与标准溶液进行比较,根据比色结果,确定产品中 Fe^{3+} 含量所对应的级别。

【注意事项】

(1) 在加 H_2SO_4 溶液溶解碎铁片或铁屑时,要用水浴;要注意补充水分,使体积保持在约 20 mL,防止 $FeSO_4$ 析出;溶解碎铁片或铁屑至无气泡产生时,应趁热过滤。

(2) 在制备过程中,要保持溶液为强酸性,否则易使 Fe^{2+} 氧化水解。若溶液出现黄色,应加 H_2SO_4 溶液和铁钉,抑制 Fe^{3+} 的出现。

(3) 蒸发过程中应用小火加热,并不断搅拌,防止暴溅。

【思考题】

(1) 在制备 $FeSO_4$ 时,为什么 Fe 需过量,溶液需调节至强酸性并用水浴加热?

(2) 能否将最后产物 $FeSO_4$·$(NH_4)_2SO_4$·$6H_2O$ 直接在蒸发皿内加热、干燥?

为什么?

(3) 检验 Fe^{3+} 时,为什么要用去氧蒸馏水溶解样品?

(4) 试比较微型实验与常规实验的利弊。

实验三十三 溶胶的制备和性质

【目的要求】

(1) 了解溶胶的制备方法。

(2) 验证溶胶的性质。

【实验原理】

溶胶的制备可用分散法和凝聚法,本实验用凝聚法制备溶胶。凝聚法是把物质的分子或离子聚合成较大的质点,通常利用一些化学反应可以实现。加热使稀 $FeCl_3$ 溶液水解以制备氢氧化铁溶胶,利用酒石酸锑钾和饱和硫化氢水溶液的复分解反应制备三硫化二锑溶胶都属凝聚法。制得的溶胶中,常会有一些相对分子质量较小的溶质及电解质等杂质,影响溶胶的稳定性,可用透析法使溶胶净化。

胶粒的大小介于溶液和悬浊液之间。当一束强光通过溶胶时,胶粒对光产生散射作用,其本身便成为一个小的发光体,从侧面可以看到由胶粒散射所形成的光路,这种现象称为 Tyndall 效应。Tyndall 效应是溶胶区别于真溶液的一个基本特征。

胶粒的另一个重要的性质是其带电荷。氢氧化铁溶胶在外加电场作用下将向负极运动,由此可见其带正电荷。胶粒带电的原因之一是其对离子的选择性吸附。通常情况下,氢氧化铁溶胶带正电荷,三硫化二锑溶胶带负电荷。胶粒带电是胶体稳定的一个重要原因。

溶胶中加入一定量电解质,会引起溶胶聚沉。电解质的聚沉能力随着引起聚沉的反离子的价数增加而增强。如氢氧化铁溶胶带正电荷,其反离子价数越高,聚沉能力越强,则聚沉能力大小为 $Na_3PO_4 > MgSO_4 > NaCl$。

【仪器与试剂】

U 形管、Tyndall 暗箱、烧杯(100 mL×3,500 mL×1)、量筒(10 mL×1,50 mL×1)、试管(10)、滴管、酒精灯、玻棒、石棉网、线、电泳仪、电炉。

$FeCl_3$ 溶液(2%)、酒石酸锑钾溶液(0.4%)、$AgNO_3$ 溶液(0.1 mol·L^{-1})、KSCN 溶液(0.5 mol·L^{-1})、HCl 溶液(0.000 1 mol·L^{-1})、NaCl 溶液(0.005 mol·L^{-1},5%)、$CaCl_2$ 溶液(0.005 mol·L^{-1})、$AlCl_3$ 溶液(0.005 mol·L^{-1})、饱和硫化氢水溶液、$CuSO_4$ 溶液(2%)、蔗糖、火棉胶。

【实验步骤】

1.溶胶的制备

(1)氢氧化铁溶胶的制备。在 100 mL 烧杯中,注入 25 mL 蒸馏水,加热至沸,然后边搅拌边逐滴加入 4 mL 2% $FeCl_3$ 溶液,继续煮沸 1~2 min 即可。观察 Tyndall 现象,并保留备用。

(2)三硫化二锑溶胶的制备。在 100 mL 烧杯中盛 20 mL 0.4% 酒石酸锑钾溶液,然后滴加饱和硫化氢水溶液,并适当搅拌,至溶液变成橙红色溶胶为止。观察 Tyndall 现象,并保留备用。

2.溶胶的净化——透析

(1)透析袋的准备。在干燥的 100 mL 烧杯中倒入约 10 mL 火棉胶溶液,慢慢转动烧杯,使火棉胶溶液浸润整个烧杯内壁,倒出多余的火棉胶溶液,倒置烧杯,使火棉胶固化成膜,取出即成透析袋。

(2)透析。将制备的氢氧化铁溶胶注入透析袋中,小心不要让溶胶污染透析袋的外面(如果外面附有溶胶,用蒸馏水洗干净),将透析袋口用线系紧,置于盛有蒸馏水的 500 mL 烧杯内,每隔 10 min 换水一次,并检查水中的 Cl^- 和 Fe^{3+}(分别用 $AgNO_3$ 和 KSCN 试剂),记录结果。哪种微粒透过了半透膜? 根据实验,溶胶中微粒的大小关系如何?

3.溶胶的性质

(1)Tyndall 效应。取 3 支试管分别装入 1/3 体积的氢氧化铁溶胶、三硫化二锑溶胶、$CuSO_4$ 溶液,对准光束,观察 Tyndall 现象。哪种液体没有 Tyndall 现象?

(2)溶胶的电学性质。于洗净的 U 形管中,注入制备的三硫化二锑溶胶,进行电泳实验,观察胶粒的迁移。胶粒向哪一极迁移? 为什么?

(3)溶胶的聚沉。

① 在 1 mL 三硫化二锑溶胶中,逐滴加入 0.005 mol · L^{-1} NaCl 溶液,边加边摇,直至试管刚出现混浊,记录所加的滴数。用 0.005 mol · L^{-1} $CaCl_2$ 溶液或 0.005 mol · L^{-1} $AlCl_3$ 溶液代替 0.005 mol · L^{-1} NaCl 溶液,重复上述实验,记录所加的滴数并比较结果,解释之。

② 在 1 支试管中,分别加入 2 mL 氢氧化铁溶胶和三硫化二锑溶胶,振摇混匀,观察所出现的现象,并解释之。

③ 将盛有 2 mL 三硫化二锑溶胶的试管加热至沸,观察现象,并解释之。

【结果记录和处理】

1.溶胶的制备

观测结果:(1)_____

(2)_____

2.溶胶的净化——透析

观测结果：_____

氢氧化铁胶粒是否透过透析袋？解释之。

3.溶胶的性质

（1）Tyndall 效应。

样品：　　氢氧化铁溶胶　　　三硫化二锑溶胶　　　$CuSO_4$溶液

观测结果：_____　　　　_____　　　　_____

（2）溶胶的电学性质。

观测结果：_____

（3）溶胶的聚沉。

0.005 mol·L^{-1}NaCl 溶液的滴数_____

0.005 mol·$L^{-1}$$CaCl_2$溶液的滴数_____

0.005 mol·$L^{-1}$$AlCl_3$溶液的滴数_____

实验三十四　　水热法制备纳米 SnO_2 微粉

【目的要求】

（1）了解水热法制备纳米材料的基本原理。

（2）了解不同外界条件对产物微晶的形成、晶粒大小及形态的影响。

（3）了解表征纳米材料的一般方法。

【实验原理】

SnO_2是一种半导体氧化物，它在传感器、催化剂和透明导电薄膜等方面具有广泛的用途。纳米 SnO_2具有很大的比表面积，是一种很好的气敏与湿敏材料。制备超细 SnO_2微粉的方法很多，有 Sol-Gel 法、化学沉淀法、激光分解法、水热法等。水热法制备纳米氧化物微粉有许多优点，如产物直接为晶态，无须经过焙烧晶化过程，因而可以减少用其他方法难以避免的颗粒团聚，同时粒度比较均匀，形态比较规则。因此，水热法是制备纳米氧化物微粉的较好方法之一。

水热法是指在温度超过 100 ℃和相应压力（高于常压）条件下利用水溶液（广义地说，溶剂介质不一定是水）中物质间的化学反应合成化合物的方法。在水热条件（相对高的温度和压力）下，水的反应活性提高，其蒸气压上升、离子积增大，而密度、表面张力及黏度下降。体系的氧化还原电势发生变化，总之，物质在水热条件下的热力学性质均不同于常态，从而为合成某些特定化合物提供了可能。水热法的主要特点：①水热条件下，反应物和溶剂的活性提高，有利于某些特殊中间态及特殊物相的形成,因此可能合成具有某些特殊结构的新化合物;②水热条件下,有利于某些晶体的生长,可获得纯度高、取向规则、形态完美、非平衡态缺陷尽可能少的晶体材料;③产物粒度较易控制,分布集中,采用适当措施可尽量减少团聚;④通过改变水热反应条件,可能形成具有不同晶体结构和结晶形态的产物,也有利于低价态、中间价态与特殊价态化合物的生成。基于以上特点,水热合成在材料领域已有广泛应用,水热合成化学也日益受到化学与材料科学界的重视。

水热反应制备纳米 SnO_2 微粉的反应机理的第一步是 $SnCl_4$ 的水解:

$$SnCl_4 + 4H_2O \longrightarrow Sn(OH)_4 + 4HCl$$

该反应形成无定形的 $Sn(OH)_4$ 沉淀,紧接着发生 $Sn(OH)_4$ 的脱水缩合和晶化作用,形成纳米 SnO_2 微粉。其反应方程式为

$$nSn(OH)_4 \longrightarrow nSnO_2 + 2nH_2O$$

本实验以水热法制备纳米 SnO_2 微粉为例,介绍水热反应的基本原理,研究不同水热反应条件对产物微晶的形成、晶粒大小及形态的影响。

【仪器与试剂】

100 mL 不锈钢压力釜(具有聚四氟乙烯衬里)、管式电炉套及温控装置、电磁搅拌器、水流抽气泵、酸度计(PB-10 型)、烧杯(100 mL×1)、布氏漏斗、滤纸、吸滤瓶。

$SnCl_4 \cdot 5H_2O(AR,s)$、$KOH(AR,s)$、乙酸（AR,l)、乙酸铵(AR,s)、乙醇溶液(95%)。

【实验步骤】

1. 原料液的配制

用蒸馏水配制 1.0 mol·L^{-1} $SnCl_4$ 溶液、10 mol·L^{-1} KOH 溶液。每次取 50 mL 1.0 mol·L^{-1} $SnCl_4$ 溶液于 100 mL 烧杯中,在电磁搅拌下逐滴加入 10 mol·L^{-1} KOH 溶液,调节反应液的 pH 值至所要求的值,制得的原料液待用。观察记录反应液的状态随 pH 值的变化。

2. 反应条件的选择

水热反应的条件(如反应物浓度、反应温度、反应介质的酸度、反应时间等)对反应产物的物相、形态、粒子尺寸及其分布和产率均有重要影响。

(1) 反应温度。反应温度低时,$SnCl_4$ 水解、脱水缩合和晶化作用慢。温度升高将促进 $SnCl_4$ 的水解和 $Sn(OH)_4$ 的脱水缩合,同时重结晶作用增强,使产物的晶体结构更完整,但也导致 SnO_2 微晶长大。本实验的反应温度以 120~160 ℃为宜。

(2) 反应介质的酸度。当反应介质的酸度较高时,$SnCl_4$ 的水解受到抑制,中间产物 $Sn(OH)_4$ 生成相对较少,脱水缩合后,形成的 SnO_2 晶核数量较少,大量 Sn^{4+} 残留在反应液中。这有利于 SnO_2 微晶的生长,但同时也容易造成粒子间的聚结,导致

产生硬团聚,这是制备纳米粒子时应尽量避免的。

当反应介质的酸度较低时,$SnCl_4$水解完全,产生大量$Sn(OH)_4$的微小颗粒。在水热条件下,经脱水缩合和晶化,形成大量纳米SnO_2微晶。此时,由于溶液中残留的Sn^{4+}数量已很少,生成的SnO_2微晶较难继续生长。因此产物具有较小的平均颗粒尺寸,粒子间的硬团聚现象也相应减少。本实验反应介质的酸度控制为pH=1.45。

(3)反应物的浓度。单独考察反应物浓度的影响时,反应物浓度越高,产物SnO_2的产率越低。这主要是由于当$SnCl_4$的浓度增大时,溶液的酸度也增大,Sn^{4+}的水解受到抑制。

当介质的pH=1.45时,反应物的黏度较大,因此反应物浓度不宜过大,否则搅拌难以进行。一般以$c(SnCl_4)=1\ mol \cdot L^{-1}$为宜。

3.水热反应

将配制好的原料液倾入具有聚四氟乙烯衬里的不锈钢压力釜内,用管式电炉套加热压力釜。用温控装置控制压力釜的温度,使水热反应在所要求的温度下进行一定时间(约2 h)。为了保证反应的均匀性,水热反应应在搅拌下进行。反应结束,停止加热,待压力釜冷却至室温时,开启压力釜,取出反应产物。

4.反应产物的后处理

将反应产物静置沉降,移去上层清液后减压过滤。过滤时应用致密的细孔滤纸,尽量避免穿滤。用大约100 mL乙酸-乙酸铵混合液(1 g乙酸铵加入100 mL 10%的乙酸中)洗涤沉淀物4～5次(防止沉淀物胶溶穿滤),洗去沉淀物中的Cl^-和K^+,最后用质量分数为95%的乙醇溶液洗涤2次,于80 ℃干燥,研细备用。

5.反应产物的表征

(1)物相分析。用多晶X射线衍射法(XRD)确定产物的物相。在JCPDS卡片集中查出SnO_2的多晶标准衍射卡片,将样品的d值和相对强度与标准卡片上的数据相对照,确定产物是否为SnO_2。

(2)粒子大小分析。由多晶X射线衍射峰的半高宽,用Scherer公式计算样品在hkl衍射峰方向上的平均晶粒尺寸:

$$D_{hkl}=\frac{K \cdot \lambda}{\beta \cdot \cos\theta_{hkl}}$$

式中:β为扣除仪器因子后hkl衍射的半高宽(弧度);K为常数,通常取0.9;θ_{hkl}为hkl衍射峰的衍射角;λ为X射线的波长。

用透射电子显微镜(TEM)直接观察样品粒子的尺寸与形貌。

(3)比表面积测定。用BET法测定样品的比表面,并计算样品的平均等效粒径。

(4)等电点测定。用显微电泳仪测定SnO_2颗粒的等电点。

【结果记录和处理】

通过适当改变反应条件,根据所得结果,将反应物浓度、反应温度、反应介质的酸度、反应时间等对反应产物的物相、形态、粒子尺寸及其分布和产率的影响进行总结。

【思考题】

（1）比较同一样品由 XRD、TEM 和 BET 法测定的粒子大小，并对各自测量结果的物理含义进行分析。

（2）水热法作为一种非常规无机合成方法具有哪些特点？

（3）用水热法制备纳米氧化物时，对物质本身有哪些基本要求？试从化学热力学和动力学角度进行定性分析。

（4）水热法制备纳米氧化物过程中，哪些因素影响产物的粒子大小及其分布？

（5）在洗涤纳米粒子沉淀物过程中，如何防止沉淀物的胶溶？

（6）从表面化学角度考虑，如何减少纳米粒子在干燥过程中的团聚？

实验三十五　茶叶中微量元素的鉴定与定量测定

【目的要求】

（1）了解鉴定茶叶中某些化学元素的方法。

（2）学会样品预处理技术。

（3）掌握配位滴定法测定茶叶中钙、镁含量的方法。

（4）掌握分光光度法测定茶叶中微量铁的方法。

【实验原理】

茶叶属植物类有机体，主要由 C、H、N 和 O 等元素组成，其中含有 Fe、Al、Ca、Mg 等微量金属元素。本实验的目的是从茶叶中定性鉴定 Fe、Al、Ca、Mg 等元素，并对 Fe、Ca、Mg 进行定量测定。

茶叶须先进行"干灰化"。所谓"干灰化"，是将试样在空气中置于敞口的蒸发皿或坩埚中加热，使有机物经氧化分解而烧成灰烬。这一方法特别适用于生物样品的预处理。灰化后，经酸溶解，即可进行定量分析。

铁、铝混合液中 Fe^{3+} 对 Al^{3+} 的鉴定有干扰，可利用 Al^{3+} 的两性，加入过量的碱使 Al^{3+} 转变为 AlO_2^- 留在溶液中，Fe^{3+} 则生成 $Fe(OH)_3$ 沉淀，经分离去除后，就可消除相互干扰。钙、镁混合液中 Ca^{2+}、Mg^{2+} 互不干扰，可直接鉴定，不必分离。

定性鉴定 Fe^{3+}、Al^{3+}、Ca^{2+}、Mg^{2+} 的特征反应如下：

$$Fe^{3+} + nKSCN(饱和) \longrightarrow Fe(SCN)_n^{3-n}(血红色) + nK^+$$

$$Al^{3+} + 铝试剂 + OH^- \longrightarrow 红色絮状沉淀$$

$$Mg^{2+} + 镁试剂 + OH^- \longrightarrow 天蓝色沉淀$$

$$Ca^{2+} + C_2O_4^{2-} \xrightarrow{HAc\ 介质} CaC_2O_4(白色沉淀)$$

Ca、Mg 含量的测定,可采用配位滴定法。在 pH=10 的条件下,以 K-B 为指示剂,EDTA 为标准溶液,直接滴定可测得 Ca、Mg 的总量。若欲测 Ca、Mg 各自的质量分数,可在 pH>12.5 时,使 Mg^{2+} 生成氢氧化物沉淀,以钙指示剂为指示剂,用 EDTA 滴定 Ca^{2+} 得其质量分数,然后用差减法即得 Mg^{2+} 的质量分数。

Fe^{3+}、Al^{3+} 的存在会干扰 Ca^{2+}、Mg^{2+} 的测定,此时,可用三乙醇胺掩蔽 Fe^{3+} 与 Al^{3+}。

茶叶中铁含量较低,可用邻二氮菲分光光度法测定。在 pH=2～9 的条件下,Fe^{2+} 与邻二氮菲能生成稳定的橙红色配合物,该配合物的 lgK_s=21.3,摩尔吸光系数 ε_{508}=1.10×10^4。在显色前,需用盐酸羟胺把 Fe^{3+} 还原为 Fe^{2+},其反应方程式如下:

$$2Fe^{3+} + 2NH_2OH \cdot HCl \Longleftrightarrow 2Fe^{2+} + 2H_2O + 4H^+ + N_2\uparrow + 2Cl^-$$

显色时,若溶液的酸度过高(pH<2),则反应较慢;若酸度太低,则 Fe^{2+} 会水解,影响显色。

【仪器与试剂】

723N 型分光光度计、比色皿(3 cm×4)、电子天平(0.01 g,0.1 mg)、电炉、研钵、蒸发皿、称量瓶、滤纸、漏斗、试管、离心机、点滴板、烧杯(150 mL×1)、量筒(20 mL×1,10 mL×2,5 mL×1)、水浴锅、酸式滴定管(50 mL×1)、锥形瓶(250 mL×3)、容量瓶(250 mL×2,50 mL×8)、移液管(25 mL×1,5 mL×3)、吸量管(10 mL×1)、洗瓶、胶头滴管、洗耳球、玻棒、表面皿。

K-B 指示剂、HCl 溶液(6 mol·L^{-1})、HAc 溶液(2 mol·L^{-1})、NaOH 溶液(6 mol·L^{-1})、$(NH_4)_2C_2O_4$ 溶液(0.25 mol·L^{-1})、EDTA 溶液(0.01 mol·L^{-1},已标定)、KSCN 溶液(饱和)、铁标准溶液(0.10 g·L^{-1})、铝试剂、镁试剂、三乙醇胺水溶液(25%)、NH_3-NH_4Cl 缓冲溶液(pH=10)、HAc-NaAc 缓冲溶液(pH=4.6)、邻二氮菲溶液(0.1%)、盐酸羟胺溶液(10%)。

【实验步骤】

1.茶叶的灰化和试液的制备

取在 100～105 ℃下烘干的茶叶 7～8 g,于研钵中捣成细末,转移至称量瓶中,用电子天平称取一定量的茶叶末,并记录其准确质量。

将盛有茶叶末的蒸发皿加热使茶叶完全灰化(在通风橱中进行),冷却后,加 10 mL 6 mol·L^{-1}HCl 溶液于蒸发皿中,搅拌溶解(可能有少量不溶物)并将溶液完全转移至 150 mL 烧杯中,加 20 mL 水,再加 10 mL 6 mol·L^{-1}NaOH 溶液,使产生沉淀,并置于沸水浴中加热 30 min,过滤,然后洗涤烧杯和滤纸。滤液直接用 250 mL

容量瓶承接，并稀释至刻度，摇匀，贴上标签，标明为 Ca^{2+}、Mg^{2+} 试液（1♯），待测。

另取一个 250 mL 容量瓶，置于长颈漏斗之下，用 10 mL 6 mol·L^{-1} HCl 溶液重新溶解滤纸上的沉淀，并少量多次地洗涤滤纸。完毕后，稀释容量瓶中滤液至刻度，摇匀，贴上标签，标明为 Fe^{3+}、Al^{3+} 试液（2♯），待测。

2. Fe、Al、Ca、Mg 元素的鉴定

从 Ca^{2+}、Mg^{2+} 试液（1♯）的容量瓶中取出 1 mL 试液置于一洁净试管中，然后从试管中取 2 滴试液于点滴板上。加镁试剂 1 滴，再加 6 mol·L^{-1} NaOH 溶液碱化，观察实验现象。

再取 2~3 滴 Ca^{2+}、Mg^{2+} 试液于另一试管中，加入 1~2 滴 2 mol·L^{-1} HAc 溶液酸化，再加 2 滴 0.25 mol·L^{-1} $(NH_4)_2C_2O_4$ 溶液，观察实验现象。

从 Fe^{3+}、Al^{3+} 试液（2♯）的容量瓶中取出 1 mL 试液于另一洁净试管中，然后从试管中取 2 滴试液于点滴板上，加 1 滴饱和 KSCN 溶液，观察实验现象。

在上述试管剩余的 Fe^{3+}、Al^{3+} 试液中，加 6 mol·L^{-1} NaOH 溶液至白色沉淀溶解为止，离心分离，取上层清液于另一试管中，加 6 mol·L^{-1} HAc 溶液酸化，加 3~4 滴铝试剂，放置片刻后，加 6 mol·L^{-1} 氨水碱化，在水浴中加热，观察实验现象。

3. 茶叶中 Ca、Mg 总量的测定

从 1♯ 容量瓶中准确吸取 25.00 mL 试液置于 250 mL 锥形瓶中，加入 5 mL 三乙醇胺，再加 10 mL NH_3-NH_4Cl 缓冲溶液，摇匀。加入少量 K-B 指示剂，用 EDTA 标准溶液滴定至溶液由紫红色恰好变为纯蓝色，即达终点。根据 EDTA 标准溶液的消耗量，可计算出茶叶中 Ca、Mg 的总量，并以 MgO 的质量分数表示。

4. 茶叶中 Fe 含量的测定

（1）标准曲线的绘制。用吸量管分别吸取铁标准溶液 0.00 mL、1.00 mL、2.00 mL、3.00 mL、4.00 mL、5.00 mL、6.00 mL 于 7 个 50 mL 容量瓶中，依次分别加入 5.00 mL 10%盐酸羟胺、5.00 mL HAc-NaAc 缓冲溶液、5.00 mL 0.1%邻二氮菲溶液，用蒸馏水稀释至刻度，摇匀，放置 10 min。用 3 cm 的比色皿，以空白溶液为参比溶液，用 723N 型分光光度计在 508 nm 波长处分别测其吸光度。以 50 mL 溶液中 Fe 的含量为横坐标，相应的吸光度为纵坐标，绘制邻二氮菲合铁（Ⅱ）的标准曲线。

（2）茶叶中 Fe 含量的测定。用吸量管从 2♯ 容量瓶中吸取 2.50 mL 试液于 50 mL 容量瓶中，依次加入 5.00 mL 10%盐酸羟胺溶液、5.00 mL HAc-NaAc 缓冲溶液、5.00 mL 0.1%邻二氮菲溶液，用水稀释至刻度，摇匀，放置 10 min。以空白溶液为参比溶液，在 508 nm 波长处测其吸光度，并从标准曲线上求出 50 mL 溶液中 Fe 的含量，然后换算出茶叶中 Fe 的含量，以 Fe_2O_3 的质量分数表示。

【注意事项】

（1）茶叶尽量捣碎，以利于灰化。

(2) 茶叶灰化后,酸溶解速度较慢时可用小火略加热,定量转移要完全。

【思考题】

(1) 应如何选择灰化的温度?

(2) 欲测该茶叶中 Al 的含量,应如何设计实验方案?

(3) 为什么 pH=7 时,能将 Fe^{3+}、Al^{3+} 与 Ca^{2+}、Mg^{2+} 分离完全?

综合性实验(一) 葡萄糖酸锌的制备及锌含量的测定

【目的要求】

(1) 了解葡萄糖酸锌的制备方法。

(2) 学会测定锌盐的含量。

【实验原理】

葡萄糖酸锌是临床上治疗人体缺锌的药物,可以通过葡萄糖酸钙与等物质的量的硫酸锌反应制得,其反应方程式为

$$Ca(C_6H_{11}O_7)_2 + ZnSO_4 =\!=\!= Zn(C_6H_{11}O_7)_2 + CaSO_4 \downarrow$$

葡萄糖酸锌中锌盐含量的测定,常用配位滴定法:用 pH=10 的 NH_3-NH_4Cl 缓冲溶液来控制溶液的酸度,以铬黑 T 作指示剂,用 EDTA 标准溶液直接滴定至溶液由紫红色(Zn^{2+} 与铬黑 T 形成的螯合物的颜色)变为纯蓝色(Zn^{2+} 与 EDTA 形成螯合物,铬黑 T 游离出来的颜色),即为终点。Zn^{2+} 与 EDTA 的反应方程式如下:

$$Zn^{2+} + H_2Y^{2-} =\!=\!= ZnY^{2-} + 2H^+$$

【仪器与试剂】

电子天平(0.01 g,0.1 mg)、水浴锅、布氏漏斗、滤纸、吸滤瓶、水流抽气泵、酸式滴定管(50 mL×1)、电炉、蒸发皿、烧杯(250 mL×1)、量筒(20 mL×1)。

葡萄糖酸钙(AR,s)、$ZnSO_4 \cdot 7H_2O$(AR,s)、乙醇溶液(95%)、NH_3-NH_4Cl 缓冲溶液(pH=10)、EDTA(约 0.1 mol·L^{-1},已标定)、铬黑 T 指示剂。

【实验步骤】

1. 葡萄糖酸锌 $Zn(C_6H_{11}O_7)_2 \cdot 3H_2O$ 的制备

量取 80 mL 蒸馏水置于 250 mL 烧杯中,加热至 80~90 ℃时加入 13.4 g $ZnSO_4 \cdot 7H_2O$ 并使其完全溶解,将烧杯放在 90 ℃ 的恒温水浴中,再逐渐加入 20 g 葡萄糖酸钙,并不断搅拌,在 90 ℃水浴上静置保温 20 min。趁热抽滤(用两层滤纸),滤液移

至蒸发皿中,将滤液在沸水浴上浓缩至黏稠状(体积约为 20 mL,如浓缩液有沉淀即 $CaSO_4$,需过滤去除),滤液冷至室温,加入 20 mL 95%乙醇溶液(降低葡萄糖酸锌的溶解度),并不断搅拌,此时有大量的胶状葡萄糖酸锌析出。用倾析法去除乙醇,再加入 20 mL 95%乙醇溶液,充分搅拌,沉淀慢慢转变成晶体状,抽滤至干,即得粗品(母液回收)。

2.重结晶

粗品加水 20 mL,加热(90 ℃)至溶解,趁热抽滤,滤液冷至室温,加入 20 mL 95%乙醇溶液,充分搅拌,结晶析出后,抽滤至干,即得精品,在 50 ℃下烘干即可。

3.含量测定

准确称取 0.8 g 葡萄糖酸锌,溶于 20 mL 水中(可微热),加 10 mL NH_3-NH_4Cl 缓冲溶液,加 4 滴铬黑 T 指示剂,用 0.1 mol·L^{-1} EDTA 标准溶液滴定至溶液由紫红色变为蓝色,即达终点。重复上述操作 2 次,记下 EDTA 标准溶液用量,按下式计算样品中锌的含量:

$$锌的含量 = \frac{c(EDTA) \times V(EDTA) \times 65}{m(样品) \times 1\,000} \times 100\%$$

【思考题】

为什么葡萄糖酸钙和硫酸锌的反应需在 90 ℃的恒温水浴中进行?

综合性实验(二)　三草酸合铁(Ⅲ)酸钾的合成及组成测定

【目的要求】

(1)了解三草酸合铁(Ⅲ)酸钾的合成原理和方法。

(2)进一步熟练掌握溶解、结晶和减压过滤等基本操作。

(3)掌握测定配位阴离子组成的原理与方法。

【实验原理】

三草酸合铁(Ⅲ)酸钾是翠绿色晶体,易溶于水而难溶于乙醇。此配合物对光敏感,见光易分解变为黄色,其反应方程式为

$$2K_3[Fe(C_2O_4)_3] \xrightarrow{光} 3K_2C_2O_4 + 2FeC_2O_4 + 2CO_2$$

因其具有光敏性,所以常用来制作化学光量计。另外,它也是一些有机化学反应良好的催化剂。其合成工艺路线有多种,方法之一是首先由硫酸亚铁与草酸反应制备草酸亚铁:

$$FeSO_4 + H_2C_2O_4 + 2H_2O == FeC_2O_4 \cdot 2H_2O \downarrow + H_2SO_4$$

然后在过量草酸根的存在下,用 H_2O_2 氧化草酸亚铁即可得到三草酸合铁(Ⅲ)酸钾,同时有氢氧化铁沉淀生成。其反应方程式为

$$6FeC_2O_4 \cdot 2H_2O + 3H_2O_2 + 6K_2C_2O_4 == 4K_3[Fe(C_2O_4)_3] + 2Fe(OH)_3 \downarrow + 12H_2O$$

加入适量草酸也可使氢氧化铁转化为三草酸合铁(Ⅲ)酸钾,即

$$2Fe(OH)_3 + 3H_2C_2O_4 + 3K_2C_2O_4 == 2K_3[Fe(C_2O_4)_3] + 6H_2O$$

三草酸合铁(Ⅲ)配位阴离子的组成可通过滴定分析方法进行测定,其中草酸根的含量可在酸性介质中直接用 $KMnO_4$ 标准溶液测定,其反应方程式为

$$5C_2O_4^{2-} + 2MnO_4^- + 16H^+ == 10CO_2 \uparrow + 2Mn^{2+} + 8H_2O$$

而 Fe^{3+} 的含量可通过用 Zn 将它还原为 Fe^{2+},再用 $KMnO_4$ 标准溶液测定,其反应方程式为

$$5Fe^{2+} + MnO_4^- + 8H^+ == 5Fe^{3+} + Mn^{2+} + 4H_2O$$

【仪器与试剂】

电子天平(0.01 g,0.1 mg)、烧杯(100 mL×1)、布氏漏斗、滤纸、吸滤瓶、水流抽气泵、蒸发皿、电磁搅拌器、酸式滴定管(50 mL×1)、容量瓶(250 mL×1)、移液管(20 mL×1)、锥形瓶(250 mL×3)、洗瓶、胶头滴管、洗耳球、玻棒。

$FeSO_4 \cdot 7H_2O(AR,s)$、H_2SO_4 溶液($3\ mol \cdot L^{-1}$)、$H_2C_2O_4$ 溶液($1\ mol \cdot L^{-1}$)、$K_2C_2O_4$ 溶液(饱和)、H_2O_2 溶液(3%)、乙醇溶液(95%)、pH 试纸、$Na_2C_2O_4$(AR,s)、$KMnO_4$(AR,s)、HCl 溶液($6\ mol \cdot L^{-1}$)、$MnSO_4$ 溶液(称取 45 g $MnSO_4$ 溶于 500 mL 水中,缓慢加入 130 mL 浓 H_2SO_4 溶液,再加入 300 mL 85% H_3PO_4 溶液,稀释到 1 L)、Zn 粉。

【实验步骤】

1. 三草酸合铁(Ⅲ)酸钾的合成

(1) $FeC_2O_4 \cdot 2H_2O$ 的制备。称取 2 g $FeSO_4 \cdot 7H_2O$ 晶体于烧杯中,加入 10 mL 蒸馏水和 4 滴 $3\ mol \cdot L^{-1}\ H_2SO_4$ 溶液,微热使其溶解,然后加入 10 mL $1\ mol \cdot L^{-1}\ H_2C_2O_4$ 溶液,边搅拌边加热直至沸腾,静置,待黄色 $FeC_2O_4 \cdot 2H_2O$ 晶体沉淀后,倾析弃去上层清液,晶体用少量蒸馏水洗涤 2~3 次。

(2) $K_3[Fe(C_2O_4)_3] \cdot 3H_2O$ 的制备。在盛有黄色 $FeC_2O_4 \cdot 2H_2O$ 晶体的烧杯中,加入 5 mL 饱和 $K_2C_2O_4$ 溶液,加热至 40 ℃左右,取下,稍冷后缓慢滴加 10 mL 3% H_2O_2 溶液,边加边搅拌,观察溶液中的现象。滴加完 H_2O_2 后将溶液加热至沸腾以除去过量的 H_2O_2,并分两次加入 4 mL $1\ mol \cdot L^{-1}\ H_2C_2O_4$ 溶液,使沉淀溶解,此时溶液呈翠绿色。加热浓缩,冷却,即有翠绿色晶体 $K_3[Fe(C_2O_4)_3] \cdot 3H_2O$ 析出。如无晶体析出,说明 $K_3[Fe(C_2O_4)_3]$ 溶液未达到饱和,可继续加热浓缩或加入少量

95%乙醇溶液，即可析出晶体，抽滤，称量，计算产率。

2.三草酸合铁(Ⅲ)配位阴离子组成的测定

(1) 0.01 mol·L^{-1} KMnO$_4$标准溶液的配制与标定(见实验十)。

(2) K$_3$[Fe(C$_2$O$_4$)$_3$]溶液的配制。称取1.0～1.2 g(称准至0.1 mg)K$_3$[Fe(C$_2$O$_4$)$_3$]·3H$_2$O晶体于烧杯中，加水溶解，定量转移至250 mL容量瓶中，定容。

(3) C$_2$O$_4^{2-}$的测定。准确吸取20.00 mL K$_3$[Fe(C$_2$O$_4$)$_3$]溶液置于250 mL锥形瓶中，加入5 mL MnSO$_4$溶液及5 mL 3 mol·L^{-1} H$_2$SO$_4$溶液，加热至75～80 ℃，立即用KMnO$_4$标准溶液滴定至溶液呈浅红色，并保持30 s内不褪色，即达终点。由消耗的KMnO$_4$溶液的体积V_1计算C$_2$O$_4^{2-}$的含量。

(4) Fe^{3+}的测定。将上述已达到滴定终点的溶液置于电炉上加热，然后向其热溶液中加入约100 mg Zn粉，继续加热至黄色消失，趁热过滤。滤液转移至另一锥形瓶中，并用热蒸馏水洗涤沉淀，将洗涤液合并至滤液中，迅速用KMnO$_4$标准溶液滴定至滤液呈浅红色且30 s内不褪色，即为终点。由消耗的KMnO$_4$溶液的体积V_2计算Fe^{3+}的含量。

【思考题】

(1) 影响三草酸合铁(Ⅲ)酸钾产率的主要因素有哪些？

(2) 三草酸合铁(Ⅲ)酸钾见光易分解，应如何保存？

(3) 用KMnO$_4$标准溶液滴定Fe^{2+}时，加入MnSO$_4$溶液的目的是什么？

综合性实验(三)　蛋壳中钙、镁含量的测定

一、配位滴定法

【实验原理】

鸡蛋壳的主要成分为CaCO$_3$，其次为MgCO$_3$、蛋白质、色素以及少量的Fe、Al。Ca、Mg含量的测定方法参见实验十二。

【仪器与试剂】

电子天平(0.01 g,0.1 mg)、烧杯(100 mL×1)、布氏漏斗、酸式滴定管(50 mL×1)、容量瓶(250 mL×1)、移液管(25 mL×1)、锥形瓶(250 mL×3)、洗瓶、胶头滴管、洗耳球。

HCl溶液(6 mol·L^{-1})、铬黑T指示剂、三乙醇胺水溶液(1∶2)、NH$_3$-NH$_4$Cl缓冲溶液(pH=10)、EDTA溶液(0.01 mol·L^{-1},已标定)。

【实验步骤】

准确称取一定量的蛋壳粉末,小心滴加 4～5 mL 6 mol·L⁻¹ HCl 溶液,微火加热至完全溶解(少量蛋白膜不溶),冷却,转移至 250 mL 容量瓶中,稀释至接近刻度线,若有泡沫,滴加 2～3 滴 95%乙醇溶液,泡沫消除后,滴加水至刻度线,摇匀。

准确吸取 25.00 mL 试液于 250 mL 锥形瓶中,分别加 20 mL 去离子水、5 mL 三乙醇胺水溶液,摇匀。再加 10 mL NH₃-NH₄Cl 缓冲溶液,摇匀。放入少许铬黑T指示剂,用 EDTA 标准溶液滴定至溶液由酒红色恰好变为纯蓝色,即达终点。根据消耗的 EDTA 溶液的体积计算 Ca^{2+}、Mg^{2+} 的总量,以 CaO 的质量分数表示。

【思考题】

(1) 如何确定蛋壳粉末的称量范围?(提示:先粗略确定蛋壳粉末中 Ca、Mg 的含量,再估计蛋壳粉末的称量范围)

(2) 蛋壳粉末溶解稀释时为何加 95%乙醇溶液可以消除泡沫?

二、酸碱滴定法

【实验原理】

蛋壳中的 $CaCO_3$ 能与 HCl 发生以下反应:

$$CaCO_3 + 2H^+ = Ca^{2+} + CO_2\uparrow + H_2O$$

过量的酸可用 NaOH 标准溶液回滴,根据实际与 $CaCO_3$ 反应消耗的 HCl 标准溶液的体积可求得蛋壳中碳酸盐的含量,以 CaO 的质量分数表示。

【仪器与试剂】

电子天平(0.1 mg,0.01 g)、酸式滴定管(50 mL×1)、碱式滴定管(50 mL×1)、锥形瓶(250 mL×3)、量筒(50 mL×1)、滴定管架、洗瓶、洗耳球、试剂瓶(500 mL×2)、烧杯(500 mL×1)。

浓 HCl(AR)、NaOH(AR,s)、酚酞指示剂。

【实验步骤】

准确称取三份经预处理的蛋壳 0.3 g 左右(精确到 0.1 mg),分别置于 3 个 250 mL 锥形瓶内,用酸式滴定管逐滴加入已标定好的 HCl 标准溶液 40 mL 左右(需精确读数),小火加热溶解,冷却,加 1～2 滴酚酞指示剂,以 NaOH 标准溶液回滴至溶液呈粉红色。

【结果记录和处理】

按滴定分析记录格式制作表格,记录数据,按下式计算 $w(CaO)$:

$$w(CaO)=\frac{[c(HCl)\times V(HCl)-c(NaOH)\times V(NaOH)]\times M(CaO)}{m(样品)\times 2\,000}\times 100\%$$

【思考题】

(1) 蛋壳溶解时应注意什么?

(2) 为什么说 $w(CaO)$ 是表示 Ca 与 Mg 的总量?

三、氧化还原滴定法

【实验原理】

利用蛋壳中的 Ca^{2+} 与草酸盐形成难溶的草酸钙沉淀,将沉淀经过滤、洗涤后溶解,用 $KMnO_4$ 法测定 $C_2O_4^{2-}$ 的含量,换算成 CaO 的含量,反应如下:

$$Ca^{2+}+C_2O_4^{2-}\!=\!=\!=\!CaC_2O_4\downarrow$$
$$CaC_2O_4+H_2SO_4\!=\!=\!=\!CaSO_4+H_2C_2O_4$$
$$5H_2C_2O_4+2MnO_4^-+6H^+\!=\!=\!=\!10CO_2+2Mn^{2+}+8H_2O$$

某些金属离子(Ba^{2+}、Sr^{2+}、Mg^{2+}、Pb^{2+}、Cd^{2+} 等)与 $C_2O_4^{2-}$ 能形成沉淀,对测定 Ca^{2+} 有干扰。

【仪器与试剂】

电子天平(0.1 mg)、干燥器、称量瓶、酸式滴定管(50 mL×1)、锥形瓶(250 mL×3)、烧杯(250 mL×2)、量筒(100 mL×1,10 mL×1)、试剂瓶(500 mL×1)、砂芯漏斗、吸滤瓶、滤纸、水流抽气泵、洗瓶、胶头滴管、洗耳球、玻棒。

$KMnO_4$ 溶液($0.01\;mol\cdot L^{-1}$)、$(NH_4)_2C_2O_4$ 溶液(5%)、氨水(10%)、HCl 溶液(浓,1:1)、H_2SO_4 溶液($1\;mol\cdot L^{-1}$)、甲基橙(0.2%)、$AgNO_3$ 溶液($0.1\;mol\cdot L^{-1}$)。

【实验步骤】

准确称取蛋壳粉末两份(每份含钙约 0.025 g),分别放在 250 mL 烧杯中,加 3 mL 1:1 HCl 溶液、20 mL 水,加热溶解,若有不溶解的蛋白质,可过滤去除。滤液置于烧杯中,然后加入 50 mL 5% $(NH_4)_2C_2O_4$ 溶液,若出现沉淀,滴加浓 HCl 溶液使之溶解,然后加热至 70~80 ℃。加入 2~3 滴甲基橙,溶液呈红色,逐滴加入 10% 氨水,不断搅拌,至溶液变黄并有氨味逸出为止。将溶液放置陈化(或在水浴中加热 30 min 陈化),沉淀经过滤、洗涤,直至无 Cl^-。将带有沉淀的滤纸铺在先前用来进行沉淀的烧杯内壁上,用 50 mL 1 mol·L^{-1} H$_2$SO$_4$ 溶液把沉淀由滤纸洗入烧杯中,再用洗瓶吹洗 1~2 次,加水稀释至溶液体积约为 100 mL,加热至 70~80 ℃,然后用 KMnO$_4$ 标准溶液滴定至溶液呈浅红色时把滤纸投入溶液中,继续滴加 KMnO$_4$ 标准溶液至浅红色,且在 30 s 内不消失为止。计算蛋壳中 CaO 的质量分数。

【思考题】

(1) 用 (NH$_4$)$_2$C$_2$O$_4$ 沉淀 Ca^{2+} 时,为什么要先在酸性溶液中加入沉淀剂,然后在 70~80 ℃时滴加氨水至溶液变黄,才能生成 CaC$_2$O$_4$ 沉淀?

(2) 为什么沉淀要洗至无 Cl$^-$ 为止?

(3) 如果将带有 CaC$_2$O$_4$ 沉淀的滤纸一起投入烧杯中,以 H$_2$SO$_4$ 溶液处理后再用 KMnO$_4$ 标准溶液滴定,这样操作对结果有什么影响?

(4) 试比较三种方法测定蛋壳中 Ca、Mg 含量的优缺点?

设计性实验(一)　钴(Ⅲ)配合物的制备及其组成的确定

本阶段实验是在进行了基本实验技能训练、综合性实验技能训练的基础上,由学生按实验要求,以"临床问题""生活中的化学问题""科研问题"为主体内容,通过查阅有关资料和灵活运用已学的知识,拟订实验方案,确定实验条件,然后独立完成实验内容,评价实验结果,书写实验小论文。通过该层次的训练使学生综合运用知识、解决实际问题的能力得到进一步的提高,并培养学生初步具备从事科学研究的能力和创新能力。

设计性实验方案的拟订包括实验原理、实验步骤、仪器、试剂、数据记录、计算方法等。方案应切实可行,建议学生自行设计的方案经师生讨论后进行探索。

【目的要求】

(1) 合成钴(Ⅲ)配合物,如二氯化一氯·五氨合钴(Ⅲ)或三氯化六氨合钴(Ⅲ)。

(2) 分析和测定配合物的组成。

【实验提要】

二价钴盐较三价钴盐稳定,而大多数三价钴配合物比二价钴配合物稳定。以二价钴盐为原料通过空气或 H$_2$O$_2$ 将 Co(Ⅱ) 氧化为 Co(Ⅲ) 可得到三价钴配合物。

以氨为配位剂,在不同条件下,可合成多种钴的氨配合物,如三氯化六氨合钴(Ⅲ)[Co(NH$_3$)$_6$]Cl$_3$(橙黄色晶体)、二氯化一氯·五氨合钴(Ⅲ)[Co(NH$_3$)$_5$Cl]Cl$_2$(紫红色晶体)和三氯化五氨·一水合钴(Ⅲ)[Co(NH$_3$)$_5$(H$_2$O)]Cl$_3$(砖红色晶体)。

【思考题】

（1）在合成[$Co(NH_3)_6$]Cl_3的过程中，NH_4Cl、活性炭、H_2O_2各起到什么作用？为什么要冷却后加入浓氨水？

（2）[$Co(NH_3)_6$]$^{3+}$与[$Co(NH_3)_6$]$^{2+}$比较，哪个更稳定？为什么？

（3）测定配离子电荷的常用方法有哪些？

（4）要使本产品（如[$Co(NH_3)_6$]Cl_3）合成产率高，哪些步骤是比较关键的？

设计性实验（二）　水样中铁含量的测定

【目的要求】

预习内容

（1）学习用 Lambert-Beer 定律测定水样中铁含量的原理和方法。

（2）熟悉 723N 型分光光度计的使用。

【实验提要】

分光光度法进行定量分析时，要经过取样、溶解、显色及测量等步骤。显色反应受多种因素的影响，为了使反应进行完全，应当确定显色剂加入量的合适范围，溶液的酸度既影响显色剂各种形式的浓度，又影响金属离子的存在状态，从而影响显色反应生成物的组成。不同的显色反应，生成稳定的有色化合物所需的时间不同，稳定后能维持的时间也不大相同。许多显色反应在室温下能很快完成，有的则需要加热才能较快进行。此外，加入试剂的顺序、离子的氧化态、干扰物质的影响等均需要加以研究，以便拟订合适的分析方案，使测定既准确又迅速。

本实验在自主学习分光光度法的基础上，针对生活中的化学问题"水样中铁含量测定"，通过 Fe(Ⅱ)-邻二氮菲显色反应的条件实验，学习如何拟订一个分光光度分析实验的测定条件，掌握通过绘制吸收曲线确定最大吸收波长和利用标准曲线进行定量分析的方法。

分光光度法是基于物质对光的选择性吸收而建立的方法，当某单色光通过溶液时，其能量就会被吸收而减弱，光能量减弱的程度和物质的浓度有一定的比例关系，符合 Lambert-Beer 定律：

$$A = \varepsilon bc \quad \text{或} \quad A = abc$$

式中：c 是溶液的浓度；ε 是摩尔吸光系数，它是吸光物质在一定波长下的特征常数；b 为液层厚度。在分光光度法中，当条件一定时，ε、b 均为常数，此时，吸光度 A 与有色物质的浓度 c 成正比。因此，以吸光度对标准溶液浓度作图，即可绘制标准曲线。通过标准曲线可获得对应的被测溶液的浓度。

邻二氮菲作显色剂测定微量铁(Ⅱ)的灵敏度高,选择性好。在 pH=2~9 的溶液中,Fe^{2+} 与邻二氮菲生成极稳定的橘红色配合物,反应方程式如下:

$$Fe^{2+}+3 \quad \text{邻二氮菲} \quad \rightleftharpoons \quad Fe^{2+}$$

邻二氮菲

该配合物的 $lgK_s=21.3(20\ ℃)$,在 508 nm 波长下有最大吸收,其摩尔吸光系数 $\varepsilon_{508}=11\ 000$。

邻二氮菲也能与 Fe(Ⅲ)生成 3∶1 的淡蓝色配合物,其 $lgK_s=14.10$。因此在显色前应先用盐酸羟胺($NH_2OH \cdot HCl$)将 Fe^{3+} 还原为 Fe^{2+},反应方程式为

$$2Fe^{3+}+2NH_2OH \cdot HCl \Longrightarrow 2Fe^{2+}+N_2\uparrow+2H_2O+4H^++2Cl^-$$

测定时,控制溶液酸度在 pH=2~9 较为适宜。酸度较高(pH<2)时,金属离子与 H_3O^+ 竞争反应,不利于配合物的生成,反应进行较慢;酸度太低,则 Fe^{2+} 水解,金属离子会形成不溶物,影响显色。

Cu^{2+}、Co^{2+}、Ni^{2+}、Hg^{2+}、Mn^{2+}、Zn^{2+} 等离子也能与邻二氮菲生成稳定配合物,在量少的情况下,不影响 Fe^{2+} 的测定,量大时可用 EDTA 掩蔽或预先分离。

该方法也可用于测定血清中铁的含量。

【思考题】

(1) 在合适波长下,为什么标准溶液的浓度还要控制在 $0.016~0.080\ mmol \cdot L^{-1}$ 之间,高于 $0.080\ mmol \cdot L^{-1}$ 或低于 $0.016\ mmol \cdot L^{-1}$ 就不理想?简要说明原因。

(2) 如果溶液为红色,表明该溶液对红色的光是吸收还是透过?

设计性实验(三) 果蔬中维生素 C 含量的测定

【目的要求】

(1) 学习果蔬中维生素 C 含量的测定方法。

(2) 查阅资料,选择测定维生素 C 含量的实验方法。

(3) 复习和巩固滴定分析法和分光光度法。

预习内容

【实验提要】

维生素 C(V_C)又称抗坏血酸,分子式为 $C_6H_8O_6$,相对分子质量为 176.12,属于

水溶性维生素。维生素 C 在医药和化学上有着非常广泛的应用。

V_C 是常用的还原剂($\varphi^{\ominus}(C_6H_6O_6/C_6H_8O_6)=0.18$ V),V_C 分子中的烯二醇基可被 I_2 氧化成二酮基,故可用 I_2 标准溶液测定。

V_C 在碱性介质中易被氧化,内环打开形成二酮古洛糖酸,二酮古洛糖酸可与2,4-二硝基苯肼反应生成红色的脎,在 500 nm 波长下,脎具有最大吸收,故也可用分光光度法测定。

【思考题】

(1) 根据维生素 C 的性质,你能设计几种分析测试方法?

(2) 维生素 C 本身是弱酸,为什么在用碘量法测定其含量时,还要加酸?

设计性实验(四)　植物中某些元素的鉴定

【目的要求】

(1) 学习样品预处理的方法。

(2) 学会茶叶或松枝的干叶中 Ca、Mg、Fe、Al、P 的分离、鉴定,紫菜或海带中碘的鉴定。

(3) 复习和巩固所学元素及化合物的性质。

【实验提要】

植物是有机体,主要由 C、H、N、O 等元素组成,此外还含有 P、I 和某些金属元素。把植物烧成灰烬并经过一系列化学处理,即可从中分离和鉴定某些元素。

本实验要求从茶叶或松枝的干叶中检出 Ca、Mg、Fe、Al 和 P 五种元素,从紫菜或海带中检出 I 元素。元素鉴定基于如下反应:

$$Ca^{2+}+C_2O_4^{2-}\longrightarrow CaC_2O_4(白色沉淀)$$

$$Fe^{3+}+K_4[Fe(CN)_6]\longrightarrow KFe[Fe(CN)_6](蓝色)+3K^+$$

$$或\ Fe^{3+}+nSCN^-\longrightarrow Fe(SCN)_n^{3-n}(血红色)(n=1,2,3,4,5,6)$$

$$HPO_4^{2-}+3NH_4^++12MoO_4^{2-}+23H^+\longrightarrow (NH_4)_3[P(Mo_3O_{10})_4]\cdot 6H_2O(黄色)+6H_2O$$

$$2I^-+Cl_2(Br_2)\longrightarrow I_2+2Cl^-(Br^-)(CCl_4层呈玫瑰红色)$$

$$Al^{3+}+铝试剂+OH^-\longrightarrow 红色絮状沉淀$$

$$Mg^{2+}+镁试剂+OH^-\longrightarrow 天蓝色沉淀$$

【思考题】

(1) 应如何选择灰化的温度?

(2) 如何分离和鉴定茶叶中的 P、海带或紫菜中的 I?

趣味性实验

【目的要求】

进一步拓宽知识面,活跃思维,激发实验兴趣,丰富学生的课余生活。

【仪器与试剂】

烧杯(50 mL×1,100 mL×1,250 mL×1)、量筒(100 mL×1)、培养皿(3)、集气瓶(50 mL×1)、胶头滴管、双孔胶塞、瓷勺、毛笔、玻璃水槽、试管(20 mL×1)、水浴锅、滤纸、白纸、沙子、石头。

$SnCl_2$ 溶液(0.5 mol·L^{-1})、$CuCl_2$ 溶液(0.5 mol·L^{-1})、$AgNO_3$ 溶液(0.5 mol·L^{-1})、NaCl 溶液(9 g·L^{-1})、浓 H_2SO_4 溶液、绿矾、乙醇、双氧水、松节油、铜片、锌片、硅酸钠(AR,s)、$CuSO_4$(AR,s)、$NiCl_2$(AR,s)、$FeCl_3$(AR,s)、$CoCl_2$(AR,s)、$MnCl_2$(AR,s)、$FeSO_4$(AR,s)、Na_2SO_4(AR,s)、KI(AR,s)、$Pb(CH_3COO)_2·3H_2O$(AR,s)、白磷、MnO_2(AR,s)、$KClO_3$(AR,s)、$KMnO_4$(AR,s)、肥皂、淀粉、萘、$Na_2SO_4·10H_2O$(AR,s)、贝壳、树枝、茶叶。

【实验步骤】

1.滤纸上金属树的制备

(1)锡树的形成。在培养皿中,均匀地贴一张被 0.5 mol·L^{-1} $SnCl_2$ 溶液润湿过的圆形滤纸(不能有气泡),滤纸中央放入一小块锌片,盖上盖子,放置 30 min,即可观察到闪光的小锡树。

(2)银树的形成。根据上述方法,以 0.5 mol·L^{-1} $AgNO_3$ 溶液润湿滤纸,并在滤纸中央放置一块铜片,即可观察到美丽发光的银树。

(3)铜树的形成。根据上述方法,用 0.5 mol·L^{-1} $CuCl_2$ 溶液代替 $SnCl_2$ 溶液,即可观察到铜树。

2.美丽的水中花园

在干净的玻璃水槽中加入 2/3 的水,并加入质量为水的 1/5 的硅酸钠粉末,用玻棒慢慢搅拌,形成无色透明的硅酸钠溶液。在水槽底部铺上一层洁净的沙子,在沙子上面放上一些色彩斑斓的石子、贝壳或玻璃弹子。然后在水槽底部不同位置分别投入 4~5 粒 $CuSO_4$、$NiCl_2$、$CoCl_2$、$MnCl_2$、$FeSO_4$ 等晶体。静置 10 min,即可观察到水槽底部开始逐渐长出不同颜色、不同形状的"枝条"来。它们的形状很像花草树木,加上周围的石子、贝壳的衬托,一个美丽的水底花园就形成了。

3.水中实验

(1) 水中火花。向 50 mL 烧杯中加入适量的盐水,并将绿豆大小的一块白磷放入烧杯中,在白磷上铺上 $KClO_3$ 晶体。然后用胶头滴管吸取浓 H_2SO_4 溶液,缓慢滴加到 $KClO_3$ 上,即可观察到水中产生了火花。

(2) 水中战场。用量筒量取浓 H_2SO_4 溶液、乙醇各 2 mL 于 250 mL 烧杯中,向烧杯中投入颗粒状的 $KMnO_4$ 固体,即可看到水中冒出火花。

(3) 水中制"黄金"。在 100 mL 烧杯中注入 50 mL 水,再加入适量 KI 和 $Pb(CH_3COO)_2 \cdot 3H_2O$ 固体,加热溶解。即将煮沸时,使其骤冷(倒入另一只空烧杯中并置于冷水浴中冷却),观察到有黄色固体析出。

4.人造雪景

在烧杯底部铺一层萘(或击碎的卫生球),取一根合适的树枝倒挂在烧杯内。将烧杯慢慢加热,稍待片刻,可观察到树枝上挂满了"霜"。

5.发射小火箭

取一个容积为 50 mL 的集气瓶并配上双孔胶塞(双孔内分别插入滴管和细玻璃管),在集气瓶中加入 MnO_2 粉末,滴管中吸入双氧水,盖上双孔胶塞。当挤压胶头滴管时,小火箭(细玻璃管)便发射出去。

6.松节油印刷

取一洁净的小烧杯,放入 4 勺水和 1 勺松节油,再加入 1 粒黄豆大小的肥皂。用玻棒轻轻搅拌混合物,至小肥皂溶解为止。把烧杯中的混合物用干净的毛笔均匀地涂到报纸的文字及插图上,接着把一张白纸盖在报纸上,用勺柄在白纸上来回摩擦,揭开白纸后,发现报纸上的文字或插图等清晰地印到白纸上。

7.茶变墨水

在一小烧杯内壁上涂一层绿矾溶液,然后把刚刚泡好的一壶茶倒入烧杯中,即可看到茶汁变成了黑色的墨水样。

【思考题】

(1) 讨论各实验的原理,写出有关化学反应方程式。

(2) 根据氧化还原概念,能否再制备几种金属树?

(3) 在松节油印刷实验中肥皂的作用是什么?

实验操作二维码

滴定管
的准备

滴定过程

容量瓶
的使用

吸量管
的使用

pH 试纸
的使用

普通电子天平
的使用

分析天平
的使用

离心机
的使用

数字式电子
电位差计

723N 型分光
光度计的使用

减压过滤

酸度计
的使用

高效液相
色谱仪介绍

原子吸收分光
光度计介绍

参加实验视频制作的学生(按姓氏拼音排序):

蔡　钦	陈世宇	高成歌	关云龙	何宗南	李龙愔	李骁晔	刘浩东
龙　进	陆官军	吕　娜	马　浪	潘伟珍	钱应仙	孙文悦	万宇航
熊超虎	杨博通	俞晨昊	张子昂	郑红菲

下　篇

英文部分

Part One　Introduction of Basic Chemistry Experiments

Chapter 1　Basic Rules and Safety Requirements

I Laboratory Objectives

Chemistry is exciting! Each day in the laboratory you are given the opportunity to confront the unknown, and to understand it. Each experiment holds many secrets. Look hard and you may see them. Work hard and you can solve them. The word "science" comes from the Latin word "scire", which means "to know". The goal of all science is knowledge. Scientists are men and women who devote their lives to the pursuit of knowledge.

In this class, you are given the opportunity to do what scientists do. The goals of laboratory work in a basic chemistry course are somewhat different from the goals of laboratory work in research. Primarily, we design laboratory "experiments" (which have predictable results) to emphasize and to reinforce important textbook concepts. Almost as important, we select laboratory "questions" to teach essential experimental skills which will be useful in your future scientific work. In addition, we also provide extended experimental investigations and problems to encourage you to apply your knowledge of chemistry in a creative and independent way.

This laboratory manual is designed to present you with experiments that are challenging, coordinated investigations related to your study of chemical principles. These experiments utilize modern techniques and apparatus and emphasize operations performed by practicing scientists. Master the scientists' skills of observation and experiment. These skills are tools to solve the secrets of the unknown. Wherever possible, they are quantitative and related to contemporary problems in pure and applied chemistry. These experiments have also been designed to be efficient, safe, economical, and nonpolluting.

II General Laboratory Rules

Please read and follow these rules before beginning to laboratory work.

(1) During the first week of classes, locker and stockroom arrangements will be explained. Since the administration of a laboratory involves coordination of the activities of many students, be sure to note and to follow requirements that may require careful attention (locker assignments, payment of fees, lock combinations, laboratory hours, etc.).

(2) You should wear a laboratory coat. Tie back long hair.

(3) Whenever you are in the chemistry laboratory, follow the directions of your instructor and the laboratory manual. Students are not permitted in laboratories unless an instructor is present.

(4) Your instructor will point out the location and proper use of the safety shower, eyewash, and fire extinguisher. Remember their locations and the locations of emergency exits from the building. Read the chapter on LABORATORY SAFETY now, and again during the middle of the semester.

(5) Read all the directions for each experiment before starting work. Note all warnings about possible dangers that may be involved.

(6) Proceed with your work thoughtfully and cautiously. It is wiser to prevent an emergency than to deal with it after it arises. Do not attempt to do experiments not specifically authorized by your instructor.

(7) Laboratory housekeeping is the responsibility of everyone in the laboratory. Carry out the following responsibilities.

① Never return chemicals to bottles of their origins. If you have taken an excess of a chemical, give it to another student, or if necessary, throw the excess away. It's better to waste a small amount of the chemical than to risk contaminating the entire contents of the bottle.

② Clean up any spills (especially in or near a balance) at once. Report any unusual spills or breakages to your laboratory instructor.

③ Dispense malodorous reagents (such as concentrated HCl and NH_3 solutions) in a fume hood if practicable. Set up and conduct all experiments that may release any toxic or flammable gas directly in a hood, so that all gaseous products enter the hood intake.

④ Never insert an unclean spatula or pipet into a reagent bottle. Don't stick objects such as pencils or eyedroppers into reagent bottles and don't lay reagent bottle stoppers down in any way that the part which goes into the bottle which comes into contact with any surface. If you need a few drops of liquid, pour a little into a beaker and then take what you need from the beaker. If a solid has packed hard in a bottle, slap the side of the bottle to loosen it. If this doesn't loosen some solid, ask the instructor to help you. Most reagent bottles for solids have hollow caps. If you need a small amount of the solid, with the cap still in the bottle, shake a little into the cap and take what you need from the cap. These techniques prevent introduction of contamination.

⑤ All chemicals in the laboratory must be clearly labeled. This applies not only to the bottles on the shelves but also to the chemicals on or in your desk.

⑥ Many reagents can be recycled, and many solid reagents cannot be safely disposed of in trash receptacles. When recycling or waste containers are provided, use them. Do not pour insoluble solids in sinks. Solutions that may be discarded in sinks should be flushed thoroughly with water.

⑦ Dispose of wastes only in the manner prescribed by your instructor. Ask him or her if you do not know. Serious cuts, fires, and explosions have resulted from improper waste disposal.

⑧ Switching reagent bottle stoppers will invariably contaminate the reagent. To avoid this, never have more than one bottle unstoppered at a time. If the stopper is the pennyhead type, hold it between the fingers of the hand you are pouring with, while pouring. If you do this, you can be certain that you are not mixing up stoppers or contaminating the reagent.

(8) Organize your laboratory time so that you have cleaned up your apparatus and be out of the laboratory at the end of the laboratory period.

(9) Report all accidents, no matter how minor, to the instructor.

(10) Do not take food into the laboratory. Don't taste or eat anything in the laboratory.

III Laboratory Notebook

A few general comments are in order about the laboratory notebook that is the primary record of your experimental work. First, although many campus bookstores sell notebooks that are specifically designed as lab notebooks, it is often sufficient to use any notebooks with tightly bound pages. Spiral and three-ring binders are inappropriate for lab notebooks because pages can be easily removed or torn out. All entries about your work must be made directly in your laboratory notebook in ink. Recording data on scraps of paper is an unacceptable practice because the paper may be lost; the practice is strictly forbidden in your laboratory.

The notebook should begin with a table of contents, set aside the first two or three pages for this purpose. The rest of the pages should be numbered sequentially, and no page should ever be torn out of a laboratory notebook. Your notebook must be written with accuracy and completeness. It must be organized and legible, but it does not need to be a work of art.

Some flexibility in format and style may be allowed, but proper records of your experimental results must answer certain questions.

(1) When did you do the work?

(2) What are you trying to accomplish in the experiment?

(3) How did you do the experiment?

(4) What did you observe?

(5) How do you explain your observations?

A lab record needs to be written in three steps: prelab, during lab, and postlab. It should contain the following sections for each experiment you do.

1. To Be Done Before You Come to the Laboratory

The basic notebook setup discussed here is designed to help you prepare for an experiment in an effective and safe fashion. It includes the date and title of the experiment or project, the balanced chemical reaction you are studying, a statement of purpose, a table of reagents and solvents, the way you will calculate the percent yield, an outline of the procedure to be used, and the answers to any prelab questions. Your instructor will undoubtedly provide specific guidelines for lab notebook procedures at your institution.

(1) Title: Use a title that clearly identifies what you are doing in this experiment or project.

(2) Date(s): Use the date on which an experiment is actually carried out. In some research labs, where patent issues are important, a witnessed signature of the date is required.

(3) Balanced chemical reaction: Write balanced chemical equations that show the overall process. Any details of reaction mechanisms go into the summary.

(4) Purpose statement: Write a brief statement of purpose for the synthesis or analysis, or state the question you are addressing, with a few words on major analytical or conceptual approaches.

(5) Table: Include all reagents and solvents. The table normally lists

molecular weights, the number of moles, and grams of reagents, as well as the densities of liquids you will be using, boiling points of compounds that are liquids at room temperature and melting points of all organic solids, and pertinent hazard warnings.

(6) Method of yield calculation: Outline the computations to be used in a synthesis experiment, including calculation of the theoretical yield.

(7) Procedure and prelab questions: Write a procedural outline in sufficient detail so that the experiment could be done without reference to your lab textbook. This outline is especially important in experiments where you have designed the procedure. Answer any assigned prelab questions.

2. To Be Done During the Laboratory Session(s)

Recording observations during the experiments is a crucial part of your laboratory record. If your observations are incomplete, you cannot interpret the results of your experiments once you have left the laboratory. It is difficult, if not impossible, to reconstruct them at a later time.

Observations must be recorded in your notebook in ink while you are doing an experiment. You must record the actual quantities of all reagents as they are used, as well as the amounts of crude and purified products you obtain. Mention which measurements (temperature, time, melting point, and so on) you took and which spectra you recorded.

Because basic chemistry is primarily an experimental science, your observations are crucial to your success. Things that seem insignificant may be important in understanding and explaining your results later. Typical laboratory observations might be as follows.

(1) A white precipitate appeared, which dissolved when sulfuric acid was added.

(2) The solution turned cloudy when it was cooled to 10 ℃.

(3) An additional 10 mL of solvent were required to completely dissolve the yellow solid.

(4) The reaction was heated at 50 ℃ for 25 min in a water bath.

(5) A small puff of white smoke appeared when sodium hydroxide was added to the reaction mixture.

Your observations may be recorded in a variety of ways. They may be written on right-hand page across from the corresponding section of the experimental outline on a left-hand page, or the page may be divided into columns with the left column used for procedure and the right column for observations. It is a good idea to cross-index your observations to specific steps in the procedure that you wrote out as part of your prelab preparation. Your instructor will probably provide specific advice on how you should record your observations during the laboratory.

3. To Be Done After the Experimental Work Has Been Completed

In this section of the notebook you evaluate and interpret your experimental results. Entries include a section on interpretation of physical and spectral data, a summary of your conclusions, calculation of the percent yield, and answers to any assigned postlab questions.

(1) Conclusions and summary: In an inquiry-based experiment or project, return to the question being addressed and discuss the conclusions you can draw from analysis of your data. For both inquiry-based experiments and those where you learned about laboratory techniques and the design of basic synthesises, discuss how your experimental results will support your conclusions. Include a thorough interpretation of analytical results, such as UV/Vis analysis. Cite any reference sources that you used and give answers to any assigned postlab questions.

(2) Percent yield: One of the most important measure of success in a chemical synthesis is the quantity of desired product synthesized. To be sure, the purity of the product is also crucial, but if a synthetic method produces only small amounts of the desired product, it is not much good. Reactions on the pages of textbooks are often far more difficult to carry out in good yield than the books suggest.

Ⅳ Laboratory Safety

Chemistry is a laboratory science. As part of your laboratory experiences, you will handle many chemical substances and manipulate specialized laboratory equipments. Many of these substances pose a health risk if handled improperly, while some of the laboratory equipments can cause severe injury if used improperly. This section is a guide to the safe laboratory practices you will use throughout this course.

1. Prevention of Fires and Explosions

(1) Keep flammable materials away from flames. A few of the flammable chemicals commonly encountered in the laboratory are:

Hydrogen	Gasoline	Benzene	Sodium	Ether
Ethanol	Carbon disulfide	Phosphorus	Sulfur	Acetone

(2) Extinguish all flames not in use. Never leave a flame unattended.

(3) Use an electric heater or a water bath for heating flammable liquids. Never

heat them over a direct flame.

(4) Avoid, wherever possible, confining mixtures of air and flammable gases or volatile liquids. Where such cannot be avoided, wrap the container with a cloth or place it behind a shield.

(5) When gases or vapors are generated by heat or chemical reaction, provide for pressure release to prevent explosion. Never cap a vessel being heated.

(6) Mixing of chemicals should always be done in small quantities as explained in your instructions. Chemicals that react vigorously can cause violent explosions if large quantities are mixed.

(7) Keep strong oxidizing agents from coming into contact with strong reducing agents.

(8) In case of fire:

① If your clothing catches fire, immediately drop to the floor and roll to smother the flames and call for help.

② If a compound or solvent catches fire, if you can, quickly cover the flames with a piece of glassware.

③ If it is feasible, use a fire extinguisher to put the fire out.

④ Do not put water on an organic chemical fire because it will only spread the fire.

⑤ If the fire is large, do not take chances, evacuate the lab and the building immediately and tell your instructor or the coordinator what has happened.

⑥ If no one in authority is available, pull the fire alarm in the hallway and call 119 from a safe phone.

⑦ If the fire alarm sounds for any reason, leave the room immediately and exit the building.

2. Prevention of Poisoning

(1) Regard all chemicals in the laboratory as poisonous and never eat, drink, or taste anything while in the chemistry laboratory. It is always possible that the bottle is mislabeled.

(2) Handle chemicals in such a way that they do not come into contact with your skin. Utilize the tools of the laboratory: spatula, pipet, funnel, and so on.

(3) When it is necessary to note the odor of a substance, waft the fumes gently with your hand toward your nose. Never smell concentrated fumes.

(4) Note before performing the experiment whether any of the chemicals are

especially poisonous. A few of the particularly poisonous chemicals commonly used in the laboratory are as follows:

Acids (especially when concentrated)　　Alkalies (such as NaOH and KOH)

Arsenic (As) and its compounds　　Hydrogen sulfide (H_2S) and sulfides

Carbon tetrachloride (CCl_4) and other chlorinated hydrocarbons

Chromium compounds (such as $K_2Cr_2O_7$)　　Iodine (I_2)　　Bromine (Br_2)

Cyanides (such as HCN, KCN, and NaCN)　　Silver salts (such as $AgNO_3$)

Lead (Pb) and its compounds　　Mercury (Hg) and its compounds

(5) Use mechanical devices for applying suction in pipetting. Never use your mouth for this purpose.

(6) Carry out all experiments involving poisonous, irritating, or objectionable gases or vapors in a fume hood.

(7) If you inhale vapors, leave the area immediately—at least into the hallway. Tell your instructor or the coordinator, they will take you outside into the fresh air, and if necessary provide first aid or take you to get medical attention.

3. Prevention of Cuts

(1) All broken glassware should be discarded immediately by placing it in containers provided for that purpose.

(2) Fire-polish all glass tubing or rods to prevent cuts from the sharp edges.

(3) When inserting glass tubing through a rubber stopper, hold the tubing very close to the rubber stopper with a towel to protect your hand and use glycerin as a lubricant.

(4) Do not attempt to force frozen glass joints, stoppers, or stopcocks. Take them to your instructor for removal.

(5) If you cut yourself, wash the wound immediately with large amount of cool water. If your neighbor has been hurt, be prepared to help him if he is unable to help himself. Apply direct pressure to stop the bleeding as necessary. If the bleeding is profuse, elevate the affected limb. Watch for evidence of shock and contact your instructor or the lab coordinator as necessary.

4. Prevention of Chemical Burns

(1) Concentrated acids and alkalies are particularly dangerous and can produce painful burns on skin and eyes, which may not be healed. These reagents must be dispensed with great care, never add them directly to other chemicals unless you are certain that it is safe to do so. Avoid all contact of the skin with these materials.

(2) Use the corks to stopper all test tubes or flasks that must be shaken, do

not use your hand or thumb as a stopper.

(3) White (yellow) phosphorus, bromine, and hydrofluoric acid can produce very painful and slow-healing burns. Handle them only with your hands adequately protected.

(4) When diluting concentrated sulfuric acid, add the acid slowly to the water. Never add water to concentrated sulfuric acid. The considerable heat evolved can cause the acid to spatter and result in serious burns.

(5) If you burn yourself, thermal burns are treated by covering the affected area with cool water or ice. After a while, you can apply a pain-relieving cream. If the burn looks like that it is more than just reddening of the skin, seek medical attention.

Chapter 2   Common Laboratory Techniques and Practices

I Glassware and Equipments List

A few of glassware and equipments commonly used in the laboratory are shown in Figure 1-1.

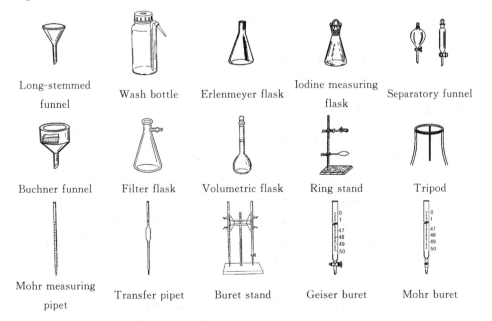

Figure 1-1   Glassware and equipments list

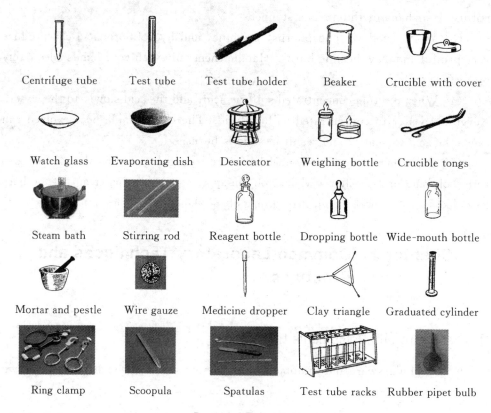

Centrifuge tube　　Test tube　　Test tube holder　　Beaker　　Crucible with cover

Watch glass　　Evaporating dish　　Desiccator　　Weighing bottle　　Crucible tongs

Steam bath　　Stirring rod　　Reagent bottle　　Dropping bottle　Wide-mouth bottle

Mortar and pestle　　Wire gauze　　Medicine dropper　　Clay triangle　Graduated cylinder

Ring clamp　　Scoopula　　Spatulas　　Test tube racks　Rubber pipet bulb

Continued Figure **1-1**

II　Cleaning and Drying Laboratory Glassware

1. Cleaning Glassware

You will be required to clean all glassware so that it will be ready for use by the next student. First, the bulk of the contents must be disposed of properly (product vial, waste bottle, or special waste container; do not dispose of anything in the sink unless instructed to do so). The proper method for cleaning depends on what was in the glassware. The list of cleaning solutions and methods for specific contaminants presented here should cover most of the glassware cleaning a technician may have to perform. If an automatic dishwasher is used, a final rinse with distilled water may be required before drying.

(1) Cleaning solutions.

① Basic permanganate solution: Dissolve 20 g of $KMnO_4$ and 50 g of NaOH in 1 L of water.

② Hot detergent mixture: Use sparingly to avoid excess foaming.

③ Acetone.

④ Chromic acid cleaning solution: A solution of $K_2Cr_2O_7$ dissolved in concentrated sulfuric acid was traditionally used for difficult cleaning tasks. This solution will not be used in this lab under any circumstances. Chromium compounds are carcinogens and their use is severely restricted.

(2) Cleaning methods.

① Stopcock grease (petroleum base): Dissolve grease in acetone, wash with detergent, rinse with tap water and then with distilled water.

② Stopcock grease (silicone base): Soak it in hot saturated NaOH in ethanol for about 15 min, and then rinse thoroughly with water. A solution of alcoholic sodium hydroxide is also our favorite cleanser for removing grease and organic residues from flasks and other glassware.

③ Fat and oil contamination: Soak in basic permanganate solution, rinse with tap water and then with distilled water.

④ Albuminous "crusts": Soak in chromic acid cleaning solution, rinse with tap water and then with distilled water.

The rinsing operation must be carried out thoroughly. If clean, the walls will retain an unbroken film of water, not droplets. The cleaning operation may be simplified by placing stained or contaminated glassware into detergent solution after use. Spectrophotometer cuvettes and other delicate glassware must be handled with extreme care and not subjected to the harsher cleaning agents.

2. Drying Glassware

(1) Oven drying of glassware. Electrically heated ovens (Figure 1-2) are commonly used in the laboratory to remove water or other solvents from chemical samples and to dry laboratory glassware. Wet glassware can be dried by heating it in an oven at 120 ℃ for 20 min. Remove the dried glassware from the oven with tongs and allow it to cool to room temperature before using it for a reaction.

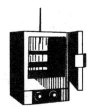

Figure 1-2   Electrically
heated oven

(2) Drying wet glassware with acetone. Glassware that is wet after washing can be dried quickly by rinsing it in a fume hood with a few milliliters of acetone. Acetone and water are completely miscible, so the water is removed from the

glassware. The acetone is collected as flammable waste, any residual acetone on the glassware is allowed to evaporate into the atmosphere. Thus there is an environmental cost, as well as the initial purchase and later waste disposal costs, in using acetone for drying glassware.

Ⅲ Water Quality Standards

Purified water is used in all industries and science-based organizations. Therefore, international and national standards authorities have established water quality standards for general types of application:

(1) The International Organization for Standardization (ISO).

(2) The American Society for Testing and Materials (ASTM).

Other representative organizations have specified criteria relevant to their particular domains. Prominent among these are:

(1) The National Committee for Clinical Laboratory Standards (NCCLS).

(2) The Pharmacopoeia.

The International Organization for Standardization specification to water for laboratory use is ISO 3696: 1987 (Table 1-1). This standard covers three grades of water as follows.

Table 1-1　International organization for standardization specification to water for laboratory use

Parameter	Grade 1	Grade 2	Grade 3
pH value inclusive range (at 25 ℃)	N/A	N/A	5.0 to 7.5
Electrical conductivity, 25 ℃, max /(μS · cm^{-1})	0.1	1.0	5.0
Oxidizable matter: Oxygen (O_2) content, max /(mg · L^{-1})	N/A	0.08	0.4
Absorbance at 254 nm and 1 cm optical path length, absorbance units, max	0.001	0.01	Not specified
Residue after evaporation on heating at 110 ℃, max /(mg · kg^{-1})	N/A	1	2
Silica (SiO_2) content, max/(mg · L^{-1})	0.01	0.02	Not specified

1. Grade 1

Essentially free from dissolved or colloidal ionic and organic contaminants. It is suitable for the most stringent analytical requirements including those of high performance liquid chromatography (HPLC). It should be produced by further treatment of grade 2 water for example by reverse osmosis or ion exchange followed by filtration through a membrane filter of pore size 0.2 μm to remove particle matter or re-distillation from a fused silica apparatu.

2. Grade 2

Very low inorganic, organic or colloidal contaminants and suitable for sensitive analytical purposes including atomic absorption spectrometry (AAS) and determination of constituents in trace quantities. It can be produced by multiple distillation, ion exchange or reverse osmosis, followed by distillation.

3. Grade 3

Suitable for the most laboratory wet chemistry work and preparation of reagent solutions. It can be produced by single distillation, by ion exchange, or by reverse osmosis. Unless otherwise specified, it should be used for ordinary analytical work.

IV Drying of Solids

There are various methods of drying solid materials. When deciding which method to use, it is important to know something of the physical properties of the material.

Although the method of air drying takes longer than the others, it is one of the safest methods for nondeliquescent solids. The damp solid, drained as dry as possible on the filter, is transferred to a watch glass and spread out evenly. This solid can be left to dry overnight in some dust-free place. If possible a second, larger watch glass should be arranged over the product as a precaution against dust, but this cover should allow free evaporation.

If the sample will not decompose by moderate heating and is not volatile, the nonessential water can be removed by placing the sample in a drying oven heated to 105 ℃ to 110 ℃. The sample is placed in a weighing bottle, which is then placed in a beaker. The weighing bottle lid should also be placed in the beaker and heated along with the sample in order to remove excess moisture from its surface. Because many drying ovens are dirty and rusty, there is always the risk that dirt may fall into your sample. Therefore, use a cover glass supported on glass hooks to cover the beaker. If a procedure does not specify the drying time, dry the sample and then weigh it, repeat the drying and weighing until the mass is constant.

Whenever a sample is dried before weighing, there is always a question whether it is really dry or not. Therefore, samples are weighed to a constant mass. They are weighed after an initial drying, and then put back in the oven and later weighed again. If the weighings are same, the sample is dry. If, however, the sample loses weight during the second drying, it should be dried a third time and reweighed. This process is repeated until two consecutive weighings give the same result.

Vacuum ovens (which may be aspirated with a vacuum pump) speed up the drying process and are especially effective for drying heat-sensitive materials since they can be used at considerably lower temperatures.

It is important to understand that even though a sample contains nonessential water, the water is a constituent of the material "as received". Unless otherwise requested, the analyst should report the percent water removed by drying and the analysis obtained on the dry sample. If an analysis is requested on an "as is" basis, the analyst does not need to dry the material at all.

Unfortunately, letting the residue reach room temperature before weighing introduces a second problem. As the object cools, it can absorb moisture from the air. This problem is solved by placing the residue in a desiccator as it cools. Many types of desiccators are in use, a typical one is shown in Figure 1-3. All have two things in common, an airtight seal which keeps the sample isolated from the outside air and a material called a desiccant which absorbs moisture.

The desiccator must be regularly recharged with fresh desiccant, and the ground-glass seal must be greased with the minimum of silicone grease, so it appears transparent. It is removed by sliding it away from you with one hand while holding the bottom portion stationary with the other. What at the bottom of the desiccator is a drying agent (often the very inexpensive $CaCl_2$) that takes up any moisture that enters when the desiccator is opened. Samples to be dried should be spread out on a watch glass and labeled with their name and date.

Any object taken from a flame or a furnace should be cooled for at least 2 min before it is placed in a desiccator. A general rule is that if heat can no longer be felt on the back of your hand when it is held 5 cm from the object, the object can be put in a desiccator. If hot objects are placed inside, a vacuum forms upon cooling, making it difficult to remove the lid. The desiccator serves as a place for dried samples to cool and be stored prior to weighing them. Transfer to and from the desiccator should normally not be by fingers but by crucible tongs or by strips of lintless paper. The way of opening a desiccator is shown in Figure 1-3 (a).

Occasionally students are tempted to carry a desiccator by the top. This usually works until the desiccator is about 1 m above the floor, and then it falls with disastrous results. The way of carrying the desiccator is shown in Figure 1-3 (b).

It is important to remember that after opening a desiccator it takes at least two hours to re-establish a dry atmosphere.

A vacuum desiccator is used to speed the drying of a sample. The sample must be covered with a second watch glass and the desiccator must be evacuated and filled slowly to avoid blowing the sample about. A vacuum desiccator must be covered with strong adhesive tape, or be enclosed in a special cage, when being evacuated and deevacuated to guard against an implosion.

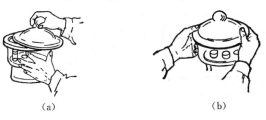

(a)   (b)

Figure 1-3 A laboratory desiccator

(a)Opening a desiccator;(b) Carrying a desiccator

V Chemicals

1. Purity and Grading

We offer wide range of products with most common grading available on each item. It includes synthesis grade, GR grade, ACS grade, grading for special applications such as HPLC grade, and biochemistry grade, etc..

The purity grade helps us to classify the large variety of reagents that exist in the market. Purity grade is expressed in the product name by means of a quality denomination that follows to the product nomenclature (i. e. ,"guarantee reagent").

Chemicals have large diversity in grading and types of use summarized as follows.

(1) Technical grade: These reagents are suitable for non-critical tasks in the laboratory such as rinsing and dissolving or are used as raw materials in production tasks.

(2) Synthesis grade: These reagents are suitable for organic synthesis and preparative applications.

(3) Chemically pure (CP) grade: This grade is almost as pure as synthesis grade, but application determines whether purity is adequate for the purpose.

(4) Guarantee reagent (GR) grade: It is the ideal quality for laboratory purposes. Batch to batch reproducibility is specially controlled to guarantee consistent analytical results. The grade is equivalent to analytical reagent (AR).

(5) ACS grade: Reagents meet the specification of American Chemical Society (ACS). Analytical reagents are found in the most laboratories and are used in a wide variety of analytical techniques for quality control, research and development.

(6) HPLC grade: Product is specially made for high performance liquid chromatography.

(7) Spectroscopy grade: Solvents display a high UV permeability and are subjected to strict IR spectroscopy tests.

(8) Biotech/Biochemistry grade: Highly pure reagents are suitable for biochemical research and analysis.

2. Labeling and Storage of Chemicals

Be certain that all chemicals are correctly and clearly labeled. Post warning signs if chemicals are flammable, highly toxic, and carcinogenic or other special problems exist. Many chemical suppliers also indicate hazards by printing the universally understandable pictograms approved at the UN-sponsored Rio Earth Summit in 1992 on the labels of their reagents (Figure 1-4). If the label on the container does not give safety information, obtain the information from some reference sources: your supervisor; a handbook such as the CRC Handbook of Laboratory Safety, Merck Index; or MSDS.

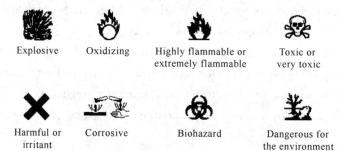

Figure 1-4 Globally Harmonized System (GHS) pictograms indicating chemical hazards

Centralized storage of bulk quantities of flammable liquids provides the best method of controlling fire hazards. The flammable liquids must be stored in fire-resistant cupboard.

Chemicals which are light-sensitive should be stored in dark bottles.

Some chemicals are incompatible with others. The incompatible chemicals should be kept segregated.

Chemicals that have high chronic toxicity, including those classified as potential carcinogens, should be stored in ventilated storage areas in unbreakable, chemically resistant containers. Storage vessels containing such substances should carry the label "CAUTION: HIGH CHRONIC TOXICITY or CANCER SUSPECT AGENT".

3. Handling Chemicals

(1) Handling solids.

Once the mass of a reagent has been determined, the reagent must be transferred to the reaction vessel without mishap. There are many local variants in each of these procedures. For example, some prefer to transfer solids with a weighing spoon, some with a finger hold bottle, and some with a paper-strap hold bottle. Students should follow the local preference, but should be aware of other acceptable options. Whatever the technique option is chosen, the procedure must be done reproducibly, if analysis quality is to be optimized.

① Hold a container with its label facing your hand. Tilt the bottle towards the vessel to which you are transferring solids, and roll the bottle back and forth until the desired amount of solids are transferred into the new vessel.

② Using a powder funnel. For reaction being run in a miniscale round-bottomed flask, a powder funnel aids in transferring the solid reagent from the weighing paper into the small neck of the flask is needed (Figure 1-5 (a)). The stem of a powder funnel has a larger diameter than that of a funnel used for liquid transfer, thus the solids will not clog it. The powder funnel serves to keep the

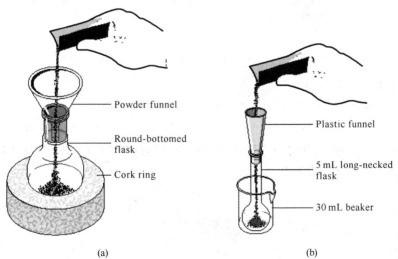

(a)   (b)

Figure 1-5   Transferring solids with a powder funnel

(a) Miniscale apparatus; (b) Williamson microscale apparatus solids from spilling and prevents any solids from sticking to the inside of the joint at the top of the flask. Use of a powder funnel is essential with Williamson microscale glassware because of the very small opening at the top of the round-bottomed flasks and reaction tubes (Figure 1-5 (b)).

③ Transferring solids to a standard taper microscale vial. To transfer solids to a standard taper microscale vial, roll the weighing paper containing the solids into a cone by overlapping two corners on the same side of the paper. Place the rolled end well down into the neck of the microscale vial and gently slide one corner of the paper away from the other to create an opening just large enough for the solids to fall into the reaction vessel, as shown in Figure 1-6. A microspatula can be used to gently push the solids through the opening in the weighing paper.

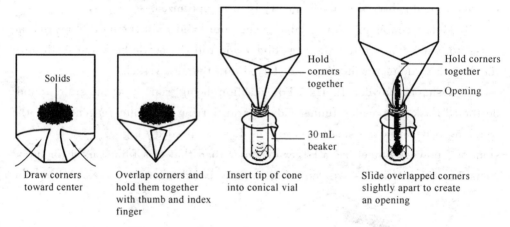

Figure **1-6** Transferring solids with a weighing paper

(2) Handling liquids.

① To dispense a liquid or solution from a reagent bottle, use the back of your fingers to remove the stopper from a reagent bottle (Figure 1-7). Hold the stopper between your fingers until the transfer of the liquid is complete. Do not place the stopper on your workbench.

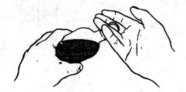

Figure 1-7 Removing a stopper from a reagent bottle

② When you are pouring a liquid from a reagent bottle into a beaker, the reagent should be poured slowly down a glass stirring rod, as shown in Figure 1-8 (a). When you are transferring a liquid from one beaker to another, you can hold the stirring rod and beaker in one hand as shown in Figure 1-8 (b). Then no drops will dribble down the outside wall of the beaker.

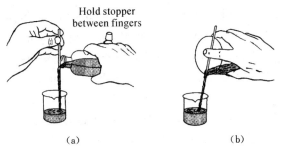

(a)   (b)

Figure **1-8**   Pouring a liquid

(a) Pour down a glass stirring rod if possible to avoid dripping;

(b) When tranferring from a beaker, hold the stirring rod in this manner

③ Medicine droppers are great for transferring liquids from one container to another. They come as two parts, a bulb and a glass pipet. They must be used in a vertical position. This means, up and down. The bulb is on top, the tip of the pipet points down (Figure 1-9). Never, I repeat NEVER, hold a filled pipet upside down. If you hold it in this way, the liquid runs into the bulb. The bulb is dirty and should not be used again.

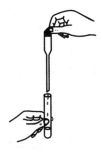

Figure **1-9**   Using a medicine dropper in this manner

Droppers from dropper bottles should not come into contact with any surface outside of the dropper bottle itself.

A very rough, but often satisfactory method for estimating volume is by counting drops delivered from a medicine dropper (20 to 25 drops per milliliter), depending on the size of the tip and the surface tension of the liquid.

④ When you are transferring a liquid to a test tube or a graduated cylinder, the container should be held at eye level. Pour the liquid slowly, until the correct volume has been transferred (Figure 1-10 (a)). When reading a volume of a liquid in a container such as a graduated cylinder, first place the cylinder on the lab bench, you will notice that the liquid is higher at the edges than in the middle and forms a phenomenon called a meniscus. The meniscus is the apparent downward curvature in the surface of a liquid contained in any narrow measuring tube, caused in part by surface tension. In graduated cylinders, and also in pipets or burets that are filled from the top, it is necessary to read the bottom of the meniscus with the eye horizontal to this surface (Figure 1-10 (b)). If the meniscus is not read at eye level, so that the front and rear parts of the graduation mark nearest the meniscus appear to coincide, parallax error in the reading will result. Determine this factor for yourself by comparing three readings of the same meniscus: one with the eye level horizontal, one with the eye directed from somewhat above, and one from somewhat below. Proper lighting is necessary to see the meniscus clearly. Each line on the graduate in Figure 1-10 (b) represents 0.1 mL. By estimating the height of the meniscus between these lines, it is possible to measure the volume of the liquid to the nearest 0.1 mL. Thus, the volume of the liquid in the Figure 1-10 (b) is 39.10 mL. The scale on your graduated cylinder may be different from that shown, but it should be divided into sufficiently small units so that the nearest 0.1 mL can be estimated accurately.

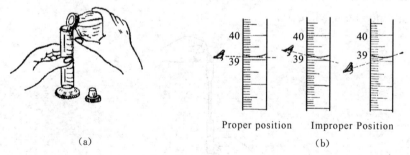

Proper position   Improper Position

(a)   (b)

Figure 1-10   A graduated cylinder

(a) Transferring a liquid to a graduated cylinder; (b) The reading of graduated cylinder

VI Heating and Cooling

1. Heating

(1) Heating devices.

Most labs use at least one type of heating device, such as ovens, hot plates, heating mantles and tapes, hot-tube furnaces, hot-air guns, muffle furnaces and microwave ovens.

① Hot plates: Hot plates work well for heating flat-bottomed containers such as beakers, Erlenmeyer flasks, and crystallizing dishes used as water baths or sand baths. Laboratory hot plates are normally used for heating solutions to 100 ℃ or above when inherently safer steam baths cannot be used. Any newly purchased hot plates should be designed in a way that avoids electrical sparks. Do not store volatile flammable materials near a hot plate.

② Heating mantles: Heating mantles are commonly used for heating round-bottomed flasks, reaction kettles and related reaction vessels. These mantles enclose a heating element in a series of layers of fiberglass cloth. Fiberglass heating mantles come in a variety of sizes to fit specific sizes of round-bottomed flasks, one size for a 100 mL flask will not work well with a flask of another size.

Both types of heating mantles have no controls and must be plugged into a variable transformer or other variable controller to adjust the rate of heating (Figure 1-11). The variable transformer is then plugged into a wall outlet.

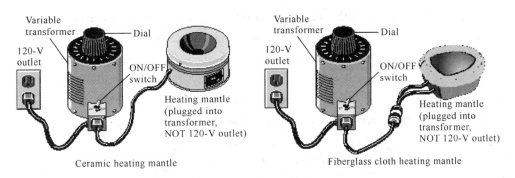

Figure 1-11   Heating mantle and variable transformer

A heating mantle with variable electronic control is used for flammable solvents that boil between room temperature and 200 ℃.

③ Heat guns: A heat gun allows hot air to be directed over a fairly narrow area (Figure 1-12 (a)). A heat gun is particularly useful as a heat source for distillations because of the high temperature near the nozzle. A heat gun usually has two heat settings as well as a cool air setting. After use, the heat gun should be suspended in a ring clamp with the heat setting on cool for a few minutes to allow the nozzle to cool before the heat gun is set on the bench (Figure 1-12 (b)).

Other uses of heat guns include the rapid removal of moisture from glassware

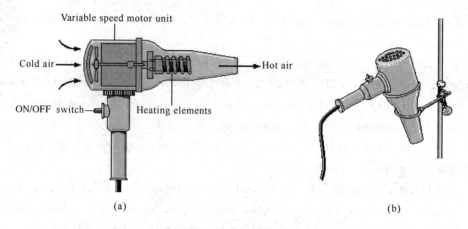

Figure **1-12**   The use of heat gun

（a）Heat gun；（b）Heat gun cooling in a ring clamp after use

where dry but not strictly anhydrous conditions are needed, and the heating of thin-layer chromatographic plates after they have been dipped in a visualizing reagent that requires heat to develop the color.

④ Laboratory jacks: Laboratory jacks are adjustable platforms that are useful for holding heating mantles, magnetic stirrers, and cooling baths under reaction flasks (Figure 1-13). The reaction apparatus is assembled with enough clearance between the bottom of the reaction or distillation flask and the bench top to position the heating or cooling device under the flask by raising the platform of the laboratory jack. At the end of the operation, the heating or cooling device can be removed easily by lowering the platform of the laboratory jack.

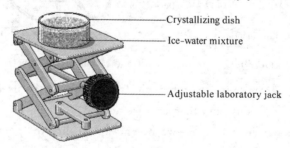

Figure **1-13**   Laboratory jack with water bath

（2）Heating methods.

① Direct heating.

Ethanol burners are usually used to heat nonflammable solvents, such as water, that boil between 100 ℃ and 200 ℃.

When heating materials in a test tube with a burner, the test tube should be held with a test-tube holder, near the upper end of the tube (Figure 1-14 (a)), the mouth of the test tube should be directed away from yourself and your neighbor, and the heating should be done gently. Fill a test tube one-third full with the liquid to be heated. The test tube must be heated gently and uniformly. Move the test tube in and out of the flame to allow time for heat transfer. Heat the area near the liquid surface slightly more than the bottom of the test tube. Heat the upper part of the test tube to prevent vapor from condensing there.

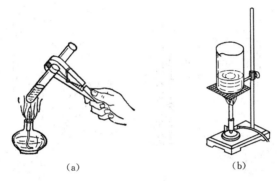

(a)   (b)

Figure 1-14   The use of ethanol burner

(a) Heating materials in a test tube;(b) Heating liquids in a beaker

CAUTION: Never point the open end of the test tube you are heating either toward yourself or anyone working nearby. Never heat the bottom of the test tube.

When heating liquids in a beaker or a flask with a burner, the container should be set on wire gauze which evenly spreads the heat from the burner (Figure 1-14 (b)). This will minimize the possibility of cracking the container or splattering the liquid. Fill a beaker one-half full with the liquid to be heated. When it is important that there is no loss whatever from splashing, it is customary to place a watch glass over the container. When acids or other solutions which emit noxious fumes are evaporated in this way, it is imperative to carry out the operation under a fume hood with strong ventilation.

CAUTION: Never heat plastic beakers or graduated glassware in a burner flame. Never let a boiling water bath boil dry, add water to it as necessary.

② Water baths.

When a temperature of less than 100 ℃ is needed, a water bath allows for closer temperature control than can be achieved with the heating methods discussed previously. The water bath can be contained in a beaker or crystallizing dish. Once the desired temperature of the water bath is reached, the water temperature can be maintained by using a low heat setting on a hot plate.

The thermometer used to monitor the temperature of a water bath should always be clamped, as shown in Figure 1-15, so that it is not touching the wall or the bottom of the vessel holding the water. The reaction vessel should be submerged in the water bath farther than the depth of the reaction mixture the reaction vessel containers.

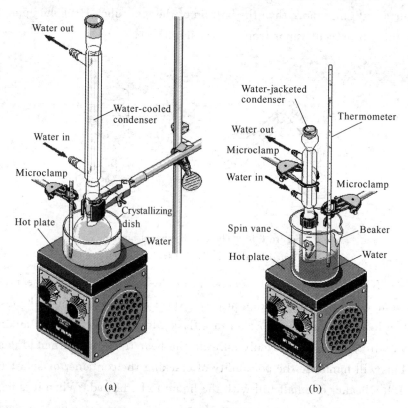

(a)   (b)

Figure **1-15**　Water baths

(a) Heating miniscale reflux apparatus in a crystallizing dish;

(b) Heating microscale reflux apparatus in a beaker

③ Oil and salt baths.

Electrically heated oil baths are often used to heat small or irregularly shaped vessels or when a stable heat source that can be maintained at a constant temperature is desired. Molten salt baths, like hot oil baths, offer the advantages of good heat transfer, commonly have a higher operating range (e. g. , 200 ℃ to 425 ℃) and may have a high thermal stability (e. g. , 540 ℃). There are several precautions to take when working with these types of heating devices:

A. Take care with hot oil baths not to generate smoke or have the oil burst into flames from overheating.

B. Always monitor oil baths by using a thermometer or other thermal sensing devices to ensure that its temperature does not exceed the flash point of the oil being used.

C. Wear heat-resistant gloves when handling a hot bath.

④ Sand baths.

A sand bath provides another method for heating microscale reactions. Sand is a poor conductor of heat, so a temperature gradient exists along the various depths of the sand, with the highest temperature occurring at the bottom of the sand and the lowest temperature near the top surface.

One method of preparing the sand bath uses a ceramic heating mantle, such as a thermowell, about two-thirds full of washed sand (Figure 1-16 (a)). A second method employs a crystallizing dish, heated on a hot plate, containing 1 cm to 1. 5 cm of washed sand (Figure 1-16 (b)); the sand in the dish should be level, not a mound. A thermometer is inserted in the sand so that the bulb is completely submerged at the same depth as the contents of the reaction vessel. The heating of a reaction vessel can be closely controlled by raising or lowering the vessel to a different depth in the sand, as well as by changing the heat supplied by the heating mantle or hot plate.

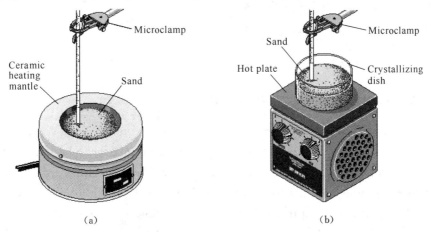

(a)   (b)

Figure 1-16   Sand baths

(a) Sand bath in a ceramic heating mantle;(b) Sand bath in a crystallizing dish on a hot plate

2. Cooling

Cooling baths are frequently needed in the organic laboratory to control exothermic reactions, to cool reaction mixtures before the next step in a procedure, and to promote recovery of the maximum amount of crystalline solids from a recrystallization. Most commonly, cold tap water or an ice-water mixture serves as the coolant. Effective cooling with ice requires the addition of just enough water to provide complete contact between the vessel being cooled and the ice. Even crushed ice does not pack well enough against the vessel for efficient cooling because the air in the spaces between the ice particles is a poor conductor of heat.

Temperatures from $-10\ ℃$ to $0\ ℃$ can be achieved by the mixing solid NaCl into an ice-water mixture. The amount of water mixed with the ice should be only enough to make good contact with the vessel being cooled.

A cooling bath of 2-propanol and chunks of solid carbon dioxide (dry ice) can be used for temperatures from $-78\ ℃$ to $-10\ ℃$. (CAUTION: Foaming occurs as chunks of solid carbon dioxide are added to 2-propanol.) The mixture of 2-propanol and dry ice is contained in a Dewar flask, a double-walled vacuum chamber that insulates the contents from ambient circumstance (Figure 1-17).

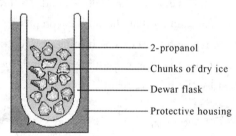

Figure **1-17** Dewar flask with a mixture of 2-propanol and dry ice

VII Crystallization and Recrystallization

Crystallization is a technique which chemists use to purify solid compounds. It is one of the fundamental procedures each chemist must master to become proficient in the laboratory. Crystallization is based on the principles of solubility: Compounds (solutes) tend to be more soluble in hot liquids (solvents) than they are in cold liquids. If a saturated hot solution is allowed to cool, the solute is no longer soluble in the solvent and forms crystals of pure compound. Impurities are excluded from the growing crystals and the pure solid crystals can be separated from the dissolved impurities by filtration.

The process of crystallization is as follows. Heat some solvent to boiling. Place the solid to be crystallized in an Erlenmeyer flask. Pour a small amount of the hot solvent into the flask containing the solid. Swirl the flask to dissolve the solid. Place the flask on the steam bath to keep the solution warm. If the solid is still not dissolved, add a tiny amount of solvent and swirl again. When the solid is all in solution, set the flask on the bench top. Do not disturb it! After a while, crystals would appear in the flask. You can now place the flask in an ice bath to finish the crystallization process. You are now ready to filter the solution to isolate the crystals. Please see the section on vacuum filtration. After your crystals are filtered from the solution, carefully scrape the crystals onto the watch glass. Let the crystals finish drying on the watch glass.

Ⅷ Separating and Purifying

1. Decantation

Sometimes adequate separation of a solid and a liquid can be achieved by decantation, especially when the solid is dense. Allow the mixture to stand until the solid has settled; then carefully decant (pour off) the liquid, leaving the solid in the original container (Figure 1-18).

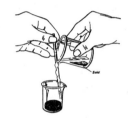

Figure 1-18   Decantation

2. Filtration

Filtration is a technique used either to remove impurities from an organic solution or to isolate a solid. The two types of filtration commonly used in chemistry laboratories are gravity filtration and vacuum or suction filtration.

(1) Gravity filtration.

Select the size of filter paper that, when folded, will be a few millimeters below the rim of your glass funnel. Fold a filter paper circle in half and then quarters. Open the folded paper to form a cone, with one thickness of the paper on one side and three thicknesses on the other, as shown in Figure 1-19 (a). Insert the conical filter paper into the funnel and wet it with a few milliliters of the solvent to be used in the following procedure. When properly set up, the liquid will fill the entire stem of the funnel, and the weight of the long liquid column will apply "suction" to speed the filtration. Place a beaker beneath the funnel to collect the filtrate. The tip of the funnel should touch the inside surface of the beaker and extend about 2 cm below the rim. Decant the liquid from the solid by pouring it down a glass stirring rod into the funnel (Figure 1-19 (b)). Be careful to keep the liquid below the top edge of the cone of filter paper at all times; the liquid must not overflow. (If the precipitate has settled, decant the clear solution to save

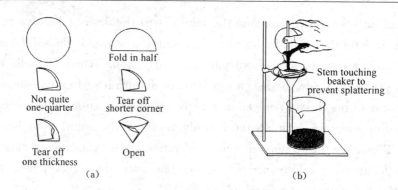

Figure **1-19** Gravity filtration

(a) Folding filter paper for gravity filtration; (b) Gravity filtration setup

filtering time. Save the decantate if desired.) Then grasp the beaker and stirring rod with one hand as shown, swirl to suspend the precipitate, and pour the suspension into the filter paper. If the filtration is slow, carefully set the beaker down and, if necessary, leave the stirring rod in the suspension (never on the bench). When all the primary suspension has been poured out of the beaker, hold the beaker and stirring rod with one hand over the filter and direct a stream of wash water into the beaker to rinse it.

(2) Vacuum filtration.

Vacuum filtration is used primarily to collect a desired solid, for instance, the collection of crystals in a recrystallization procedure. Vacuum filtration is faster than gravity filtration, because the solvent or solution and air are forced through the filter paper by the application of reduced pressure. The reduced pressure requires that they should be carried out in special equipment (Figure 1-20 (a)): Buchner or Hirsch funnel; heavy-walled, side arm filtering flask; rubber adaptor or stopper to seal the funnel to the flask when under vacuum; vacuum source.

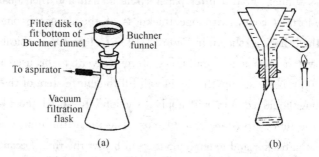

Figure **1-20** Vacuum filtration and hot gravity filtration

(a) Vacuum filtration; (b) Hot gravity filtration

Procedure for vacuum filtration is as follows.

① Assemble the apparatus. Check the side arm flask carefully for cracks, since cracks could cause the flask to break when vacuum is applied. Then, clamp the flask securely to a ring stand. Add an adaptor and a Buchner funnel. Place a piece of filter paper in the funnel that is small enough to remain flat but large enough to cover all of the holes in the filter. Connect the side arm flask to a vacuum source always with thick-walled tubing, since Tygon tubing will collapse under reduced pressure.

Whenever you use a water aspirator, you run the risk of sucking water from the aspirator into your vacuum filtration unit. The water-trap placed in-line will catch any such water. If you do not need the filtrate, but only need the solid matter collected on the Buchner funnel, this presents no problem. Most of the time this is the case, and usually students do not need a water-trap.

② Wet the filter paper with a small amount of the solvent to be used in the filtration. Turn on the vacuum source.

③ Filter the solution. Pour the mixture to be filtered onto the filter paper. The vacuum should rapidly pull the liquid through the funnel. Watch that particulates do not creep under the edges of the filter paper. If this happens, start over and carefully pour portions of the solution onto the very center of the filter paper.

④ Rinse the solids. Rinse the cake with a small amount of fresh and cold solvent to help remove impurities that were dissolved in the filtrate. Disconnect the rubber tubing before turning off the water aspirator. This prevents water from being sucked into the vacuum flask. Carefully remove the filter paper and solid from the Buchner funnel. Usually you will set it on a watch glass and let it dry in the air for a while.

Note: Do not use vacuum filtration to filter a solid from a liquid if it is the liquid that you want and if the liquid is low boiling point. Any solvent which boils at about 125 ℃ or lower will boil off under the reduced pressure in the vacuum flask.

(3) Hot gravity filtration.

A filtration procedure called "hot gravity filtration" is used to separate insoluble impurities from a hot solution. Hot filtration (Figure 1-20 (b)) requires fluted filter paper and careful attention to the procedure to keep the apparatus warm but covered so that solvent does not evaporate.

3. Centrifugation

A centrifuge substitutes centrifugal force for gravity in the separation of solids from liquids (Figure 1-21). Whenever the centrifuge is used, it must be balanced,

or else it may become damaged. Therefore, before centrifuging a mixture contained in a test tube or a centrifuge tube, prepare another tube to balance it in the centrifuge by filling an identical tube with water until the liquid levels in both tubes are the same. Insert the tubes

Figure 1-21　Electric centrifuge for separating a precipitate from a liquid

in opposite positions (at 180°) in the centrifuge, close the cover, and set the machine in motion. The time required for centrifugation depends on the particle size of the solid being separated; for example, crystalline solids require less time than colloidal precipitates. Allow the centrifuge to come to rest before removing the tubes. Keep the cover closed and your hands away from the top of the centrifuge while it is rotating.

The solution is either quickly decanted from the tube without disturbing the precipitate or withdrawn by means of a medicine dropper.

IX Application of Digital Electronic Potentiometer

1. Calibration

Zero point calibration: The function is selected to the "external standard" position, and the "external standard" interface is short circuited. Set the electromotive force shift knob to the zero of electromotive force indication, press the "calibration" button, and the balance indication will be zero.

The standard battery is connected to the "external standard", the function selection is set to the "external standard" position, and the electromotive force shift knob is set to the electromotive force indicating the potential value of the standard battery. Press the "calibration" button, and the balance indication will be zero.

2. Measurement

Set the function selection to "measure" position, connect the battery to be measured cell, adjust the electromotive force shift knob until the balance indication is close to zero, and the reading is "electromotive force" when it is stable (Figure 1-22).

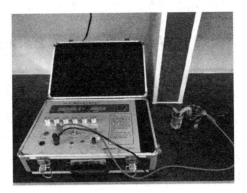

Figure 1-22   Digital electronic potentiometer

X Test Papers

Wide range test papers (pH, lead acetate, potassium iodide-starch, etc.) enable quick and costeffective semi-quantitative testing in the laboratory.

1. pH Test Paper

Indispensable for lab work! Simply dip paper wick into liquid or wet surface to measure acidity or alkalinity level. This measurement can be determined by the use of papers with color changes, solutions with color changes or pH meters that read pH in digital or analog numbers. Wide range pH test strips provide a distinct color for each pH unit from 1 to 14. Short range pH test strips show a distinct color change for each half pH unit. For instance, strong acids like sulfuric acid and nitric acid test around 1 (red), while weak acids like acetic acid and carbonic acid test around 6 (yellow). A pH of 7 (green) is neutral (distilled water). Weak bases like calcium hydroxide test around 8 (blue), while strong bases like sodium hydroxide test around 14 (purple). pH also indicates relative hydrogen ion concentration (increases with acidity).

2. Lead Acetate Test Paper

Used to test for hydrogen sulfide (H_2S) vapors. Paper must be moistened with water prior to use.

3. Potassium Iodide-Starch Test Paper

Used to test for free iodine in solution. Color varies from white through blue to black, depending on iodine concentration.

Chapter 3　Weighing with Balances

The analytical balance is the most accurate and precise instrument in a laboratory. Objects of up to 100 g may be weighed to 6 significant figures. Early analytical balances were entirely mechanical with two weighing pans, one for the chemical, and the other one for the counterweight. Now, most analytical balances are hybrid mechanical and electronic with a single pan for the substance to be weighed. These balances use the substitution method of weighing. That is to say, the counterweight is fixed (hidden within the balance), and removable weights are mechanically added or subtracted from the sample side of the lever and fulcrum.

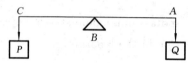

Figure 1-23　Schematic sketch of the two pans balance

A very schematic sketch of the two pans balance is shown in Figure 1-23. The mass of the product times the distance from the balance point to the fulcrum determines the moment about the fulcrum. When these are equal for both sample and standard (i. e. , mass), the pans will be level and the balance beam will be horizontal.

$$m_Q \times l_{AB} = m_P \times l_{BC}$$

Most laboratories have two different types of balance available for measuring the mass of an object. The first type is the general-purpose balance, such as a DA/DTA electronic top-loading balance or the tray balance, which is usually capable of measuring to two decimal places (i. e. , to 0. 01 g). The second type is the analytical balance, which is usually electronic in more modern laboratories, and mechanical in older facilities.

I DA/DTA Electronic Balance

Use a top loading balance to weigh solid materials when a precision of 0. 1 g is adequate. For more accurate mass measurements or small amounts, use a DA/DTA electronic balance (Figure 1-24).

(1) Check if the balance is turned on. If not, press the ON/OFF button and wait until the display reads 0. 0 g.

(2) Place a container or a large and creased weighing paper on the balance pan. Push tare button to zero the balance.

(3) Use a spatula to add small portions of the reagent to the container or paper until the desired mass is shown on the digital display. Record the actual amount you use in your notebook.

(4) Clean-up: Use the brush provided to clean any spills. Discard any disposable tare containers, weighing paper, or Kimwipes in the nearest wastebasket.

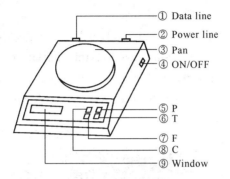

① Data line
② Power line
③ Pan
④ ON/OFF

⑤ P
⑥ T

⑦ F
⑧ C
⑨ Window

Figure 1-24   DA/DTA electronic balance

Ⅱ Analytical Balance

In certain instances, the less precise (and quicker) top loading or triple beam balances should be used. However, since every analysis involves at least one, accurate weighing step, it is essential that you are able to use the analytical balance accurately and reproducibly. Analytical balance can measure to four or five decimal places (i. e. , to 0. 000 1 g or 0. 000 01 g).

1. General Rules for Use of the Analytical Balance

(1) The balance should be located on a hard, stable, and level surface which is free of vibrations and excessive air drafts.

(2) Keep the balance clean. Remove dust, etc. from the pans with a camel hair brush.

(3) Learn the capacity of your balance, and never exceed this capacity.

(4) Objects to be weighed should be at room temperature.

(5) Strategies must be developed to ensure that moisture is not transferred to the object being weighed during handling.

(6) Chemicals are never placed directly on the balance pan. Use a weighing bottle, beaker, watch glass, etc. .

(7) After you have completed weighing, check the following things:

① You have recorded your results correctly.

② The balance pan is clean.

③ There are no objects left on the pan.

(8) Corrosive liquids and solids are always placed in a vapor tight, pre-weighed container before weighing on an analytical balance.

(9) Report and record anything unusual.

2. The Electronic Analytical Balance

The single pan electronic analytical balance (Figure 1-25) is fast and convenient. Its rapid digital readout obscures the subtlety of its operation. It is the device with the highest precision that you will use in the laboratory. It is both delicate and expensive. Some simple rules must be followed in its use.

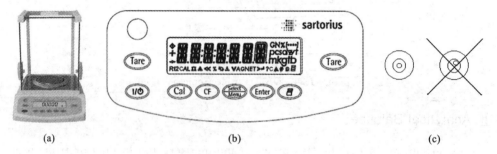

Figure **1-25** Electronic analytical balance

(a) Analytical balance;(b) Display area and operation key;(c) Horizontal-level bubble gauge

(1) Powdered and liquid materials must never be placed directly on the balance pan.

(2) Spills should be avoided by not transferring materials into containers while they are on the balance.

(3) If they do occur, they should be cleaned up at once (carefully).

(4) Do not try to calibrate an analytical balance. If in doubt, ask an instructor to check it.

An analytical balance is one which weighs to ± 0.1 mg and has a maximum capacity of 200 g. A number of companies produce reliable and reproducible analytical balances. The balances in the laboratory are produced by the Changshu Bailing Company. They are accurate to ± 0.1 mg and have a maximum capacity of 100 g.

3. Procedure for Obtaining the Mass of an Object

Using analytical instrumentation correctly requires practice. This exercise will give you the opportunity to develop confidence in your weighing skills.

(1) Check the zero load before and after each weighing.

(2) Determine the mass of a clean and dry weighing bottle (without lid) to within $+0.1$ mg.

CAUTION: Do not handle the glassware with your fingers (or thumbs or toes) unless otherwise instructed.

(3) Determine the mass of the weighing bottle lid to within $+0.1$ mg.

(4) Determine the total mass of the weighing bottle plus lid to within $+0.1$ mg.

(5) Repeat steps (2) to (4) at least two more times to demonstrate the reproducibility of these measurements.

(6) Make sure you have recorded all your data in your laboratory notebook. Compare the sum of the mass of the weighing bottle and lid determined separately with the mass of the lid and bottle determined together. Explain any discrepancies between the masses that you find. Suggest using a value that is most likely to be closest to the "real true mass" in your data for this series of experiments.

4. Weighing Out Samples and Using Weighing Bottles

Weighing bottles are small glass bottles with ground glass tops. Weighing bottles are to be used only for drying, storing, and weighing solid standards and unknowns. Weighing bottles should be numbered in pencil on the ground glass surface. Samples to be dried are placed in the weighing bottle without the stopper and placed in a beaker with a watch glass cover and a piece of paper with your name. This entire apparatus is then placed in the oven for the specified time. Upon removal from the oven, the weighing bottle is allowed to cool until it can be easily handled and then transferred to the desiccator. The weighing bottle should not be inserted until the bottle has come to room temperature in the desiccator.

The best way to manipulate the weighing bottle is to use a band of dry paper pulled firmly around the bottle (Figure 1-26). Do not use your fingers directly on the weighing bottle as the moisture from your fingers will affect the mass. If the weighing bottle stands for several hours in the desiccator before taking the next sample, its mass should be rechecked.

Figure 1-26   The use of weighing bottle

5. Weighing by Addition

Samples can be added to a clean and dry container, often a weighing boat, which has been previously weighed or tared on the balance. Extreme care must be taken when samples are transferred from this container to insure that no material is lost. Normally, the solvent should be used to wash any residue from the boat into the container at the end of the transfer. Steps in weighing by addition are as follows.

(1) Check to ensure that the horizontal position of the balance is level. Each balance is equipped with a level indicator. If not level, ask an instructor to adjust it.

(2) Clean the balance pan with a brush.

(3) Place a weighing boat, small beaker may also be used, on the center of the balance pan and be sure to close the balance doors.

(4) Tare the balance and wait until it reads 0.000 0 g.

(5) Remove the weighing boat from the balance. Gently add solid sample to the weighing boat. Never add reagent while the weighing boat is in the balance!

(6) Return the weighing boat to the balance and close the balance doors. Record the mass to the nearest 0.1 mg (i. e., four places after the decimal).

(7) Remove the weighing boat and sample. Transfer the sample to the appropriate container.

6. Weighing by Difference

The preferred method is known as weighing by difference. Determine the amount of solid you wish to weigh first. This is called the target value. Your task is to hit this target value within about 10%, then record the mass to the nearest 0.000 1 g. With practice you can learn to "tap" the solid from your weighing bottle into the flask or beaker outside the balance (Figure 1-26). Start by tapping less than the amount you will need. Reweigh the weighing bottle and calculate the mass transferred by subtracting the previous mass. Estimate how much more solid you will need to add to reach the target value. Tap in a bit less than that amount, and calculate the new mass transferred. If necessary, do a third tap. With practice you can hit your value (plus or minus 10%) in three tries. Don't waste time trying to hit your target value exactly.

This technique is useful when several duplicate masses of a material must be weighed out. Steps in weighing by difference are as follows.

(1) Check to ensure that the horizontal position of the balance is level. Each balance is equipped with a level indicator. If not level, ask an instructor to adjust it.

(2) Clean the balance pan with a brush.

(3) Place a weighing bottle on the center of the balance pan and be sure to close the balance doors.

(4) Tare the balance and wait until it reads 0.000 0 g.

(5) Remove the weighing bottle from the balance. Place 1 g to 4 g of the

material to be measured into the weighing bottle. Never add reagent while the weighing bottle is in the balance!

(6) Return the weighing bottle to the balance and close the balance doors. Record the mass to the nearest 0. 1 mg (i. e. , four places after the decimal).

(7) Carefully remove some material from the weighing bottle and place it in an appropriate container. Reweigh the weighing bottle. The difference between the original mass and the final mass is equal to the mass of sample taken. Repeat as necessary.

Chapter 4   Basic Operation of Volumetric Glassware

The apparatus for the precise measurement of volume are burets, pipets and volumetric flasks.

I Buret

A buret is a common piece of equipment used to deliver known volumes of liquids. It is a slender glass tube of uniform bore with graduation marks along its length. A 50 mL buret usually has the milliliter marks numbered, with unnumbered 0.1 mL subdivisions in between. To obtain maximum precision, volumes are estimated to 0. 01 mL.

Two kinds of burets are illustrated in Figure 1-27. Geiser buret for use with stopcock is useful for acid solutions or oxidation solutions, and Mohr buret for use with pinchcock is useful for basic solutions.

1. Cleaning a Buret

A scrupulously cleaned buret is one that drains smoothly to leave an unbroken invisible film of liquid on its walls, droplets indicate dirty walls and a buret unfit for accurate work. Cleaning is best accomplished by the use of liquid detergent solution and scrubbing with a buret brush with a long wire handle.

Either chromic acid or alkaline permanganate can be used; the latter reagent is generally preferred, but it must be used to be hot (near the boiling point) and repeatedly. To clean a buret, turn it upside down and immerse it in the boiling alkaline permanganate in a beaker. Suck up the permanganate into the buret by placing a rubber pipet bulb over the tip. To retain the solution in the buret simply close the stopcock (Figure 1-28). Let the solution stand until cool, drain and wash

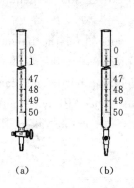

Figure 1-27　Buret

(a) Geiser buret;

(b) Mohr buret for use with pinchcock

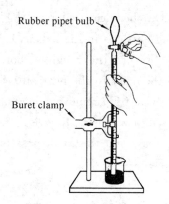

Figure 1-28　Cleaning buret with

cleaning solution

the buret thoroughly with tap water and then with distilled water.

In cleaning a Mohr buret, remove the glass bead inside the rubber tube, replace the rubber tube, and suck the cleaning solution into the buret by placing a rubber pipet bulb over the tip of the buret which has been inverted and immersed in the hot alkaline permanganate. To retain the solution in the buret, place a pinch cock on the rubber tubing. Do not suck the cleaning solution up into the rubber tubing.

2. Cleaning and Lubricating a Stopcock

A buret stopcock must be regreased after the buret is cleaned. The technique for cleaning and lubricating a stopcock is demonstrated in Figure 1-29.

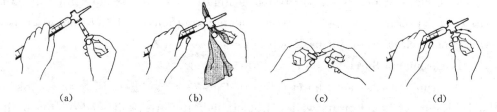

Figure 1-29　Cleaning and lubricating a stopcock

(a) Removing stopcock; (b) Cleaning plug; (c) Lubricating stopcock; (d) Oscillating plug

(1) Remove stopcock.

(2) Remove all old grease. Clean and dry the plug also.

(3) Apply a thin film of stopcock grease to the plug on each side of the bore.

(4) Distribute the grease by oscillating the plug slightly, making sure that there is a uniform film of grease over all the stopcock.

If there is grease in the buret tip, fill the buret with water, open the valve and lower the tip into the beaker of hot water. Do not use a shortcut method of heating the tip with a match.

3. Checking a Buret for Leakage

To check your buret for leakage, clamp your buret on a buret stand and fill it to above the "0" mark with distilled water. After eliminating any air bubbles from the tip, lower the meniscus to approximately "0" mark or a bit below. Let the buret stand for 5 min. If the meniscus drops, the stopcock leaks and it must be adjusted or replaced.

4. Filling a Buret

Before it is filled, the buret should always be rinsed three or more times with small portions of the solution to be filled. Rinse the buret with the solution to be used by taking a portion of about 5 mL from a beaker or flask (not a large reagent bottle), pouring it into the buret, tilting the buret horizontal and rocking and rotating it until all its walls have been washed. Then turn the buret upright and let the solution drain through the tip (not the open end). Repeat rinsing, and then fill the buret with solution above the "0" mark. Last, open the stopcock or pinchcock and shake the buret to remove any air that may be trapped in the tip. If you are using a pinchcock-type buret, a good way to remove air is to aim the tip upward and to allow a little liquid to flow through (Figure 1-30). Air being less dense that the liquid should flow out before the liquid does. If you are using a stopcock-type buret, a good way to remove air is to use a rubber pipet bulb to exert pressure on the liquid and to increase the rate of flow. Adjust the solution level until it is at or below the "0" mark. Clamp the buret with a buret clamp.

5. Reading a Buret

Water will wet a clean glass surface, the top surface of a water column in a glass cylinder is a concave-upward meniscus. Two readings are necessary to measure a dispensed volume. If both readings are made in a consistent fashion, volumes can be measured to ± 0.02 mL with a 50 mL buret. To make a reading, place a white paper with a black band just below the curved meniscus (a match box or even a finger can serve this purpose). Sight along a line horizontal with the meniscus, you should see the white paper directly behind the meniscus and the black surface reflected in the curved meniscus itself. In this way the meniscus is clearly outlined and the liquid level can be read along its flat bottom surface (Figure 1-31). Repeat this technique every time you read a buret, always remember to sight along a horizontal line. Always record readings to ± 0.01 mL, if the meniscus is at 7 mL, record it as 7.00 mL, not 7 mL.

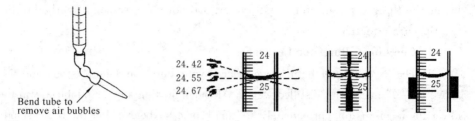

Bend tube to
remove air bubbles

24.42
24.55
24.67

Figure 1-30　Removing air bubbles　　　　　　Figure 1-31　Reading a buret

The buret tip should be handled in the same way as the pipet tip. It should be wiped with a tissue; then, after a bit of liquid is withdrawn, it should be touched to some wet glass surface before the initial reading is taken or before a measured volume is withdrawn. After the desired volume is withdrawn, the tip should again be touched to the wet receiver wall before the final buret reading is taken.

6. Titration

The most satisfactory method of manipulating the rate of delivery from a buret is to use the left hand to turn the stopcock (this is assuming you are right-handed), the right hand is used to swirl the titration flask. With the scale of the buret facing the operator, the handle of the stopcock is on the operator's right. With the base of the left hand to the left of the buret, the thumb and first two fingers encircle the buret to control the handle of the plug, and the last two fingers against the left of the tip. This braced position of the hand leads to maximum control of the stopcock. It also makes it possible to keep constant pull on the plug into a secure position in the seat (this technique was developed for glass stopcocks to keep the stopcock from being pulled out). This is essential with glass stopcocks to avoid leakage. Although this technique may seem awkward at first, a little practice will remove the strangeness and you will find you can titrate more rapidly than other procedures. The technique for titrating with a Geiser buret is shown in Figure 1-32(a).

In the following discussion, we shall assume that you have followed the instructions in the preceding section for rinsing, filling, and preparing the buret for use. After recording the initial buret reading to the nearest 0.01 mL, the titrant may be added rapidly at first to the titration vessel (usually an Erlenmeyer flask). Remember a buret cannot be drained too rapidly or too much liquid will adhere to the walls—a rate of 0.2 mL $\cdot$ s^{-1} is satisfactory. The technique for titrating with a Mohr buret is shown in Figure 1-32 (b). Using the right hand to swirl the flask and the left hand to control the buret, pinch tube just above bead to release liquid, and add liquid at a rapid and uniform rate. Reaction in the localized region of mixing

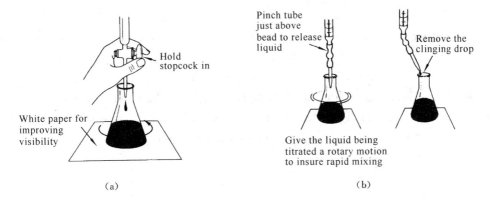

Figure 1-32 Titration

(a) Titrating with a Geiser buret; (b) Titrating with a Mohr buret

produces an indicator change. The addition of the titrant is periodically stopped and the rapidity with which the indicator returns to its color in the first solution is observed. Using this as a guide, the addition of the titrant is continued at a gradually decreasing rate. The tip of the buret and the walls of the flask are washed down with a small volume of distilled water from the wash bottle. The process of addition and rinsing is continued until the end has been located within a drop or within a partial drop. After a suitable drainage period, the buret is read.

Near the end of the titration, the rate of addition should be decreased until the titrant is being added drop by drop. Very near the endpoint partial drops of titrant can be added in several ways (a typical drop is 0. 05 mL).

(1) Let part of a drop form on the tip of the buret and wash it into the flask with water from your wash bottle.

(2) Let a partial drop form on the tip and detach it by touching the tip to the inside surface of the flask. Then rinse the sides of the flask with the wash bottle.

(3) Very rapidly flip the buret stopcock through 180°. This will deliver a partial drop directly into the flask. This technique should be practised before the endpoint is reached, for the speed of the flip determines the volume of titrant added.

When the endpoint is first observed, the walls of the flask should be rinsed with a stream of distilled water from a wash bottle. If necessary, additional partial drops of the titrant should then be added.

Ⅱ Pipet

The transfer and accurate measurement of relatively small volumes of liquids are often carried out by means of pipets. Two kinds of pipets are illustrated in

Figure 1-33. The ungraduated form is called a "volumetric" or "transfer" pipet, and the other is called a "graduated" pipet or Mohr measuring pipet. The use of a volumetric pipet will be described. A volumetric pipet has a single calibration mark and delivers the volume printed on the bulb of the pipet at the temperature specified (a graduated pipet has calibrations along the length of the pipet). Volumes can be measured more accurately with a volumetric pipet than with a graduated pipet. The techniques of handling them may be summarized as follows.

(a)   (b)

Figure 1-33   Pipets

(a) Transfer pipet;(b) Mohr measuring pipet

The pipet should be clean and rinsed three times with the liquid to be pipeted. The liquid to be pipeted is sucked into a clean pipet by means of a rubber pipet bulb, not by mouth. A right-handed person should hold the upper end of the pipet in the right hand between the thumb and other fingers, leaving the index finger free (Figure 1-34 (a)). The rubber pipet bulb should be held in the left hand and compressed before connecting it to the upper end of the pipet, and the connection should be just secure enough so as to avoid air leakage (Figure 1-34 (b)). The tip of the pipet should be placed below the surface of the liquid to be dispensed. As soon as the liquid level rises to a bit above the desired graduation mark, the bulb is slipped off to one side and the end of the index finger is quickly placed over the end of the pipet (Figure 1-34 (c)). The tip of the pipet is withdrawn from the supply of liquid and the outside of the lower stem is wiped dry with a cleaning tissue. Pressure from the index finger is relieved slightly to permit the liquid meniscus to descend to the desired graduation mark, and then increased again so as to hold the liquid at this position. Persons with very dry skin may have a difficult time holding the meniscus at a fixed position unless they first moisten the index finger. When the meniscus is at the mark, the pipet tip is touched to a wet glass wall of

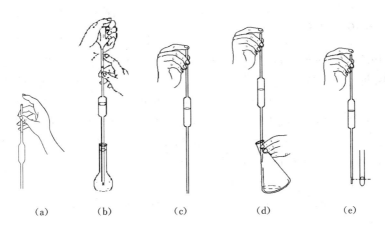

(a)   (b)   (c)   (d)   (e)

Figure **1-34**   Operation of a pipet

something like a beaker in order to detach the drop or partial drop of liquid held there. The filled pipet with its carefully adjusted meniscus must not be subjected to sudden, jerky motions that may result in loss of some of the liquid from the tip. When using the volumetric pipet, the full contents of the pipet are allowed to flow into the desired container. After waiting a few seconds for draining, the pipet tip is touched to the wet container wall to remove the drop or partial drop held there and in the capillary end of the pipet (Figure 1-34 (d)). Do not blow out the remaining liquid, the small amount that stays behind is reproducible and has been allowed for in the calibration of the pipet (Figure 1-34 (e)). A left-handed person should hold the pipet in the left hand and the bulb in the right. Because it seriously hampers control of the pipet, you should not control the flow of liquid from the pipet by means of your thumb. When the liquid drains from the walls of the pipet, there should be left a continuous invisible film of liquid, not droplets. If droplets appear, the pipet must be cleaned before use with liquid detergent solution followed by copious rinsing, first with tap water and then with distilled water.

When using the graduated pipet, the handling techniques are the same as for the volumetric pipet except that instead of draining the entire contents, the meniscus is allowed to drop only to the desired level. The partial drop hanging at the tip is also removed as before. For reproducibly accurate work, the pipet must not be drained too fast; minimums of 20 s for a 10 mL pipet and 30 s for a 50 mL pipet are recommended. Pipets which meet the standards set by the National Bureau of Standards will have errors that do not exceed 0. 02 mL for a 10 mL pipet or 0. 03 mL for a 25 mL pipet.

Ⅲ Volumetric Flask

A volumetric flask is commonly used in the preparation of chemical solutions. Because it has a narrow and clearly-marked neck, it is possible to fill it in a reproducible way and minimize the error of measurement. When the flask is filled, the bottom of the meniscus (the curved line of the water surface) should appear to lie in the plane that passes through the circular line etched on the neck of the flask. The eyes of the observer must be in this same plane. The error that results when the eyes are above or below this plane is called parallax error. The close-fitting stopper prevents evaporation and permits the vigorous shaking needed for good mixing in the preparation of solutions.

As with other volumetric ware, the walls must be scrupulously cleaned so that no drops will cling to the neck above the mark. Care must also be taken to insure that no significant amount of liquid is trapped by the stopper. During the filling process, the flask should be held only by the neck above the mark, otherwise the heat of your hand will raise the temperature of the liquid which will expand and fill the flask with less liquid than is required at room temperature. Volumetric flasks should never be placed on a flame or hot plate to dissolve a solute. This can cause permanent changes in the volume of the flask.

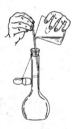

Figure 1-35　Transferring the solution

If a solute is difficult to dissolve, carry out the dissolution in a beaker or a flask and then quantitatively transfer the solution to the volumetric flask by the stirring rod (Figure 1-35). Solvent is added until the bulb of the flask is about three-quarters filled and a uniform solution is obtained by swinging the flask in a small circle to promote swirling of the liquid without bringing it into the neck. Mixing at this time allows volume changes which accompany dilution to take place before the solution is made up to volume. Solvent is now added to bring the solution to the calibration mark. The last few drops may be added with a medicine dropper. After the final dilution, remember to mix your solution thoroughly, by inverting the flask and shaking. Since a uniform solution has been prepared, solution that is now removed on the stopper in no way changes the concentration of the solution.

According to the minimum standards set by the National Institute of Standards and Technology, a first-class 50 mL flask should be in error by no more than 0. 05 mL; a 250 mL flask by no more than 0. 12 mL. For very accurate work, the volumetric flask should be calibrated so that a suitable correction can be made. In any case, it is important to realize that the volumetric flask will contain the volume for which it is marked, not deliver it.

Chapter 5   pH Meter

I Principles of Operation

One of the most common instruments in any laboratory is the pH meter. The pH meter consists of a voltaic cell and a device to measure the EMF (electromotive force) derived from the cell. The EMF is dependent upon the concentration of hydrogen ions in the solution. Therefore the pH meter allows us to measure the hydrogen ion concentration indirectly by measuring the EMF produced by the pH-sensitive cell.

The cell is a combination of two half-cells as shown in Figure 1-36. The overall cell can be represented as

Ag, AgCl | Cl$^-$ | glass | H$^+$ (variable) ∥ Cl$^-$ (saturated) | Hg$_2$Cl$_2$(s), Hg, Pt

One half-cell consists of a reference electrode designed to give a constant potential regardless of the hydrogen ion concentration. The other half-cell consists of the measuring electrode and the sample solution into which it dips. The EMF of the measuring electrode is dependent on the pH. Electrical contact between two cells is provided by a fiber plug (this serves the same purpose as a salt bridge) in the reference electrode.

A calomel electrode is commonly used as the reference electrode (Figure 1-36 (b)). The half-cell reaction is

$$Hg_2Cl_2(s) + 2e^- \rightleftharpoons 2Hg(l) + 2Cl^-$$

(Constant concentration present from saturated KCl solution)

$$\varphi_{SCE} = \varphi^\ominus - 0.059\ 16 \lg [Cl^-] = 0.241\ 2\ V$$

Hg$_2$Cl$_2$ and mercury metal are placed in the inner tube of the electrode, and the inner tube is in contact with the surrounding solution of chloride ions (Cl$^-$). A constant [Cl$^-$] is maintained by filling the electrode with a saturated solution of

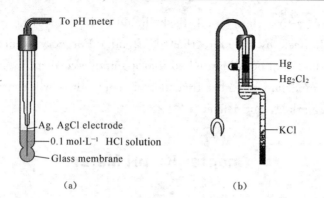

Figure 1-36   Electrodes for a pH meter

(a) Glass measuring electrode; (b) Calomel reference electrode

KCl. A few crystals of solid KCl keep the solution saturated. Because the concentrations of all species involved in the half-cell reaction are constant (provided that the temperature does not change), the EMF value of the half-cell remains constant.

The pH-measuring electrode is called a glass electrode (Figure 1-36 (a)). What at the end of this electrode is a thin bulb made of special glass membrane which develops a potential if the $[H^+]$ is different in solutions contacting the two sides of the glass. The mechanism responsible for this potential is complicated and we don't need concern here. The application of the Nernst equation to the half-reaction has the form:

$$\varphi_G = \varphi_G^\ominus + \frac{2.303RT}{F} \lg \frac{[H^+]_{outside}(variable)}{[H^+]_{inside}(constant)} = \varphi_G^\ominus - 0.05916 pH_x$$

If the bulb of the glass electrode is filled with a solution of HCl, the $[H^+]$ inside, cannot change. The internal electrode of the glass electrode assembly is a silver-silver chloride electrode whose potential likewise does not change. The overall cell voltage then only depends on the $[H^+]$ in the unknown solution:

$$E_{obs} = \varphi_{SCE} - \varphi_G = \varphi_{SCE} - \varphi_G^\ominus + \frac{2.303RT}{F} pH_x = E^* + \frac{2.303RT}{F} pH_x$$

In this form of the Nernst equation, we have used the symbol E^* to indicate a constant term, the value of which will depend upon the constant conditions of the particular electrode assembly. The equation shows that E_{obs} depends directly on the pH of the solution. The scale of the meter can be marked in volts or directly in pH units. Calibration of the meter is accomplished by dipping the electrode assembly into a standard solution of known pH and adjusting the circuit to make the meter reading agree with the known pH of the solution.

II Details of Operation

1. pH Meter PB-10 Setup

The setup of pH meter PB-10 is shown in Figure 1-37.

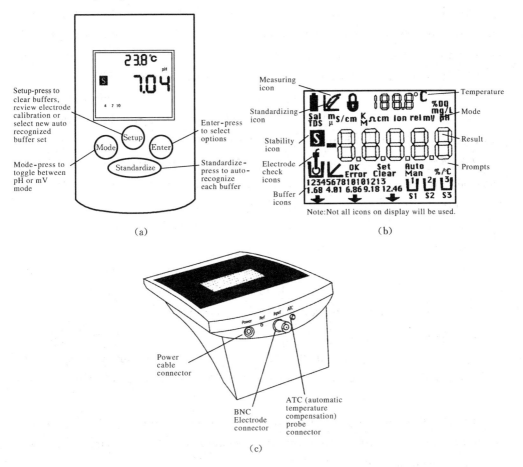

Figure **1-37**   pH meter PB-10

(a) Front panel controls; (b) Digital display; (c) Rear panel connectors

2. Digital pH Meter Operating Instructions

(1) Connect power cable to meter power jack and to AC power source.

(2) Remove the shorting cap on the BNC connector. Install the combination glass pH/ATC electrode by plugging it into the input connection (push on and twist to lock) and the ATC connector into the ATC jack.

(3) Press the Mode button to select pH.

(4) Press the Setup button, and then press the Enter button to clear the existing standardization.

(5) Press the Setup button, and then press the Enter button to select a new set of buffers "1. 68 4. 01 6. 86 9. 18 12. 46".

(6) Remove the electrode from the bottle of storage solution. Rinse with distilled water. Blot dry electrode (do not wipe). Immerse the electrode in pH 6. 86 buffer. Swirl the solution to fully saturate the electrode with buffer. Allow the electrode to reach a stable value and the digital display indicates "S".

(7) Press the Standardize button. The meter recognizes the buffer and flashes a buffer icon. When the signal is stable, or when you press the Enter button, the buffer is entered and the digital display indicates "6. 86".

(8) Remove the electrode from the pH 6. 86 buffer, rinse and blot dry the electrode. Immerse the electrode in the pH 4. 01 buffer and swirl. Press the Standardize button again to calibrate with this buffer. The meter will display a calibration slope and the two buffer icons, "4. 01 6. 86", and then return to the measure screen.

(9) Now the meter should be calibrated and ready to use for measuring the pH of any solution. Immerse the electrode in the solution to be measured, stir, allow time for the electrode to stabilize, and record the display.

3. Notes

(1) Before first use of your glass electrode, or whenever the electrode is dry, soak over night in an electrode filling solution, KCl solution or electrode storage solution.

(2) Rinse and blot dry the electrode between each measurement (do not wipe). Rinse the electrode with distilled water or deionized water, or part of the next solution to be measured.

(3) The pH meter allows automatic standardization using up to three buffers. When you enter a fourth buffer, the buffer farthest away is replaced by the pH of new buffer.

(4) The pH meter performs automatic temperature compensation. If an ATC probe is used, the meter continually adjusts for temperature. Therefore, buffers may vary slightly from the nominal values because of temperature. Default temperature is 25 ℃.

Chapter 6　Instructions for 723N Spectrophotometer

Ⅰ Principles of Operation

Incident radiation of radiant power I_0 passes through a solution of an absorbing species at concentration c and path length b, and the transmitted radiation has radiant power I. This radiant power is the quantity measured by spectrometric detectors. Bouguer in 1729 and Lambert in 1760 recognized that when electromagnetic energy is absorbed, the power of the transmitted energy decreases geometrically (exponentially). Since the fraction of radiant energy transmitted decays exponentially with path length, we can write it in exponential form:

$$T=\frac{I}{I_0}=10^{-abc}$$

It is more convenient to omit the negative sign on the right-hand side of the equation and to define a new term:

$$A=-\lg T=\lg\frac{I_0}{I}=abc$$

where A is the absorbance. This is the common form of Lambert-Beer's law. Note that it is the absorbance that is directly proportional to the concentration. The path length b is expressed in centimeters and the concentration c in grams per liter. The constant a is called the absorptivity and is dependent on the wavelength and the nature of the absorbing material. In an absorption spectrum, the absorbance varies with wavelength in direct proportion to a (b and c are constants). The product of the absorptivity and the molecular weight of the absorbing species is called the molar absorptivity ε. Thus,

$$A=\varepsilon bc$$

where c is now in moles per liter.

Ⅱ Details of Operation

1. 723N Spectrophotometer Setup

723N spectrophotometer (Figure 1-38) measures the amount of visible light absorbed by a colored solution. It boasts a 320 nm to 1 100 nm visible range, a 2 nm bandwidth, absorbance, transmittance, concentration, and factor modes, and an easy-to-read LED.

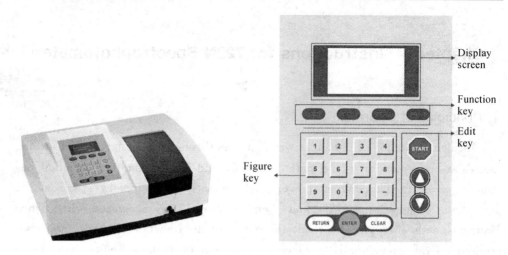

Figure 1-38   723N spectrophotometer

2. 723N Spectrophotometer Operating Instructions

(1) Check that the instrument is turned on. Allow 20 min for warming up after the instrument-self check.

(2) Obtain a cuvette. Make sure it is clean inside and out. Rinse the cuvette in with small amounts of the blank. Then fill the cuvette about three-quarters full. Dry the outside of the cuvette carefully, and insert it into the sample compartment with its transparent sides aligned with the light path. Close the cover.

(3) Set the measurement mode: Press "set" key, and then press "up or down (∧ or ∨)" key to select the mode as "photometric mode", finally press "enter" key to confirm.

(4) Set wavelength: Press "Go λ" key, and then press "number" key to enter the wavelength, finally press "enter" key to confirm.

(5) Calibration blank: Place the "reference solution (blank)" cuvette in the light path, and press "zero" key to calibrate 0.000Abs/100.0%T.

(6) To analyze your sample, insert sample cuvette and read the absorbance value on the LED.

(7) Turn off the instrument when finished.

3. Notes

(1) Sample cuvettes have two opposite sides that are cloudy and two opposite sides that are transparent, for the light to pass through. Place your cuvette in the sample compartment, with the transparent sides aligned with the light path.

(2) Never touch the transparent sides of the cuvette, since this will disrupt the

path of the light beam.

(3) Rinse the cuvette thoroughly with distilled water and then with the liquid to be filled.

Chapter 7   Evaluation of Experimental Data

I Uncertainty in Measurement: Significant Figures

1. Types of Errors

Because of the limitation of the measuring device and the limited power of observation of the individual making the measurement, every measurement carries a degree of uncertainty or error. Even when very elaborate measuring devices are used, some degree of uncertainty is always present.

Any measurement has an associated uncertainty that we call "error", which means the difference between the true value and the observed or calculated value. Errors that can be determined and eliminated are called determinate or systematic errors. The second class of errors includes the indeterminate errors, often called accidental or random errors, which affect the distribution of measurements around a central value.

(1) Determinate errors.

Errors affecting the accuracy of an analysis are called determinate errors and are characterized by a systematic deviation from the true value; that is, all the individual measurements are either too large or too small. A positive determinate error results in a central value that is larger than the true value, and a negative determinate error leads to a central value that is smaller than the true value. Both positive and negative determinate errors may affect the result of an analysis, with their cumulative effect leading to a net positive or negative determinate error. It is possible, although not likely, that positive and negative determinate errors may be equal, resulting in a central value with no net determinate error.

Determinate errors may be divided into four categories: instrumental errors, operative errors, method errors, and measurement errors.

Systematic errors can be avoided, or at least taken into account, through calibration of the measuring device, that is, by comparing it with a known standard.

(2) Indeterminate errors.

Indeterminate errors do not affect the accuracy of an analysis (random errors affect the precision of a measurement). These errors are revealed by small differences in successive measurements made by the same analyst under virtually identical conditions, and they cannot be predicted or estimated. These accidental errors will follow a random distribution; therefore, mathematical laws of probability can be applied to arrive at some conclusion regarding the most probable result of a series of measurements. It is apparent that there should be few very large errors; there should be an equal number of positive and negative errors; and small errors occur much more frequently than large errors.

Random errors are always present, cannot be corrected. These errors can be reduced by taking more measurements.

2. Precision and Accuracy

Realizing that our data for the measurement can be characterized by a measure of central tendency and a measure of spread suggests two questions. First, does our measure of central tendency agree with the true, or expected value? Second, why are our data scattered around the central value? Errors associated with central tendency reflect the accuracy of the analysis, but the precision of the analysis is determined by those errors associated with the spread.

(1) Accuracy.

The term accuracy describes the nearness of an experimental value (X_i) or a mean ($\overline{X}$) to the ture value (μ). It is usually expressed as either an absolute error

$$E = X_i - \mu \quad \text{or} \quad \overline{X} - \mu$$

or a percent relative error (E_r)

$$E_r = \frac{E}{\mu} \times 100\%$$

The mean, $\overline{X}$, is obtained by dividing the sum of the individual measurements by the number of measurements:

$$\overline{X} = \frac{X_1 + X_2 + X_3 + \cdots + X_n}{n} = \frac{\sum_{i=1}^{n} X_i}{n}$$

where X_1, X_2, X_3, $\cdots$, X_n are the individual values, n is the number of values, and $\sum_{i=1}^{n} X_i$ is the sum of values of X_i.

(2) Precision.

Precision, a term often mistakenly used in place of accuracy, refers to the agreement between values in a set of data. The fact that the values of replicate measurements all agree well does not necessarily mean that they are close to the true value. Precision may be expressed as the average deviation, or the standard deviation.

The average deviation $(\overline{d})$ is found by summing the individual deviations and dividing by the number of measurements. Thus the average deviation from the mean is given by

$$\overline{d} = \frac{|X_1 - \overline{X}| + |X_2 - \overline{X}| + |X_3 - \overline{X}| + \cdots + |X_n - \overline{X}|}{n}$$

$$= \frac{|d_1| + |d_2| + |d_3| + \cdots + |d_n|}{n} = \frac{\sum\limits_{i=1}^{n} |X_i - \overline{X}|}{n}$$

where $d_1, d_2, d_3, \cdots, d_n$ are the individual deviations.

Historically, average deviation has been used extensively as a measure of precision, but it is not preferred, primarily because, unlike other estimates of precision, it is not statistically interpretable and it gives equal weight to large and small deviations, which are not equally probable.

The standard deviation (s) or the root-mean-square deviation as it is sometimes called, is the preferred measure of precision and is calculated from the equation.

$$s = \sqrt{\frac{\sum\limits_{i=1}^{n} (X_i - \overline{X})^2}{n-1}}$$

where X_i is one of individual values, and $\overline{X}$ is the mean.

Both average and standard deviations can also be expressed in relative terms to facilitate comparison between data sets:

Relative average deviation $\overline{d}_r = \dfrac{\overline{d}}{\overline{X}} \times 100\%$

Relative standard deviation $s_r = \dfrac{s}{\overline{X}} \times 100\%$

(3) Proper use of accuracy and precision.

The terms "accuracy" and "precision" often are used incorrectly, by interchanging their meanings. Errors and deviations, the respective measures of accuracy and precision, are not always numerically related to one another. That is, the precision of the data in a set can be excellent while the overall accuracy is terrible. Examine the rifle targets in Figure 1-39 and assume that the holes (marked by "×") are equivalent to individual values and the bull's-eye is the true value. Target in Figure 1-39 (a) represents good precision (holes close to each other) and good accuracy (holes close to true value), while target (b) represents good precision but poor accuracy. The precision in target (c) is poor because the individual holes are not close to each other but the accuracy of the mean is good. Both the precision and the accuracy are poor in target (d). The reasons for the different distributions and placements of shots in these targets are impotent because they indicate whether a numerical relationship exists between the accuracy and the precision and how the accuracy may be improved.

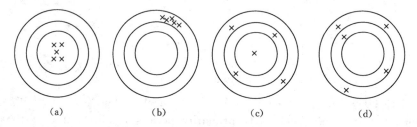

(a)　　　　　　(b)　　　　　　(c)　　　　　　(d)

Figure 1-39　Targets illustrating the differences between accuracy and precision

(a) Good precision and good accuracy; (b) Good precision but poor accuracy;

(c) Good accuracy but poor precision; (d) Poor precision and poor accuracy

3. Significant Figures

Because measurements are never exact, two types of information must be conveyed whenever a numerical value for a measurement is recorded: the magnitude of the measurement and the precision or uncertainty of the measurement. The magnitude is indicated by the digit values. The precision is indicated by the number of significant figures recorded. Significant figures are the digits in any measurement that are known with certainty plus one digit that is uncertain. The number of significant figures in a measurement depends upon the measuring device.

(1) Guidelines for determining significant figures.

① In any measurement, all nonzero digits are significant.

② Zeros may or may not be significant because zeros can be used in two ways: to position a decimal point, and to indicate a measured value. Zeros that are to position a decimal point are not significant, and zeros that are to indicate a measured value are significant. When zeros are present in a measured number, we follow these rules.

A. Leading zeros, those at the beginning of a number, are never significant.

0. 014 1 has three significant figures.

0. 000 000 004 8 has two significant figures.

B. Confined zeros, those between nonzero digits, are always significant.

3. 063 has four significant figures.

0. 001 004 has four significant figures.

C. Trailing zeros, those at the end of a number, are significant if a decimal point is present in the number.

56. 00 has four significant figures.

0. 050 50 has four significant figures.

D. Trailing zeros, those at the end of a number, are not significant if the number lacks an explicitly shown decimal point.

59 000 000 has two significant figures.

6 010 has three significant figures.

③ Exact numbers. Some numbers are called exact numbers because they have no uncertainty associated with them. Some exact numbers are part of a unit definition: there are 60 minutes in 1 hour, 1 000 micrograms in 1 milligram, and 2. 54 centimeters in 1 inch. Other exact numbers result from actually counting individual items: there are exactly 3 quarters in my hand, 26 letters in the English alphabet, and so forth. Since they have no uncertainty, exact numbers do not limit the number of significant figures in the answer. Put another way, exact numbers have as many significant figures as a calculation requires.

(2) Significant figures and mathematical operations.

When measurements are added, subtracted, multiplied, or divided, consideration must be given to the number of significant figures in the computed result.

① Rounding off numbers.

Rounding off is the process of deleting unwanted (nonsignificant) digits from calculated numbers. There are three rules for rounding off numbers.

A. If the digit removed is more than 5, the preceding number is increased by 1: 5. 379 rounds to 5. 38 if three significant figures are retained and to 5. 4 if two significant figures are retained.

B. If the digit removed is less than 5, the preceding number is unchanged: 0. 241 3 rounds to 0. 241 if three significant figures are retained and to 0. 24 if two significant figures are retained.

C. If the digit removed is 5, the preceding number is increased by 1 if it is odd and remains unchanged if it is even: 17. 75 rounds to 17. 8, but 17. 65 rounds to 17. 6. If the 5 is followed only by zeros, rule C is followed; if the 5 is followed by nonzeros, rule A is followed: 17. 650 0 rounds to 17. 6, but 17. 651 3 rounds to 17. 7.

② Operational rules.

Significant-figure considerations in mathematical operations that involve measured numbers are governed by two rules, one for multiplication and division, and the other one for addition and subtraction.

A. In multiplication and division, the number of significant figures in the answer is the same as the number of significant figures in the measurement that contains the fewest significant figures. For example,

$$6. 038 \times 2. 57 = 15. 517 66 \quad \text{(calculator answer)}$$
$$= 15. 5 \quad \text{(correct answer)}$$

The calculator answer is rounded to three significant figures because the measurement with the fewest significant figures (2. 57) contains only three significant figures.

B. In addition and subtraction, the answer has no more digits to the right of the decimal point than are found in the measurement with the fewest digits to the right of the decimal point. For example,

$$
\begin{array}{r}
9. 333 \\
+1. 4 \\
\hline
\end{array}
$$

10. 733 (calculator answer)

10. 7 (correct answer)

The calculator answer is rounded to the tenths place because the uncertainty in the number 1. 4 is in the tenths place.

Note the contrast between the rules for multiplication and division and for addition and subtraction. In multiplication and division, significant figures are counted; in addition and subtraction, decimal places are counted. It is possible to gain or lose significant figures during addition or subtraction, but never during multiplication or division. In our previous sample addition problem, one of the input numbers (1. 4) has two significant figures and the correct answer (10. 7) has three significant figures. This is allowable in addition (and subtraction) because we are counting decimal places, not significant figures.

③ Logarithms and antilogarithms.

In changing from logarithms to antilogarithms, and vice versa, the number being operated on and the logarithm mantissa have the same number of significant figures. Suppose, for example, we wish to calculate the pH of a 2.0×10^{-3} mol · L^{-1} solution of HCl from pH $= -\lg [H^+]$. Then,

$$pH = -\lg(2.0 \times 10^{-3}) = -(-3 + 0.30) = 2.70$$

The -3 is the characteristic (from 10^{-3}), a pure number determined by the position of the decimal. The 0.30 is the mantissa for the logarithm of 2.0 and therefore has only two digits. So, even though we know the concentration to two significant figures, the pH (the logarithm) has three significant figures. If we wish to take the antilogarithm of a mantissa, the corresponding number will likewise have the same number of digits as the mantissa. The antilogarithm of 0.072 (contains three digits in mantissa .072) is 1.18, and the logarithm of 12.1 is 1.083 (1 is the characteristic, and the mantissa has three digits, .083).

Ⅱ Evaluation of Experimental Data

1. Tables

Large amounts of data that do not easily display in "figures" can be reported in tabular form. Tables should be numbered in the order in which they are cited in the text. Each table should be given a number, followed by a caption (legend) that appears above the table and gives the title of the table and clearly describes its content. Be sure to include the appropriate units in the table.

2. Graphs

Graphs are "figures" (Figure 1-40). Figures include a variety of illustrations such as diagrams, photographs and schematics. Like tables, they should be given

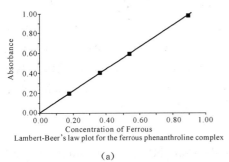

(a)

(b)

Figure 1-40 Sample graphs

numbers in their order of citation in the text. Do not include figures (or tables) that are not cited in the text of your report. The most important figure for introductory laboratory reports is the graph, which may offer an efficient way of displaying data, especially when you want to emphasize trends and patterns.

(1) Plotting. Usually there are two variables to be considered: ① the independent variable (e. g. , time or any variable that you change in order to change the result) is plotted on the x-axis (horizontal); ② the dependent variable (something that changes because of the change in the independent variable) is plotted on the y-axis (vertical). Plots can be done by hand or by computer. If you do a plot by hand, draw any straight lines with a straight-edge.

(2) Scale. For your scale use units for which interpolation is easy. For example, a scale from 0 to 10 would be conveniently broken down into 10 unit portions, or perhaps 20 one-half unit portions; a breakdown into 37 units each of 0. 270 3 would not be useful. The x-axis scale need not be the same as the y-axis. It is not necessary to start either scale from zero. For example, if your data points range between 22 and 78, your lower and upper limits will usually be 20 and 80, respectively. If the axis were extended from 0 to 100, part of your graph would be empty; and even worse, the data being communicated would be restricted to a smaller area and hence harder to interpret. When you set up your scale, be sure that the intervals between tick marks are identical.

(3) Legends. Each graph should have a descriptive legend located beneath the graph that clearly states what information the graph conveys.

(4) Labels. The axes should be clearly labeled and the units of measurement should be shown. Show a key to the special symbols (e. g. , ○, △, ◆, □, ★) that depict the different curves.

(5) Clarity. The simplest graph compatible with its objective is the most effective. The graph should be big enough to be easily interpreted. If appropriate, several curves can be drawn on the same graph; however, the points of each curve should be denoted by a unique symbol. Never plot a point that is not an actual data point without an important reason; if you do so, be sure that it is clearly labeled as "not a data point".

3. Creating Graphs with Excel

Open excel. In the spreadsheet, enter the data for the x-axis in column A, and the data for the y-axis in column B. Point to cell A_1 with the mouse, and then click and hold the mouse button down. Drag the pointer over your data to highlight these cells and release the mouse button. Point to the toolbar at the top of the screen and click on the icon that looks like a column chart. In the pop-up menu window that appears, choose XY (scatter) for the type of chart. Make sure the first chart sub-type at the right is selected (the one with no lines through the points); if not, select it by clicking on it. Click Next> at the bottom of the window. In the next pop-up window just click Next> at the bottom of the window. In the next pop-up window, enter the chart title, as well as the title for the x-axis and y-axis (don't forget units) in the appropriate fields. At the top of the window select the Gridlines tab. Remove check marks in all boxes by clicking on them. Click the Legend tab, and remove the check in the Show Legend box. Click Finish at the bottom of the window, and then the chart appears in your spreadsheet. To add a best fit line, point to any of your data points and click once, and they should all become highlighted. Go to the Chart menu at the top of the screen and choose Add Trendline... In the pop-up window that appears, choose the fit type you want for your data by clicking on it (usually Linear). Click on the Options tab. Near the bottom, click in the box next to Display equation on chart to place a check mark in it. Click OK at the bottom of the window. The graph is finished. Go to the File menu at the top of the page and choose Print... In the pop-up menu that appears, make sure the dot next to Selected Chart is filled in. If not, click on it. Click Print.

Ⅲ Laboratory Reports

Complete your laboratory reports as directed by your instructor. Work independently in performing calculations and in completing your laboratory reports, even if you collect data with a partner. A typical laboratory report includes four sections.

(1) A cover sheet with your name, section, course number, and instructor's name. Write the title of the experiment and a concise statement of the experimental objectives on the cover sheet; do not copy or paraphrase the text of the laboratory manual, but add any deviations from the procedures in the laboratory manual.

(2) Data sheets.

(3) Data interpretation: calculations, results, graphs, and so on. Include the conclusions you have drawn from the experiment. If interpretations of your results are called for (such as identification or explanation of a particular result or the error or uncertainty of a result), state and justify your interpretations. If appropriate, evaluate the experimental arrangement and make suggestions.

(4) Assigned problems or questions.

Submit your report at the next laboratory session, late reports will be penalized.

Laboratory reports are graded on the following bases.

(1) Clarity of statements of objectives, conclusions, interpretations, and suggestions. Use concise and declarative sentences in the active voice: Say "I observed ..." instead of "It was observed that ...".

(2) Neatness, completeness, and accuracy of data recording and calculating.

(3) Error treatment: significant figures, error estimations, uncertainty limits, quantitative discussion of uncertainties. Note: Misreading a balance, spilling a sample, and errors in calculation are not experimental errors but blunders. (Experimental error is the error which presents when careful techniques have been followed.)

(4) Complete references to any books or written procedures you have followed.

Part Two   Experiments in Basic Chemistry

Experiment 1   Measurements, Common Laboratory Techniques and Practices

I Learning Objectives

(1) Understand glassware and equipment.

(2) Learn the method of cleaning and drying laboratory glassware.

(3) Understand the meaning of "accuracy" and "precision".

(4) To apply significant digits.

II Principles

All glassware to be used in experiments must be cleaned before and after use. It is each student's responsibility to properly clean all glassware that she/he uses.

A common laboratory requirement is to clean glassware. If clean, the walls will retain an unbroken film of water, not droplets. This can usually be achieved most simply and safely by scrubbing the wet walls with some common commercial scouring powder and an appropriate brush, followed by rinsing with tap water and finally with distilled water. Never use scouring powder on glassware which is inaccessible to scrubbing such as the inside of a transfer pipet. For this type of glassware use a liquid detergent in place of the scouring powder. Occasionally, specific chemical deposits are completely unaffected by these general cleaning methods, but if the chemical nature of the deposit is known, a specific reagent may be selected for cleaning, ask your instructor for advice in this circumstance. CAUTION: The proper method for cleaning depends on what was in the glassware.

Wet glassware can be dried by methods as follows: ① placing it on the drying rack (or inverting on a paper towel); ② placing it in the drying oven (for items that are water-wet only, no flammable solvents); ③ rinsing with a solvent such as acetone, methanol or ethanol and then gently blowing compressed air into the vessel until it is dry. The first method is preferred for drying quantitatively clean glassware. Volumetric glassware and cuvettes are never to be placed in drying ovens, even if they are not quantitatively clean. The third method is acceptable only when the compressed air supply is known to be free oil and other contaminants.

Ⅲ Apparatus and Reagents

Geiser buret (50 mL×1), Mohr buret (50 mL×1), reagent bottles (white, 500 mL×2), reagent bottle (brown, 500 mL×1), glass-stopped bottles (250 mL ×3), Erlenmeyer flasks (250 mL×3, 50 mL×2), volumetric flasks (100 mL×2, 50 mL×5), beakers (500 mL×1, 300 mL×3, 100 mL×2, 50 mL×2, 10 mL× 5), transfer pipets (25 mL×1, 20 mL×1), Mohr measuring pipets (10 mL×1, 5 mL×1, 2 mL×1, 1 mL×1), graduated cylinder (100 mL×1), graduated cups (25 mL×1, 10 mL×1), dropping bottles (2), wash bottle, rubber pipet bulb, crucible (porcelain with cover), watch glass, stemmed funnels (9 cm, 7 cm), thermometer (−10 ℃ to 200 ℃), evaporating dish, Buchner funnel, filter flask, test tubes (4), wire gauze, stirring rod and medicine droppers (2).

Detergent, soap and distilled water.

Ⅳ Procedure

(1) A typical student desk contains an assortment of beakers, Erlenmeyer flasks, filter flasks, thermometers, graduated cylinders, test tubes, funnels, and a variety of other items. Your desk or drawer will probably have most, if not all, of the equipment items shown in desk equipment. Make sure all glassware is clean and has no chips or cracks. Replace damaged glassware.

(2) Cleaning options.

① Clean the glassware, e. g. , two tubes and a beaker, with soap or detergent. Rinse first with tap water and then with small amounts of distilled (or deionized) water once or twice.

② If necessary, rinse with acetone to remove water-insoluble materials.

(3) Drying options.

① Invert clean glassware on a paper towel to dry. (Air dry on a drying rack.)

② Remove excess water, and then place in the drying oven.

③ Hold carefully over a burner flame until it is dry.

④ Dry glassware with heat gun starting from the bottom.

V Questions

(1) How to tell if glassware is clean?

(2) Why should the tube be tilted when drying?

(3) Why couldn't the volume measurement apparatus be dried by heating?

Experiment 2   Determination of the Gas Constant

I Learning Objectives

(1) To experimentally determine the value of the gas constant, R.

(2) Illustrate the ideal gas equation and Dalton's law of partial pressures.

II Principles

From the ideal gas equation, $pV = nRT$, you can see that it is possible to determine the value for R if you can isolate a sample of gas for which P, V, T and n are all known. In this experiment, you will accomplish this by collecting hydrogen gas formed in the reaction of magnesium metal with hydrochloric acid. The equation is

$$\text{Mg (s)} + 2\text{HCl (aq)} = \text{MgCl}_2 \text{(aq)} + \text{H}_2 \text{(g)}$$

When you collect the hydrogen gas you will also measure the temperature, pressure and volume of the gas collected. From the data, the value for R can be calculated.

Since the hydrogen gas will be collected over water in a buret, it will be saturated with water vapor. According to Dalton's law, the total pressure of the gas mixture is the sum of the partial pressure of H_2 plus the partial pressure of the water vapor. The partial pressure of the water vapor can be looked up in tables in the CRC, and subtracted from the total pressure to find the pressure of the H_2. The volume of the gas will be measured directly from the buret (Figure 2-1).

Ⅲ Apparatus and Reagents

Analytical balance (0.1 mg), buret, latex tubing, ring stand, and funnel. HCl solution (2 mol • L^{-1}) and magnesium ribbon.

Ⅳ Procedure

(1) Cut a piece of magnesium ribbon weighing approximately 0.03 g. Record the exact mass in your notebook.

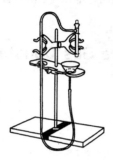

Figure 2-1   Experimental apparatus for determining the gas constant

(2) An apparatus should be set up as shown in Figure 2-1. Make sure the system is airtight. Record the level of the water in the buret (to two decimal places, as usual). The level should be at or below the zero mark.

(3) To test the apparatus for gas leaks, proceed as follows. With the stopper of the tube removed, lower the water level in the buret to near the bottom, insert the stopper tightly in the tube, and raise the funnel until the water level height difference in the buret and funnel is about "0" cm. Read the position of the meniscus in the buret and repeat this reading after 5 min. If the two readings differ by more than 2 mm and the temperature has remained constant, there is a leak that must be repaired. The leak test should then be repeated.

(4) For each sample proceed as follows: Fold the magnesium ribbon into a strip that will comfortably fit lengthwise into the mouth of the tube. Using a funnel, carefully add approximately 5 mL of 2 mol • L^{-1} HCl solution to the tube. Be sure not to spill any of the HCl solution, otherwise the reaction between the HCl and the magnesium will begin prematurely and you will have to start the experiment again. Carefully insert a stopper into the mouth of the tube. The leak test should then be repeated. Adjust the funnel so that the water level inside the buret is the same as the water level in the funnel, as shown in Figure 2-1. Record the water level in the buret to the nearest 0.1 mL. Make sure you are reading the scale correctly.

Start the reaction by tilting the tube so that the HCl sink toward the magnesium ribbon. Gently swirl the tube so that a complete reaction occurs. Hydrogen gas will be evolved and will be collected in the buret. This will cause the water level in the buret to fall. At the same time continually lower the funnel to follow the sinking level in the buret so as to minimize the effect of any potential leak. Continue to swirl the flask for at least 10 min, by which time the water level in the buret should have stabilized. Readjust the funnel, equalize the water levels in the buret and funnel and wait 5 min to 10 min to permit temperature equilibrium to establish itself. Record the final water level in the buret.

Record the room temperature. This should be the same as the temperature of the gas in the buret. Repeat the experiment two more times. Obtain the atmospheric pressure.

V Data

Items	I	II	III
$m(Mg)/g$			
T/K			
p/kPa			
$R = pV/(nT)$			
$\bar{R}$			
$\bar{d}_r/(\%)$			

Experiment 3   Determination of the Relative Molecular Weight of Solute by Freezing Point Depression

I Learning Objectives

(1) Determine the relative molecular weight by freezing point depression.

(2) Review the method of analytical balance weighing.

II Principles

Adding a nonvolatile solute to a solvent changes the properties of the solution. Compared to the pure solvent, the solution will have a lower freezing point and a higher boiling point. In this experiment you will investigate the phenomenon of freezing point depression and determine the relative molecular weight of an unknown solute. The relationship between the lowering of the freezing point and the concentration of a solution is given by the following:

$$\Delta T_f = T_f^0(\text{pure solvent}) - T_f(\text{solution}) = K_f b_B$$

where K_f is the molal freezing point depression constant (a property of a given solvent) and b_B is the molality of solute in the solution. Molality of a solute is defined as follows:

$$b_B = \text{moles of solute / mass of solvent(kg)}$$

Thus,

$$\Delta T_f = K_f \frac{m_B/M_B}{m_A} \times 1\,000$$

$$M_B = \frac{K_f m_B}{m_A \Delta T_f} \times 1\,000$$

where M_B is the relative molecular weight of solute, m_B is the mass of solute, m_A is the mass of water, and K_f for water is 1.86 K · kg · mol^{-1}.

III Apparatus and Reagents

Analytical balance (0.01 g), thermometer (0.1 ℃), test tube (40 mm×150 mm), beaker (500 mL×1), transfer pipet (50 mL×1), rubber pipet bulb and stirring rod.

Ice, salt, glucose (AR, s) and distilled water.

IV Procedure

1. Preparation of Ice Bath

Fill the large beaker 3/4 full with ice. Cover the ice with 1/4 to 1/2 inches of table salt. Stir this ice-salt mixture with a stirring rod and make sure the temperature drops to at least −10 ℃.

2. Determination of the Freezing Point of Glucose Solution

Weigh out accurately 4.2-5.1 g of glucose with an analytical balance and put it into a dry large test tube, and then add 50.00 mL of distilled water to it. After the glucose has dissolved completely, install the stopper with thermometer and stirrer. Put the tube into a beaker of ice, stir gently and observe carefully as the temperature is rising (Figure 2-2). When the temperature no longer rises, record the temperature (T_f). Take out the test tube and allow the ice to thaw (it is acceptable to use your hands to let the solvent thaw quicker). Repeat the above procedures twice and when the difference of two results does not exceed 0.05 ℃, take the average value ($\overline{T}_f$).

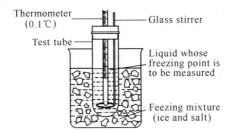

Figure 2-2　Experimental set up for measuring freezing point

3. Determination of the Freezing Point of Distilled Water

Wash the large test tube carefully, add 50.00 mL of distilled water to it with a pipet. Repeat the above procedures twice, take the average value ($\overline{T_f^0}$) as the freezing point of distilled water.

V Questions

(1) Why can the mixture of ice and salt be used as the coolant?

(2) 2.0 g of an unknown solute is added to 65.0 g of camphor and the freezing point depression is measured to be 7.39 ℃. How much is the relative molecular weight of the unknown solute?

Experiment 4　Preparation and Comparison of Acid and Base Standard Solutions

I Learning Objectives

(1) Learn the procedure for cleaning volumetric apparatus.

(2) Understand the principles of acid-base titration.

(3) Learn the method of the preparation of acid and base standard solutions.

(4) Learn to use the buret and judge the endpoint of the titration.

II Principles

In an acid-base titration, the standard solutions cannot be prepared directly because common acids and bases contain some impurities and are unstable. At first, prepare solutions of the approximate concentrations required, and then standardize these solutions.

All acid-base reactions are expressed as:

$$H_3O^+ + OH^- \mathop{=\!=\!=} 2H_2O$$

When hydrochloric acid reacts with sodium hydroxide completely, the amount of substance of each will be equal (this is known as the equivalence point of the titration):

$$n(HCl) = n(NaOH)$$

or

$$c(HCl) \times V(HCl) = c(NaOH) \times V(NaOH)$$

To find out the equivalence point, you can use an indicator such as methyl orange that changes from yellow in base solution to orange in acid solution. As in this experiment, if an acid solution is progressively added to a base solution in the presence of methyl orange, the point at which the first orange color appears is taken as the equivalence point. At this point, called the endpoint, neglecting the small amount of reagent required in excess to bring about the color change, you can assume that equal numbers of acid and base have been mixed. By measuring the volumes of the two solutions mixed and knowing the concentration of one, you can calculate the concentration of the other.

Note that the pH at the equivalence point is somewhat less than 7.0, the methyl orange is still a very satisfactory indicator. However, if the pH at the equivalence point is somewhat higher than 7.0, methyl orange will not be as a good indicator for the titration as, for example, phenolphthalein, whose color changes from colorless to pink as the pH changes from about 8.0 to 10.0. Ordinarily, indicators will be chosen so that their color change occurs at about the pH at the equivalence point of a given acid-base titration.

In this experiment, you will first prepare two solutions of the sodium hydroxide and the hydrochloric acid, and then determine the volume ratio of HCl solution to NaOH solution by comparative titration of the two solutions. If the concentration of HCl solution is accurately known, the accurate concentration of NaOH solution can be calculated with the above equation.

Ⅲ Apparatus and Reagents

Geiser buret (50 mL×1), Mohr measuring buret (50 mL×1), Erlenmeyer flasks (250 mL×3), beakers (50 mL×1, 250 mL×1), graduated cylinders (10 mL×1, 100 mL×1), reagent bottles (500 mL×2), wash bottle, label, rubber pipet bulb and stirring rod.

HCl solution (2. 0 mol · L^{-1}), NaOH solution (2. 0 mol · L^{-1}) and methyl orange indicator.

IV Procedure

1. Preparation of Approximate 0. 1 mol · L^{-1} HCl Solution and 0. 1 mol · L^{-1} NaOH Solution

(1) Preparation of 0. 1 mol · L^{-1} HCl solution. Measure out about 25 mL of 2 mol · L^{-1} HCl solution and add about 475 mL of distilled water. Stir thoroughly and finally label the bottle.

(2) Preparation of 0. 1 mol · L^{-1} NaOH solution. Measure out about 25 mL of 2 mol · L^{-1} NaOH solution and add about 475 mL of distilled water. Stir thoroughly and finally label the bottle.

2. Determination of the Volume Ratio of NaOH Solution to HCl Solution

(1) Clean the buret and check the tip for leakage. If no leakage is observed, rinse your cleaned buret once with distilled water and two or three times with the prepared 0. 1 mol · L^{-1} HCl solution (about 10 mL each time). Add the acid solution into the buret and work air bubbles out.

(2) Treat the other buret with 0. 1 mol · L^{-1} NaOH solution in the similar manner. Add the NaOH solution into the buret.

(3) Adjust the meniscus surface of the liquid to the zero mark or lower and remain for one minute. Record the initial reading (the volume is read to the nearest 0. 01 mL).

(4) Run out about 25 mL of the base solution from the buret into a clean 250 mL Erlenmeyer flask (but not necessarily dry). Add 2 drops of methyl orange indicator solution. Place a sheet of white paper under the flask to aid in the detection of any color change. The solution shows yellow.

(5) Titrate the base solution in the flask with the acid solution from the buret, note the solution color as the drops of acid hit the base solution. Swirl the liquid in the flask gently and continuously as you add the HCl solution. When the orange color begins to change, slow down the rate of addition of the HCl solution. Rinse down the inside of the flask with a jet of distilled water from your wash bottle just before the termination of the titration. In the final stage of the titration, add the HCl solution drop by drop, stirring between drops, until the orange color persists for about 30 s. If you go past the endpoint and obtain a red solution, add a few drops of the NaOH solution to remove the color, and then add HCl solution a drop

at a time until the orange color persists. Carefully record the final readings on the HCl and NaOH burets.

(6) Repeat the titration two more times. Calculate the volume ratio of the NaOH solution to the HCl solution and relative average deviation ($\bar{d}_r$). $\bar{d}_r$ must be less than 0.2%.

V Data

Items		I	II	III
HCl	Final buret reading/mL			
	Initial buret reading/mL			
	$V(HCl)/mL$			
NaOH	Final buret reading/mL			
	Initial buret reading/mL			
	$V(NaOH)/mL$			
$V(NaOH) : V(HCl)$				
Average of $V(NaOH) : V(HCl)$				
$\bar{d}_r/(\%)$				

VI Questions

(1) The initial reading should be set at or very close to the zero mark in each titration. Why?

(2) The buret must be rinsed by the solution to be filled. Why?

(3) The Erlenmeyer flask cannot be rinsed by the solution to be titrated. Why?

(4) Methyl orange was used as the indicator in this experiment. What is the role of the indicator? Why was methyl orange used and not phenolphthalein indicator?

Experiment 5   Determination of the Ionization Degree and Ionization Constant of Acetic Acid

I Learning Objectives

(1) Learn the method of determination of the ionization degree and ionization constant of a weak acid.

(2) Understand the principles of potentiometric determination of pH and learn the operation of a pH meter.

II Principles

Acetic acid is a weak acid. The equilibrium acid ionization constant, K_a, expresses the ratio of concentrations for the reaction:

$$HAc + H_2O \rightleftharpoons Ac^- + H_3O^+$$

$$K_a = \frac{[H_3O^+][Ac^-]}{[HAc]} = \frac{[H^+][Ac^-]}{[HAc]}$$

To calculate the ionization constant, K_a, for an acetic acid, it is necessary to experimentally determine the equilibrium concentrations of H^+, Ac^-, and HAc. The most straight forward of these is $[H^+]$, because you know that the pH $= -lg[H^+]$. So if you measure the pH of the equilibrium solution, you will not only know the concentration of the hydrogen ion, $[H^+]$, but also the concentration of the weak acid's conjugate, $[Ac^-]$, as well.

However, you still need to determine the equilibrium concentration of HAc. Unfortunately, it is difficult to determine since most methods of analysis will change the concentration of the HAc and cause the equilibrium to shift. Since you can not directly determine the $[HAc]$, you need to find the initial concentration of HAc. To do this you need to neutralize all of the HAc present by titrating it with a strong base of known concentration. Then you can calculate the equilibrium concentration of HAc, by subtracting the equilibrium $[H^+]$ from the initial HAc concentration:

$$[HAc] = [HAc]_{initial} - [H^+]$$

Now you have all of the equilibrium concentrations necessary to calculate the K_a for your weak acid!

For an aqueous solution of a weak acid we denote the degree of ionization by the symbol α(alpha), and define it as

$$\alpha = \frac{[H^+]}{c_a}$$

where c_a is the initial concentration of the weak acid.

III Apparatus and Reagents

Mohr buret (50 mL×1), pH meter (PB-10), volumetric flasks (50 mL×3), Erlenmeyer flasks (250 mL×3), beakers (50 mL×4), Mohr measuring pipet (10 mL×1), transfer pipets (25 mL×1, 10 mL×1), wash bottle, rubber pipet bulb and medicine dropper.

NaOH solution (0.1 mol · L^{-1}, standardized solution), phenolphthalein indicator, HAc solution (approximately 0.2 mol · L^{-1}) and standard buffer solutions (pH=4.00 and pH=6.86).

Ⅳ Procedure

(1) Determination of initial weak acid concentration. Using a pipet, transfer 10.00 mL of acetic acid to a clean 250 mL Erlenmyer flask. Add 2-3 drops of phenolphthalein indicator to the flask. Then titrate with the NaOH standard solution until a faint pink color remains for 30 s. Repeat the titration with two other 10.00 mL solutions and calculate the concentration of the acetic acid solution.

(2) Preparation of acetic acid solutions at different concentrations. Transfer 25.00 mL, 5.00 mL and 2.50 mL of the standardized acetic acid solution, respectively, into three 50 mL volumetric flasks with the pipets. Dilute with distilled water to the mark of each flask. Mix the solutions thoroughly.

(3) Measurement of the pH of the above four solutions. Take out about 25 mL of the above acetic acid solutions into four dry 50 mL beakers, respectively. Measure the pH values of the acetic acid solutions successively from dilute to concentrated with a pH meter, record the pH value and the temperature of the unknown acid solution.

(4) According to the equations $\alpha = \dfrac{[H^+]}{c_a}$ and $K_a = \dfrac{[H^+][Ac^-]}{[HAc]}$, calculate the K_a for this acid at different concentrations.

Ⅴ Data

1. Titration of Acetic Acid Solution

Items		Ⅰ	Ⅱ	Ⅲ
NaOH	Final buret reading/mL			
	Initial buret reading/mL			
	$V(NaOH)$/mL			
Concentration of standardized NaOH/(mol · L^{-1})				
$c(HAc)$/(mol · L^{-1})				
$\bar{c}(HAc)$/(mol · L^{-1})				
$\bar{d}_r$/(%)				

2. Determination of the Ionization Constant of HAc

Items	I	II	III	IV
$c(HAc)/(mol \cdot L^{-1})$				
pH				
$c(H_3O^+)/(mol \cdot L^{-1})$				
α				
K_a				
$\overline{K}_a$				
Temperature/℃				

VI Questions

(1) Do the acetic acid solutions at different concentrations have the same ionization degree and ionization constant at the same temperature?

(2) How will the ionization degree and ionization constant change if the HAc solution has an obvious change in temperature at the same concentration?

(3) Phenolphthalein was used as the indicator in this experiment. What is the role of the indicator? Why was phenolphthalein used and not some other indicators?

Experiment 6 Determination of a Rate Law and Activation Energy

I Learning Objectives

(1) Testify the influence of concentration, temperature and catalyst on the rate of chemical reactions.

(2) Determine the rate law for a chemical reaction.

(3) Use graphical techniques in the analysis of experimental data.

II Principles

In this experiment you will determine the rate equation for the reaction of potassium persulfate, $K_2S_2O_8$, with potassium iodide. The reaction is

$$S_2O_8^{2-} + 2I^- = 2SO_4^{2-} + I_2 \qquad (1)$$

The rate law for this reaction is rate $= k[S_2O_8^{2-}]^m[I^-]^n$. The rate can be measured conveniently by following the rate of formation of the I_2 product.

$$v = \frac{\Delta[I_2]}{\Delta t} = k[S_2O_8^{2-}]^m[I^-]^n$$

This is done indirectly by adding a constant known amount of thiosulfate ion $(S_2O_3^{2-})$ to each reaction mixture. The thiosulfate ion reacts rapidly with the I_2 as it is formed from reaction (1).

$$2S_2O_3^{2-} + I_2 \Longrightarrow S_4O_6^{2-} + 2I^- \tag{2}$$

The amount of thiosulfate added is kept small. Once all the $S_2O_3^{2-}$ is used up, reaction (2) can no longer occur and the I_2 still being formed in reaction (1) will appear in the solution as a dark color. The color can more readily be seen by adding a small amount of starch which forms an intense blue-black color with the I_2. Note that the reaction between the thiosulfate ion and the iodine molecule is a 2 : 1 reaction. Therefore, each mole of $S_2O_3^{2-}$ used is equivalent to 1/2 mole of I_2 formed.

$$v = \frac{\Delta[I_2]}{\Delta t} = \frac{\Delta[S_2O_3^{2-}]}{2\Delta t} = k[S_2O_8^{2-}]^m[I^-]^n$$

In logarithmic form this equation becomes $\lg v = m\lg[S_2O_8^{2-}] + n\lg[I^-] + \lg k$

In order to determine the value of m, you will measure the rate of a series of reactions for a constant iodide ion concentration as the persulfate ion concentration is changed and plot $\lg(\text{rate})$ vs. $\lg[S_2O_8^{2-}]$. The value of m is the slope of this plot. The value of n is determined through a similar series of reactions in which $[I^-]$ is varied while $[S_2O_8^{2-}]$ is kept constant.

Using the same reaction,

$$S_2O_8^{2-} + 2I^- \Longrightarrow 2SO_4^{2-} + I_2$$

but you allow the reaction to proceed at different temperatures to investigate the temperature effect on the reaction rate. The temperature effect is best described by the activation energy, E_a, defined in the Arrhenius equation:

$$k = Ae^{-E_a/(RT)} \quad \text{or} \quad \lg k = \frac{-E_a}{2.303RT} + \lg A$$

A plot of $\lg k$ vs. $1/T$ yields a straight line with a slope of $-\dfrac{E_a}{2.303R}$ and an intercept of $\lg A$.

Furthermore, you also investigate the effect of a catalyst on the reaction rate. You determine the change in activation energy when the catalyst $CuSO_4$ is added.

III Apparatus and Reagents

Mohr measuring pipets (10 mL×5), buret (10 mL×1), beakers (100 mL×2), rubber pipet bulb, stopwatch and thermometer.

KI solution (0. 2 mol · L^{-1}), $Na_2S_2O_3$ solution (0. 01 mol · L^{-1}), $(NH_4)_2SO_4$ solution (0. 2 mol · L^{-1}), $(NH_4)_2S_2O_8$ solution (0. 2 mol · L^{-1}), starch solution (2 g · L^{-1}) and $Cu(NO_3)_2$ solution (0. 02 mol · L^{-1}).

Ⅳ Procedure

1. Determination of the Reaction Rate Law in the Absence of a Catalyst (Experiments 1-5)

The table below summarizes the preparation of the test solutions. Measure the volumes to ±0. 05 mL using either a pipet or a buret.

Experiment No.	Solution A				Solution B
	0. 2 mol · L^{-1} KI	2 g · L^{-1} starch	0. 01 mol · L^{-1} $Na_2S_2O_3$	0. 2 mol · L^{-1} $(NH_4)_2SO_4$	0. 2 mol · L^{-1} $(NH_4)_2S_2O_8$
1	10 mL	4 mL	8 mL	0 mL	10 mL
2	10 mL	4 mL	8 mL	5 mL	5 mL
3	10 mL	4 mL	8 mL	7. 5 mL	2. 5 mL
4	5 mL	4 mL	8 mL	5 mL	10 mL
5	2. 5 mL	4 mL	8 mL	7. 5 mL	10 mL

(1) Prepare solution A in a 100 mL beaker. Stir the solution thoroughly and record its temperature.

(2) The reaction begins when solution B is poured into solution A, therefore, be prepared to start timing the reaction in seconds with a stopwatch. Place the reaction vessel on a white sheet of paper so that the color change is more easily detected.

2. The Effect of Temperature on the Reaction Rate (Experiments 6 and 7)

(1) Experiment 6: Repeat experiment 1 at a lower temperature (5-10 ℃). Prepare an ice water bath in a crystallizing dish and prepare two necessary solutions. Cool two solutions in the ice water bath until two are at 5-10 ℃. Quickly take the solutions out of the ice water bath, pour the solutions together and place the reaction beaker back in the ice bath. Record the data and temperature.

(2) Experiment 7: Repeat experiment 1 at a higher temperature, above 40 ℃, using a hot water bath. Record the data and temperature.

3. The Effect of Copper Ion as a Catalyst (Experiment 8)

Repeat experiment 1, except that 3 drops of 0. 02 mol · L^{-1} $Cu(NO_3)_2$ solution is added to the iodide-starch-$S_2O_3^{2-}$ mixture as a catalyst.

V Data

(1) Using experiments 1, 4, and 5 plot $\lg k$ vs. $\lg[\text{I}^-]$. Determine n from this plot.

(2) Using experiments 1, 2, and 3 plot $\lg k$ vs. $\lg[\text{S}_2\text{O}_8^{2-}]$. Determine m from this plot.

(3) Using the n and m, substitute into the rate equation for each experiment and determine k. Calculate the average of k.

(4) A plot of $\lg k$ vs. $1/T$ to calculate activation energy.

(5) Calculate the rate constant, k, for the reaction in the presence of the Cu^{2+} catalyst.

VI Questions

(1) What would appear in solution if the $\text{Na}_2\text{S}_2\text{O}_3$ solution was omitted?

(2) How would the recorded time for the blue color to appear be affected if the solutions being mixed at the temperatures above room temperature cooled after mixing? Explain it.

Experiment 7　Determination of the Purity of an Unknown Acid

I Learning Objectives

(1) Learn the method of standardization of sodium hydroxide with the primary standard.

(2) Determine the purity of an unknown acid, oxalic acid dihydrate ($\text{H}_2\text{C}_2\text{O}_4 \cdot 2\text{H}_2\text{O}$) by means of an acid-base titration with NaOH.

II Principles

This analysis consists of two parts. In the first section you prepare and standardize a solution of NaOH. In the second section you apply the method to the analysis of an unknown acid.

In this experiment, you will standardize a solution of NaOH. To do this you will use potassium hydrogen phthalate, $\text{KHC}_8\text{H}_4\text{O}_4$, as a primary standard acid.

The balanced equation for the acid-base reaction involved in the standardization procedure is

$$KHC_8H_4O_4 + NaOH \Longrightarrow KNaC_8H_4O_4 + H_2O$$

From the titration volume and the mass of $KHC_8H_4O_4$, calculate the concentration of the NaOH.

$$c(NaOH) = \frac{m(KHC_8H_4O_4)}{V(NaOH) \times M(KHC_8H_4O_4)} \times 1\ 000$$

You will then use the standardized solution of NaOH to determine the purity of the oxalic acid dihydrate, $H_2C_2O_4 \cdot 2H_2O$. The reaction is shown below:

$$H_2C_2O_4(aq) + 2NaOH(aq) \Longrightarrow Na_2C_2O_4(aq) + 2H_2O(l)$$

Note that this is a 1 : 2 titration. Two moles of base will titrate one mole of acid. The endpoint of the titration will be determined by an indicator, phenolphthalein. It is colorless under acidic conditions and changes to a pink color under basic conditions. Therefore, the first persistent presence of color indicates that you are beginning to titrate the indicator and have reached the endpoint. From the titration volume and the mass of $H_2C_2O_4 \cdot 2H_2O$, calculate the purity of the $H_2C_2O_4 \cdot 2H_2O$.

$$w(H_2C_2O_4 \cdot 2H_2O)(\%) = \frac{c(NaOH) \times V(NaOH) \times \dfrac{M(H_2C_2O_4 \cdot 2H_2O)}{2 \times 1\ 000}}{m(sample) \times \dfrac{25.00}{250.00}} \times 100\%$$

Ⅲ Apparatus and Reagents

Analytical balance (0. 1 mg), Mohr buret (50 mL×1), beakers (50 mL×1, 250 mL × 1), transfer pipet (25 mL × 1), Erlenmeyer flasks (250 mL × 3), graduated cylinder (10 mL×1), wash bottle, stirring rod, volumetric flask (250 mL×1), weighing bottle, rubber pipet bulb and medicine dropper.

NaOH (AR, s), phenolphthalein indicator, potassium hydrogen phthalate (AR, s), unknown organic acid ($H_2C_2O_4 \cdot 2H_2O$, s).

Ⅳ Procedure

1. Standardization of 0. 1 mol · L⁻¹ NaOH solution

(1) Prepare 500 mL of approximately 0. 1 mol · L^{-1} NaOH solution for standardization. Use 50% NaOH solution (1. 53 g · mL^{-1}) which has been filtered or allowed to settle. (You must calculate the amount of this solution needed.) The solution should be stored in a polyethylene bottle since NaOH dissolves silica from

glass containers. The slow diffusion of CO_2 through the plastic will not be a problem during the duration of the experiment. Minimize the exposure of this solution to air. Mix the solution thoroughly before using. The solution may settle between labs, so always mix thoroughly before using.

(2) Standardization of NaOH solution. Weigh accurately an appropriate amount of $KHC_8H_4O_4$ into a titration flask (weigh by difference from the weighing bottle. 20-30 mL of NaOH standard solution will be consumed), dissolve it in about 25 mL of distilled water and add 2 drops of phenolphthalein indicator. (You may begin to titrate before all of the solid is dissolved, but insure that it is all dissolved at the endpoint.) Titrate with NaOH standard solution to a faint pink and the color should persist for at least 30 s. Repeat the titration two more times. Then calculate the concentration of NaOH solution.

2. Determination of the Purity of an Unknown Diprotic Acid

Your instructor will give you a portion of an unknown solid acid in a stoppered test tube. Accurately weigh about 1.7-1.9 g (± 0.1 mg) of unknown organic acid into a clean 150 mL beaker, dissolve it by adding the appropriate volume of distilled water. Transfer the solution into a 250 mL volumetric flask, dilute to the mark and mix the solution thoroughly. Pipet 25.00 mL of this solution to a 250 mL Erlenmeyer flask, add 2 drops of phenolphthalein indicator, titrate the sample with NaOH standard solution to a faint pink and the color should persist for at least 30 s. Repeat the titration two more times. Then calculate the purity of $H_2C_2O_4 \cdot 2H_2O$.

Ⅴ Data

1. Standardization of 0.1 mol · L^{-1} NaOH Solution

Items		I	Ⅱ	Ⅲ
	Mass of $KHC_8H_4O_4$/g			
NaOH	Initial buret reading/mL Final buret reading/mL V(NaOH)/mL			
	c(NaOH)/ (mol · L^{-1})			
	$\bar{c}$(NaOH)/ (mol · L^{-1})			
	$\bar{d}_r$/(%)			

2. Determination of Purity of Unknown Organic Acid

Items		I	II	III
Mass of unknown organic acid/g				
NaOH	Initial buret reading/mL			
	Final buret reading/mL			
	V(NaOH)/mL			
$w/(\%)$				
$\bar{w}/(\%)$				
$\bar{d}_r/(\%)$				

Ⅵ Questions

(1) Why must you prepare the NaOH solution in a plastic container rather than a glass container?

(2) What is a primary standard, and what are its characteristics?

Experiment 8　Determination of Aspirin in Aspirin Tablets

Ⅰ Learning Objectives

(1) Review the methods and principles of acid-base titration.

(2) Grasp the methods and principles of determining aspirin in commercial aspirin tablets.

Ⅱ Principles

Aspirin, acetylsalicylic acid, is both an organic ester and an organic acid (pK_a =3.5). It is used extensively in medicine as a pain killer and fever reducing drug. The quantitative reaction of aspirin with a standardized NaOH solution occurs according to the following reaction. The equivalence point may be determined by titration using phenolphthalein indicator (in the pH range 8.3-10).

$$\text{C}_6\text{H}_4\begin{matrix}-\text{COOH}\\-\text{OCOCH}_3\end{matrix} + \text{NaOH} \rightleftharpoons \text{C}_6\text{H}_4\begin{matrix}-\text{COONa}\\-\text{OCOCH}_3\end{matrix} + \text{H}_2\text{O}$$

Aspirin is a weak acid that also undergoes slow hydrolysis; i. e. , each aspirin molecule reacts with two hydroxide ions. To overcome this problem, this reaction must be taken place in ethanol solution and the temperature must be kept under 10 ℃.

$$\underset{\text{COOH}}{\underset{\text{OCOCH}_3}{\bigcirc}} + 2NaOH \rightleftharpoons \underset{\text{COONa}}{\underset{\text{OH}}{\bigcirc}} + H_2O + CH_3COONa$$

Ⅲ Apparatus and Reagents

Analytical balance (0.1 mg), graduated cylinder (50 mL × 1), Erlenmeyer flasks (250 mL × 3), beaker (250 mL × 1), Mohr buret (50 mL × 1), stirring rod, wash bottle, mortar and pestle.

Aspirin tablets, NaOH solution (0.1 mol · L^{-1}, standardized solution), phenolphthalein indicator and ethanol.

Ⅳ Procedure

Accurately record the mass of a group of three aspirin tablets so that you can determine an average tablet mass. Use a mortar and pestle to crush enough tablets to produce about 1.5 g tablet powder. Using a clean dry weighing bottle, weigh accurately by difference, triplicate 0.4-0.5 g samples of tablet, into labeled 250 mL Erlenmeyer flasks. To each flask, add 20 mL of ethanol (measured by graduated cylinder) and 3 drops of phenolphthalein indicator. Keep the temperature under 10 ℃. Swirl gently to dissolve. (The ethanol helps the aspirin dissolve. Note that an aspirin tablet contains other compounds in addition to aspirin. Some of these are not very soluble. Your solution will be cloudy due to insoluble components of the tablet.) Clean, rinse, and fill a buret with the standardized about 0.1 mol · L^{-1} NaOH solution. Titrate the first aspirin sample with NaOH standard solution to a faint pink and the color should persist for at least 30 s. Repeat the titration two more times. Then calculate the percentage of $C_9H_8O_4$.

$$w(C_9H_8O_4) = \frac{c(NaOH) \times V(NaOH) \times M(C_9H_8O_4)}{m(sample) \times 1\ 000} \times 100\%$$

Ⅴ Data

Items		Ⅰ	Ⅱ	Ⅲ
NaOH	Final buret reading/mL			
	Initial buret reading/mL			
	V(NaOH)/mL			

continued

Items	I	II	III
$c(NaOH)/(mol \cdot L^{-1})$			
Mass of aspirin tablet/g			
$w(C_9H_8O_4)/(\%)$			
$\bar{w}(C_9H_8O_4)/(\%)$			
$\bar{d}_r/(\%)$			

VI Question

This titration reaction must be taken place in ethanol solution and the temperature must be kept under 10 ℃. Why?

Experiment 9   Determination of the Composition of a Carbonate-Bicarbonate Mixture

I Learning Objectives

(1) Learn the method of standardization of hydrochloric acid with primary standard.

(2) Learn to determine the composition of carbonate mixtures.

II Principles

You can have a solid mixture of NaOH, Na_2CO_3, and $NaHCO_3$, but in solution a maximum of two of these species can co-exist at one time. In the present laboratory, you will receive a mixture containing sodium carbonate (Na_2CO_3) and sodium bicarbonate ($NaHCO_3$). For determination of this mixture, the methods applied and their fundamental principles are given below and the necessary adaptations have been made.

1. Double Endpoint Method

This procedure involves two titrations. The addition of acid (V_1) to the sample will convert the carbonate to bicarbonate until no carbonate remains. The addition of further acid (V_2) will convert the bicarbonate to carbonic acid until no bicarbonate remains. The carbonate and carbonic acid equivalence points may be determined either by titration using indicators.

The first endpoint determined (in the pH range 8. 3-10) represents the completion (equivalence point or stoichiometric endpoint) of the following reaction:

$$CO_3^{2-} + H^+ = HCO_3^-$$

i. e. , the carbonate has been neutralized by the acid-forming bicarbonate ions.

In the pH range 3. 2-4. 5, all of the bicarbonate ions initially present in the sample, together with all of those produced from the reaction of the carbonate ions, will be neutralized. The resulting alkalinity is known as the total alkalinity.

$$HCO_3^- + H^+ = H_2CO_3$$

It is relatively simple to determine the composition of a mixture by titrating separate aliquots to a phenolphthalein endpoint and to a methyl orange endpoint.

$$\rho(NaHCO_3) = \frac{(V_2 - V_1) \times c(HCl) \times M(NaHCO_3)}{V_s}$$

$$\rho(Na_2CO_3) = \frac{V_1 \times c(HCl) \times M(Na_2CO_3)}{V_s}$$

2. BaCl₂ Method

This procedure involves two titrations. First, total alkalinity ($[HCO_3^-] + 2[CO_3^{2-}]$) is measured by titrating the mixture with HCl standard solution (V_3) to a orange endpoint:

$$HCO_3^- + H^+ = H_2CO_3$$

$$CO_3^{2-} + 2H^+ = H_2CO_3$$

A separate unknown aliquot is treated with excess NaOH standard solution (V_1) to convert HCO_3^- to CO_3^{2-}:

$$HCO_3^- + OH^- = CO_3^{2-} + H_2O$$

Then all the carbonate is precipitated with BaCl₂:

$$Ba^{2+} + CO_3^{2-} = BaCO_3(s)$$

The excess NaOH is immediately titrated with HCl standard solution (V_2) to determine how much HCO_3^- is present.

From the total alkalinity and bicarbonate concentration, you can calculate the original carbonate concentration.

$$\rho(NaHCO_3) = \frac{[c(NaOH) \times V_1 - c(HCl) \times V_2] \times M(NaHCO_3)}{V_s}$$

$$\rho(Na_2CO_3) = \frac{\{c(HCl) \times V_3 - [c(NaOH) \times V_1 - c(HCl) \times V_2]\} \times M(Na_2CO_3)}{2V_s}$$

Ⅲ Apparatus and Reagents

Analytical balance (0.1 mg), Geiser buret (50 mL×1), transfer pipets (20 mL×2), Erlenmeyer flasks (250 mL×3), wash bottle and rubber pipet bulb.

Unhydrous Na_2CO_3 (AR, s), mixture, phenolphthalein indicator, methyl orange indicator, $BaCl_2$ solution (1%), HCl solution (0.1 mol · L^{-1}) and NaOH solution (0.1 mol · L^{-1}, standardized solution).

Ⅳ Procedure

1. Preparation and Standardization of 0.1 mol · L^{-1} HCl Solution

Prepare a hydrochloric acid solution by adding 3.5 mL of concentrated HCl solution to 400 mL of distilled water. Mix thoroughly.

Accurately weigh about 0.15-0.20 g of unhydrous Na_2CO_3 (dried at 110 ℃ to 120 ℃ for 2 h.) into a 250 mL Erlenmeyer flask, add 20-30 mL of distilled water and 2 drops of methyl orange indicator, and titrate with 0.1 mol · L^{-1} HCl solution until the color changes from yellow to orange. Record the buret reading. Repeat the titration two more times. Then calculate the concentration of HCl solution.

2. Determination of a Carbonate-Bicarbonate Mixture

(1) Double endpoint method.

Pipet 20.00 mL of the unknown solution into a 250 mL Erlenmeyer flask, add 2 drops of phenolphthalein indicator, and titrate with HCl standard solution (V_1) until the color changes from red to colorless. Then add 2 drops of methyl orange indicator and continue the titration until the color changes from yellow to orange. The volume of HCl solution is V_2. Repeat this procedure with two more 20.00 mL unknown samples.

(2) $BaCl_2$ method.

Pipet 20.00 mL aliquot of the unknown solution into a 250 mL Erlenmeyer flask, add 2 drops of methyl orange indicator, and titrate with HCl standard solution (V_3) until the color changes from yellow to orange. Repeat this procedure with two more 20.00 mL aliquots.

Pipet 20.00 mL of the unknown solution into a 250 mL Erlenmeyer flask and add (using a volumetric pipet) standardized NaOH solution (V_1). Swirl and add 1% $BaCl_2$ solution to precipitate $BaCO_3$. Add 2 drops of phenolphthalein indicator, and immediately titrate (to a faint pink endpoint) with standard 0.1 mol · L^{-1} HCl solution (V_2). Repeat this procedure with two more 20.00 mL unknown samples.

V Questions

(1) Compare the two methods of determination of a carbonate-bicarbonate mixture.

(2) What is the effect on the result of the concentration of HCl solution if small amount of moisture is absorbed in primary standard Na_2CO_3?

Experiment 10 Determination of Hydrogen Peroxide in Nosocomial Disinfector

I Learning Objectives

(1) Learn the method of preparation and standardization of $KMnO_4$ solution.

(2) Learn to determine H_2O_2 by redox titration.

II Principles

Most nosocomial disinfectors of hydrogen peroxide are about 3% H_2O_2. In this experiment, you will analyze an unknown solution by titrating it with $KMnO_4$ solution. In acid solution, MnO_4^- oxidizes H_2O_2 to form O_2 and colorless Mn^{2+}. The reaction is

$$5H_2O_2 + 2MnO_4^- + 6H^+ = 2Mn^{2+} + 8H_2O + 5O_2\uparrow \qquad (1)$$

Thus, when a solution of $KMnO_4$ is added dropwise to an acidified solution of H_2O_2, each drop is decolorized until all the H_2O_2 is used up. The next drop added remains colored (endpoint). By knowing the concentration of the $KMnO_4$ solution and the volume needed to react with all the H_2O_2, you will be able to calculate the number of moles of H_2O_2 oxidized.

$KMnO_4$ is easily reduced by dust and other organic matter, and because of its instability, it is not available as a primary standard. Therefore, standard solutions are prepared approximately and then standardized by a primary standard reagent. In neutral solution, the reduction product of $KMnO_4$ is insoluble MnO_2. The $KMnO_4$ solution is boiled to react with any impurities and then filtered to remove MnO_2 before standardization.

One of the primary standards used for standardization of $KMnO_4$ is sodium oxalate ($Na_2C_2O_4$) which reacts as shown in Equation (2):

$$5C_2O_4^{2-} + 2MnO_4^- + 16H^+ = 2Mn^{2+} + 10CO_2 \uparrow + 8H_2O \qquad (2)$$

This reaction proceeds somewhat slowly for a useful titration, and various methods are used to accelerate it. One of the simplest method, used in this procedure, is to heat the solution to 80-90 ℃ and maintain it above 60 ℃ throughout the titration.

Ⅲ Apparatus and Reagents

Analytical balances (0. 1 mg, 0. 01 g), desiccator, weighing bottle, Geiser buret (50 mL×1), transfer pipets (10 mL×1, 25 mL×2), volumetric flasks (250 mL×2), Erlenmeyer flasks (250 mL×3), beakers (100 mL×1, 250 mL×1), graduated cylinder (100 mL×1), reagent bottle (500 mL×1), Buchner funnel, wash bottle, medicine dropper, rubber pipet bulb and stirring rod.

$KMnO_4$ (AR, s), $Na_2C_2O_4$ (AR, s), H_2SO_4 solution (6 mol · L^{-1}) and H_2O_2 solution (about 3%).

Ⅳ Procedure

1. Preparation and Standardization of 0. 02 mol · L^{-1} $KMnO_4$ Solution

(1) Weigh out about 1. 5 g of $KMnO_4$ and dissolve it in 500 mL of distilled water. Boil for about 1 h, cover, and let stand overnight. Filter through a Buchner funnel, and store the $KMnO_4$ solution in a clean and glass-stoppered bottle. $KMnO_4$ solution should be stored in the dark.

(2) Transfer 3 g of $Na_2C_2O_4$ to a weighing bottle, and dry at 110-120 ℃ for 1 h. Cool in a desiccator. Accurately weigh 1. 6-1. 7 g (±0. 1 mg) of $Na_2C_2O_4$ into a clean 150 mL beaker, dissolve it by adding the appropriate volume of distilled water. Transfer the solution into a 250 mL volumetric flask with a stirring rod. Rinse the beaker with distilled water for two or three times and add the rinsing to the volumetric flask. When the distilled water is added nearly to the calibration mark, distilled water is added with a medicine dropper until the bottom of the meniscus reaches the calibration mark. Stopper the flask, and mix the solution well.

(3) With a transfer pipet, transfer 25. 00 mL of $Na_2C_2O_4$ solution to a 250 mL Erlenmeyer flask. Add 15 mL of 6 mol · L^{-1} H_2SO_4 solution. Heat to 80-90 ℃. Titrate slowly with $KMnO_4$ solution (rapid addition of $KMnO_4$ solution may allow MnO_4^- to react with Mn^{2+} forming some brown MnO_2). Maintain the temperature

above 60 ℃. Then add the KMnO₄ solution dropwise, swirling after each addition, until one drop produces a pink color that persists for at least 30 s (the color is more readily seen if there is a piece of white paper under the flask). Record the buret reading. (Because KMnO₄ is so intensely colored, it is difficult to observe the meniscus. The surface level is normally read.) Repeat the titration twice. From the titration volume and the mass of $Na_2C_2O_4$, calculate the concentration of the KMnO₄ solution.

$$c(KMnO_4) = \frac{2}{5} \times \frac{m(Na_2C_2O_4) \times 1\,000 \times 25.00}{250.0 \times V(KMnO_4) \times M(Na_2C_2O_4)}$$

2. Determination of Hydrogen Peroxide

(1) Transfer 10.00 mL of H_2O_2 solution into a 250 mL volumetric flask with transfer pipet, and dilute it to the calibration mark with distilled water. With a transfer pipet, transfer 25.00 mL of diluted peroxide solution to a 250 mL Erlenmeyer flask. Add 15 mL of 6 mol · L⁻¹ H_2SO_4 solution. Swirl to mix.

(2) Titrate by running a few milliliters of KMnO₄ solution into the flask and swirling. Continue successive addition of KMnO₄ solution until one drop produces a pink color that persists for at least 30 s. Record the buret reading.

(3) Repeat the titration on a duplicate sample twice. From the titration volume, calculate the content of H_2O_2 in the sample.

$$\rho(H_2O_2) = \frac{5}{2} \times \frac{c(KMnO_4) \times V(KMnO_4) \times M(H_2O_2)}{10.00 \times \frac{25.00}{250.0}}$$

V Data

1. Preparation and Standardization of 0.02 mol · L⁻¹ KMnO₄ Solution

Items		I	II	III
	Mass of $Na_2C_2O_4$/g			
KMnO₄	Initial buret reading/mL			
	Final buret reading/mL			
	$V(KMnO_4)$/mL			
$c(KMnO_4)$/(mol · L⁻¹)				
$\bar{c}(KMnO_4)$/(mol · L⁻¹)				
$\bar{d}_r$/(%)				

2. Determination of Hydrogen Peroxide

Items		I	II	III
KMnO$_4$	Initial buret reading/mL Final buret reading/mL $V(KMnO_4)/mL$			
$\rho(H_2O_2)/(g \cdot L^{-1})$				
$\bar{\rho}(H_2O_2)/(g \cdot L^{-1})$				
$\bar{d}_r/(\%)$				

VI Notes

It may take 30-45 s since the reaction is not instantaneous. In your titrations, you can add KMnO$_4$ solution at a rate of 25-30 mL per minute until you are within 2-3 mL of the equivalence point. Let the solutions stand to see if the color disappears. If so, proceed slowly to the endpoint. If you have passed the endpoint, throw it out and start again.

VII Questions

(1) The titrant in this experiment is _____ and the analyte is _____.

(2) The color (if any) of the titrated solution at the equivalence point is

_____.

Experiment 11　Iodimetric Determination of Glucose in Nosocomial Injection

I Learning Objectives

(1) Learn the method of preparation and standardization of sodium thiosulfate and iodine solution.

(2) Learn to determine glucose by iodimetric.

II Principles

An oxidation-reduction reaction in which iodine is produced from iodide by the action of an oxidizing agent has many applications in analytical chemistry. Any method that uses a redox titration involving iodine is called iodometry. This method is used when an oxidizing agent cannot be titrated directly with a solution of a reducing agent.

In this experiment, you will determine the percentage of glucose in nosocomial injection. The iodine reacts with NaOH to yield NaIO. IO^- oxidizes glucose to gluconic acid. In an acidic solution, the excessive NaIO can form iodine. The iodine can then be titrated with a solution of sodium thiosulfate ($Na_2S_2O_3$) of known concentration. The equations for these reactions are as follows:

$$I_2 + C_6H_{12}O_6 + 2NaOH = C_6H_{12}O_7 + 2NaI + H_2O$$
$$3IO^- = IO_3^- + 2I^-$$
$$IO_3^- + 5I^- + 6H^+ = 3I_2 + 3H_2O$$
$$I_2 + 2S_2O_3^{2-} = S_4O_6^{2-} + 2I^-$$

Sodium thiosulfate, $Na_2S_2O_3$, is often called "hypo" and is used in the photographic industry to dissolve the unactivated and undeveloped silver halide from photographic negatives and prints. This compound is usually obtained as the white crystalline pentahydrate, $Na_2S_2O_3 \cdot 5H_2O$, with a formula weight of 248.19. Unfortunately, this form of sodium thiosulfate effloresces (loses water) readily and a standard solution of this compound is difficult to prepare by weight. Instead, a solution of approximately the desired concentration is prepared and then standardized.

Potassium dichromate ($K_2Cr_2O_7$), potassium iodate (KIO_3), potassium bromate ($KBrO_3$), and copper (Cu) are examples of primary standards that can be used to standardize sodium thiosulfate solutions. Each industrial laboratory will have a preference as to which primary standard is used. The reactions involved in the standardization with potassium dichromate are as follows:

$$Cr_2O_7^{2-} + 6I^- + 14H^+ = 2Cr^{3+} + 3I_2 + 7H_2O$$
$$I_2 + 2S_2O_3^{2-} = S_4O_6^{2-} + 2I^-$$

Ⅲ Apparatus and Reagents

Analytical balance (0.01 g), Geiser buret (50 mL×1), Mohr buret (50 mL×1), transfer pipets (20 mL×2), Erlenmeyer flasks (250 mL×3), reagent bottles (500 mL×2), beakers (100 mL×1, 250 mL×1), wash bottle, rubber pipet bulb and stirring rod.

HCl solution (2 mol · L^{-1}, 1∶1), NaOH solution (0.2 mol · L^{-1}), starch solution (5 g · L^{-1}), $Na_2S_2O_3 \cdot 5H_2O$ (AR, s), KI (AR, s), I_2 (AR, s), $K_2Cr_2O_7$ solution (0.016 67 mol · L^{-1}) and glucose solution (5%).

IV Procedure

1. Preparation and Standardization of 0.05 mol · L^{-1} Na$_2$S$_2$O$_3$ Solution

Boil about 1 L of distilled water for at least 10 min. Allow the water to cool to room temperature. Weigh out sufficient sodium thiosulfate to make a 0.05 mol · L^{-1} solution. Weigh out about 0.1 g solid sodium carbonate (Na$_2$CO$_3$). Stir the sodium carbonate first, and then add the sodium thiosulfate to the cooled water. Continue stirring until the solid sodium thiosulfate is completely dissolved. Store the sodium thiosulfate solution in the freshly prepared dark bottle. Allow the sodium thiosulfate solution to stand for 24 h before it is standardized.

Pipet 25.00 mL of 0.016 67 mol · L^{-1} K$_2$Cr$_2$O$_7$ solution into a 250 mL Erlenmeyer flask, add 1 g of KI and 3 mL of HCl solution (1 ∶ 1). Swirl the solution gently. Let it stand in dark place for 5 min. Add 100 mL distilled water. Titrate immediately with Na$_2$S$_2$O$_3$ solution until the solution has lost its initial reddish-brown color and has become pale yellow. Add 2 mL of starch indicator and complete the titration. Repeat the titration twice. From the titration volume, calculate the concentration of the Na$_2$S$_2$O$_3$ solution.

$$c(\text{Na}_2\text{S}_2\text{O}_3) = \frac{6 \times c(\text{K}_2\text{Cr}_2\text{O}_7) \times V(\text{K}_2\text{Cr}_2\text{O}_7)}{V(\text{Na}_2\text{S}_2\text{O}_3)}$$

2. Preparation and Standardization of 0.025 mol · L^{-1} I$_2$ Solution

Weigh about 7.3 g of KI into a 100 mL beaker, add 2 g of I$_2$ and 5 mL of distilled water, stir for several minutes, introduce an additional 10 mL of distilled water, and stir again for several minutes, carefully decant the bulk of the liquid into a storage bottle, and then dilute to 300 mL.

Pipet 20.00 mL of I$_2$ solution into a 250 mL Erlenmeyer flask, add 100 mL of distilled water. Titrate immediately with Na$_2$S$_2$O$_3$ solution until the solution has lost its initial reddish-brown color and has become pale yellow. Add 2 mL of starch indicator and complete the titration. Repeat the titration twice. From the titration volume, calculate the concentration of the I$_2$ solution.

$$c(\text{I}_2) = \frac{c(\text{Na}_2\text{S}_2\text{O}_3) \times V(\text{Na}_2\text{S}_2\text{O}_3)}{2 \times V(\text{I}_2)}$$

3. Determination of the Content of the Glucose

Pipet 1.00 mL of 5% glucose solution into a 100 mL volumetric flask, dilute it to the mark and mix thoroughly. Transfer 20.00 mL of this solution into a 250 mL Erlenmeyer flask, add 20.00 mL of I$_2$ standard solution. Add 0.2 mol · L^{-1} NaOH solution dropwise until the dark brown of the iodine in solution has diminished and the solution is a pale yellow color. Allow the solution to stand for 10-20 min, and then add 6 mL of 2 mol $\cdot$ L^{-1} HCl solution. Titrate immediately with 0. 05 mol $\cdot$ L^{-1} Na$_2$S$_2$O$_3$ solution until the solution has become pale yellow. Add 2 mL of starch indicator and continue the titration until the intense blue of the starch-iodine complex just disappears. Repeat the titration twice. From the titration volume, calculate the content of the glucose.

Content of C$_6$H$_{12}$O$_6$

$$= \frac{[2c(I_2) \times V(I_2) - c(Na_2S_2O_3) \times V(Na_2S_2O_3)] \times M(C_6H_{12}O_6) \times 100}{2\ 000 \times 20.\ 00}$$

V Questions

(1) Why is the excessive KI added when preparing I$_2$ solution?

(2) Why should the NaOH solution be added slowly when the glucose is oxidized?

Experiment 12　Determination of Water Hardness Using Complexometric Titration

I Learning Objectives

(1) Learn complexometric titration.

(2) Learn to determine water hardness.

II Principles

In nature, water is hardened by the passage of rainwater containing dissolved carbon dioxide through layers of stone such as chalk, gypsum, or limestone. Hard water contains multiply charged ions such as calcium, magnesium, and heavy metal ions, which replace sodium and potassium ions in soaps and detergents to form precipitates. These precipitates interfere with cleaning action and leave bathtub rings and scum. Calcium carbonate (CaCO$_3$) is the most common precipitate. It is water insoluble and is the main component that clogs pipes. Concentrations of Mg^{2+} and Ca^{2+} are much higher than any other ions responsible for hardness, and total water hardness is defined as the sum of the calcium and magnesium concentrations. Total water hardness is usually expressed as the milligrams of $CaCO_3$ equivalent to the total amount of calcium and magnesium present in one liter of water ($mg \cdot L^{-1}$). Water hardness may range from zero to hundreds $mg \cdot L^{-1}$, depending on the source. The classification of degree of water hardness according to the US Geological Survey is as follows:

Soft　　　　　　　　　0-60 $mg \cdot L^{-1}$ $CaCO_3$ equivalents

Moderately hard　　　61-120 $mg \cdot L^{-1}$ $CaCO_3$ equivalents

Hard　　　　　　　　121-180 $mg \cdot L^{-1}$ $CaCO_3$ equivalents

Very hard　　　　　$\geqslant$181 $mg \cdot L^{-1}$ $CaCO_3$ equivalents

Complexometric titration is based on the formation of a complex ion. Ethlyenediaminetetraacetic acid (EDTA or H_4Y, where $Y = C_{10}H_{12}N_2O_8$) is a complexing agent designed to bind metal ions quantitatively, forming stable, water soluble complexes with a 1 : 1 stoichiometry for most metal ions (i. e. , 1 mole of EDTA binds to 1 mole of metal ion). EDTA binds to both calcium and magnesium, but binds more tightly to calcium, thus:

$$Ca^{2+} + H_2Y^{2-} \rightleftharpoons [CaY]^{2-} + 2H^+$$
$$Mg^{2+} + H_2Y^{2-} \rightleftharpoons [MgY]^{2-} + 2H^+$$
$$Ca^{2+} + [MgY]^{2-} \rightleftharpoons [CaY]^{2-} + Mg^{2+}$$

As a sample is titrated with EDTA, the calcium ions in the sample are preferentially complexed by the EDTA, while magnesium complexes with the indicator. EDTA-metal complexes are generally uncolored; however, metallochromic indicators change color depending on whether they are bound or unbound. After all the free calcium and magnesium are bound by EDTA, additional EDTA extracts the magnesium ions from the eriochrome black T indicator, restoring it to its uncomplexed blue color, and an endpoint is observed.

$$[MgIn]^- (wine\ red) + H_2Y^{2-} \rightleftharpoons [MgY]^{2-} + HIn^{2-} (blue) + H^+$$

Eriochrome black T does not give a sharp color change for water containing calcium, but no magnesium. To make sure that there is some magnesium present in the sample, we add a small amount of Mg-EDTA (Magnesium already complexed with EDTA). Since we add the same amount of EDTA as Mg^{2+}, the addition of Mg-EDTA to the sample has no net effect on the subsequent titration.

Both EDTA and the metallochromic indicators are weak acids and their actions are very pH dependent; thus we use a pH 10 buffer solution to hold the solutions at an appropriate pH for both the EDTA and the eriochrome black T indicator to work well. Some metal ions interfere with this titration by causing indistinct endpoints, or by complexing with EDTA and/or the indicator more strongly than the metals of interest. We will look at an example of a chemical masking agent that is used to counteract such occurrences.

In this experiment, you will use EDTA complexometric titration to determine the hardness of a sample of water brought from your home. Both the total hardness and the individual calcium and magnesium hardnesses will be measured. EDTA and the metallochromic indicators used are involved in complexation reactions with the magnesium and calcium ions that are responsible for water hardness. A color change is observed when EDTA replaces the indicator molecule as the ligand in the divalent ion complex. Solubility products will be used to our advantage when determining the calcium hardness. You are encouraged to bring your own water sample to study.

III Apparatus and Reagents

Analytical balances (0.1 mg, 0.01 g), weighing bottles (2), Geiser buret (50 mL×1), transfer pipets (20 mL×1, 100 mL×1), Mohr measuring pipets (20 mL ×1, 10 mL×1), volumetric flask (250 mL×1), Erlenmeyer flasks (250 mL×3), beakers (100 mL×1, 250 mL×1, 400 mL×1), graduated cylinders (100 mL×1, 50 mL×1, 10 mL×1), reagent bottle (500 mL×1), wash bottle, medicine dropper, rubber pipet bulb, stirring rod, watch glass and hot plate.

EDTA (AR, s), $CaCO_3$ (GR, s), HCl solution (1 : 1), eriochrome black T indicator, NH_3-NH_4Cl buffer solution (pH = 10), Mg-EDTA solution (0.01 $mol \cdot L^{-1}$) and water sample.

IV Procedure

1. Preparation and Standardization of 0.02 $mol \cdot L^{-1}$ EDTA Solution

Weigh about 9.3 g of $Na_2EDTA \cdot 2H_2O$ into a clean 400 mL beaker. Dissolve it and transfer it to a clean 500 mL bottle. Dilute to about 500 mL. Mix the solution thoroughly and label the bottle.

Obtain dried $CaCO_3$ stored in the desiccator at the front of the lab. Accurately weigh about 0.5 g in a 250 mL beaker. Dissolve the solid completely (clear solution) in the minimum amount of 1 : 1 HCl solution. Heat on a hot plate to evaporate to dryness. Then dissolve the residue in distilled water. Transfer to a 250 mL volumetric flask and dilute to the mark.

Transfer 20.00 mL of the primary standard Ca^{2+} solution into a 250 mL

Erlenmeyer flask. Add 50 mL of distilled water, 5 mL of pH 10 buffer solution, 2 mL of Mg-EDTA solution, and 3 drops of eriochrome black T indicator (purple-red) and mix well. Titrate carefully with the 0. 02 mol • L^{-1} EDTA solution until the color changes from wine red to pure blue. Repeat the titration two more times. Calculate the concentration of the EDTA solution.

2. Determination of Water Hardness

Transfer 100. 00 mL water sample into a 250 mL Erlenmeyer flask. Add 5 mL of pH 10 buffer solution and 3 drops of eriochrome black T indicator. Titrate carefully with the 0. 02 mol • L^{-1} EDTA solution until the color changes from wine red to pure blue. Repeat the titration two more times. Calculate the total hardness of your water sample as mg • L^{-1} of $CaCO_3$ equivalents, using the molecular weight of $CaCO_3$ in your calculation.

V Questions

(1) Why did you use a pH = 10 buffer solution for your total water hardness titrations?

(2) Considering solubility products, explain the function of the sodium hydroxide when you analyze calcium ions. Why didn't you use eriochrome black T indicator for the calcium determination?

(3) EDTA or other chelating agents can be found in many products such as shampoos, soaps, cleaning products, plant foods, salad dressings, canned foods, etc.. Choose such a product and suggest the function of EDTA in that product.

Experiment 13   The Common Ion Effect and Precipitation Equilibrium

I Learning Objectives

(1) Observe the common ion effect on solubility.

(2) Understand the precipitation equilibrium and the shift of the equilibrium.

(3) Judge the formation, dissolution and transformation of the precipitates.

II Principles

The common ion effect is an example of Le Chatelier's principle which states that a system at equilibrium, subjected to a disturbance or stress, adjusts so as to reduce the effect of the disturbance. For example, HAc in equilibrium with Ac^- (aq) and H_3O^+ (aq) is described by

$$HAc + H_2O \Longrightarrow H_3O^+ + Ac^-$$

The equilibrium was disturbed by the addition of Ac^-, a shift in the equilibrium will occur that will reduce the concentration of Ac^-. The degree of ionization of HAc is decreased by the addition of NaAc. Consequently, the $[H^+]$ of the solution is reduced. The NaAc has Ac^- in common with HAc, so the influence is known as the common ion effect.

When an excess of a slightly soluble ionic compound is mixed with water, an equilibrium occurs between the solid compound and the ions in the saturated solution.

$$A_m B_n \Longrightarrow m A^{n+} + n B^{m-}$$

The equilibrium constant for this solubility process is called the solubility product constant of a slightly soluble ionic compound. It is written:

$$K_{sp} = [A^{n+}]^m [B^{m-}]^n$$

Precipitation is expected to occur if the ion product (IP) for a solubility reaction is greater than K_{sp}. If the ion product is less than K_{sp}, precipitation will not occur (the solution is unsaturated with respect to the ionic compound). If the ion product equals K_{sp}, the reaction is at equilibrium (the solution is saturated with the ionic compound).

If IP $< K_{sp}$, precipitation will not occur. (Unsaturated solution)

If IP $= K_{sp}$, the reaction is at equilibrium. (Saturated solution)

If IP $> K_{sp}$, precipitation is expected to occur. (Supersaturated solution)

When two anions form sparingly soluble compounds with the same cation or when two cations form sparingly soluble compounds with the same anion, the less soluble compound will precipitate first on the addition of a precipitant to a solution containing both. An additional quantity of the less soluble compound will precipitate along with the precipitation of the more soluble compound if addition of the precipitant is continued (coprecipitation).

Ⅲ Apparatus and Reagents

Centrifuge, beakers (100 mL×4), centrifuge tubes (2) and test tubes (10).

NaAc (AR,s), NaAc (0. 1 mol · L^{-1}), NH_4Cl (s), HAc solution (0. 1 mol · L^{-1}), HNO_3 solution (6 mol · L^{-1}), NaOH solution (0. 2 mol · L^{-1}, 0. 002 mol · L^{-1}),

$NH_3 \cdot H_2O$ solution (0.1 mol $\cdot$ L^{-1}, 2 mol $\cdot$ L^{-1}), HCl solution (0.1 mol $\cdot$ L^{-1}, 6 mol $\cdot$ L^{-1}), $Pb(NO_3)_2$ solution (0.1 mol $\cdot$ L^{-1}, 0.001 mol $\cdot$ L^{-1}), KI solution (0.1 mol $\cdot$ L^{-1}, 0.001 mol $\cdot$ L^{-1}), NH_4Cl solution (1 mol $\cdot$ L^{-1}), $CdCl_2$ solution (0.1 mol $\cdot$ L^{-1}), $FeCl_3$ solution (0.1 mol $\cdot$ L^{-1}), K_2CrO_4 solution (0.1 mol $\cdot$ L^{-1}), Na_2S solution (0.1 mol $\cdot$ L^{-1}), Na_2CO_3 solution (0.1 mol $\cdot$ L^{-1}), NaCl solution (1 mol $\cdot$ L^{-1}, 0.1 mol $\cdot$ L^{-1}), $MgCl_2$ solution (0.2 mol $\cdot$ L^{-1}), $(NH_4)_2C_2O_4$ solution (saturated solution), $AgNO_3$ solution (0.1 mol $\cdot$ L^{-1}), $CuSO_4$ solution (0.1 mol $\cdot$ L^{-1}), $CaCl_2$ solution (0.1 mol $\cdot$ L^{-1}), $BaCl_2$ solution (0.3 mol $\cdot$ L^{-1}), pH test papers (5.5-9.0), methyl orange indicator and phenolphthalein indicator.

Ⅳ Procedure

1. The Common Ion Effect

(1) Add 5 mL of 0.1 mol $\cdot$ L^{-1} HAc solution to a test tube. Observe the color of the solution when 1 drop of methyl orange indicator is added. Then add a little amount of solid NaAc to it. What color appears? Please draw a conclusion from that change.

(2) Take two test tubes containing 2 mL of 0.1 mol $\cdot$ L^{-1} $NH_3 \cdot H_2O$ solution and 1 drop of phenolphthalein indicator. Observe the color of the solutions. Add a little amount of solid NH_4Ac to one tube. Please compare it with the other tube without NH_4Ac. Explain the reason of change.

(3) Add 15 mL of 0.1 mol $\cdot$ L^{-1} HAc solution and 15 mL of 0.1 mol $\cdot$ L^{-1} NaAc solution to a beaker to prepare a HAc-NaAc buffer solution. Using pH test paper, determine the pH of the solution. Then divide the solution into three tubes. To one test tube add 10 drops of 0.1 mol $\cdot$ L^{-1} HCl solution, to the second one add 10 drops of 0.1 mol $\cdot$ L^{-1} NaOH solution, to the third one add 10 drops of H_2O, redetermine all the pH.

2. The Application of the Solubility Product

(1) Formation of the precipitates.

Add 1 mL of 0.1 mol $\cdot$ L^{-1} $Pb(NO_3)_2$ solution to a test tube, and then add 1 mL of 0.1 mol $\cdot$ L^{-1} KI solution. Observe if there are precipitates forming. Explain the reason.

Add 1 mL of 0.001 mol $\cdot$ L^{-1} $Pb(NO_3)_2$ solution to a test tube, and then add 1 mL of 0.001 mol $\cdot$ L^{-1} KI solution. Observe if there are precipitates forming. Explain the reason.

Add 2 drops of 0.1 mol $\cdot$ L^{-1} CuSO$_4$ solution and 6 drops of 0.1 mol $\cdot$ L^{-1} CdCl$_2$ solution to a centrifuge tube. Dilute it with 2 mL of distilled water. Then add 3 drops of 0.1 mol $\cdot$ L^{-1} Na$_2$S solution. Observe the color of the precipitate that first appears (black or yellow). Centrifuge any precipitate (that's the solid) that form, decant and save the supernatant (that's the liquid). Then add 0.1 mol $\cdot$ L^{-1} Na$_2$S solution dropwise to the supernatant until the precipitate forms. Observe the color of the precipitate. Interpret your results in terms of solubility product.

(2) Dissolution of the precipitates.

Add 5 drops of 0.3 mol $\cdot$ L^{-1} BaCl$_2$ solution to a test tube, and then add 3 drops of (NH$_4$)$_2$C$_2$O$_4$ saturated solution. White precipitate is forming. Now add 6 mol $\cdot$ L^{-1} HCl solution to the precipitate. What happens? Write the reaction equation.

Add 10 drops of 0.1 mol $\cdot$ L^{-1} AgNO$_3$ solution to a test tube, and then add an equal volume of 0.1 mol $\cdot$ L^{-1} NaCl solution to the tube. White precipitate is forming. Now add 2 mol $\cdot$ L^{-1} NH$_3$ $\cdot$ H$_2$O solution to the precipitate. What happens? Write the reaction equation.

To one test tube mix 5 drops of 0.1 mol $\cdot$ L^{-1} FeCl$_3$ solution with 5 drops of 0.2 mol $\cdot$ L^{-1} NaOH solution to form precipitate Fe(OH)$_3$. To the other, mix 5 drops of 0.1 mol $\cdot$ L^{-1} Na$_2$CO$_3$ solution with 5 drops of 0.1 mol $\cdot$ L^{-1} CaCl$_2$ solution to form precipitate CaCO$_3$. Add 6 mol $\cdot$ L^{-1} HCl solution dropwise to the each precipitate mentioned above. What happens? Write the reaction equation.

Add 10 drops of 0.2 mol $\cdot$ L^{-1} MgCl$_2$ solution to a test tube, and then add 2 drops of 2 mol $\cdot$ L^{-1} NH$_3$ $\cdot$ H$_2$O solution. What sign of a reaction do you observe? Now add 10 drops of 1 mol $\cdot$ L^{-1} NH$_4$Cl solution to the precipitate. What happens then? Write the reaction equation.

Add 5 drops of 0.1 mol $\cdot$ L^{-1} CuSO$_4$ solution to a test tube containing 5 drops of 0.1 mol $\cdot$ L^{-1} Na$_2$S solution. What sign of a reaction do you observe? Then add 10 drops of 6 mol $\cdot$ L^{-1} HNO$_3$ solution and heat slightly. What happens? Write the reaction equation.

(3) Transformation of precipitates.

Add 5 drops of 0.1 mol $\cdot$ L^{-1} K$_2$CrO$_4$ solution to a test tube containing 10 drops of 0.1 mol $\cdot$ L^{-1} AgNO$_3$ solution. What sign of a reaction do you observe? Then add 10 drops of 0.1 mol $\cdot$ L^{-1} NaCl solution. What happens? Explain the reason.

Add 10 drops of 0.1 mol $\cdot$ L^{-1} Pb(NO$_3$)$_2$ solution and 10 drops of 1 mol $\cdot$ L^{-1}

NaCl solution to a centrifuge tube. Centrifuge any precipitate (that's the solid) that forms, decant and save the precipitate. Then add $0.1 \text{ mol} \cdot \text{L}^{-1}$ KI solution dropwise to the precipitate. Observe the color of the precipitate. Write the reaction equation.

3. Predict the Value of the Solubility Product of Mg(OH)$_2$

Add 25 mL of $0.2 \text{ mol} \cdot \text{L}^{-1}$ MgCl$_2$ solution to a 50 mL beaker which is underlaid a piece of black paper at the bottom. Then add $0.002 \text{ mol} \cdot \text{L}^{-1}$ NaOH solution to MgCl$_2$ solution drop by drop. Stir constantly until precipitate is forming. (Please observe on the blazing sunshine directly.) Note that NaOH solution should not be excessive. (Why?) Determine the value of the pH of the solution with pH test paper. Calculate $[OH^-]$ and K_{sp}.

V Questions

(1) Is the common ion effect in the precipitation equilibrium as same as that in the ionization equilibrium?

(2) What happened to the pH of the Mg(OH)$_2$ saturated solution after MgCl$_2$ solution was added? Explain in terms of Le Chatelier's principle.

(3) What is the condition of the formation of the precipitate?

(4) What is the common ion effect? What is a buffer solution?

Experiment 14   Preparation and Properties of Buffer Solutions

I Learning Objectives

(1) Learn the properties of buffer solutions.

(2) Learn the preparation of buffer solutions.

II Principles

A buffer solution is defined as a solution that resists a change in pH when a small amount of an acid or base is added to it or when the solution is diluted. A buffer solution consists of a mixture of a weak acid (HB) and its conjugate base (B$^-$). The pH value of a buffer solution can be calculated by the following equation:

$$pH = pK_a + \lg \frac{c(B^-)}{c(HB)}$$

K_a is the acid ionization constant.

From the equation you can see that the pH value of a buffer solution depends upon the value of the ionization constant of conjugate acid and the concentration ratio of the conjugate acid to its conjugate base at equilibrium.

When a buffer solution is prepared by mixing equal concentrations of conjugate acid and conjugate base, the equation can be expressed as:

$$pH = pK_a + \lg \frac{V(B^-)}{V(HB)}$$

Colorimetry may be used to measure the pH value of buffer solutions. Prepare standard colorimetric series with a suitable indicator (a series of buffer solutions of known pH, and then add the same kind and amount of indicator into a sample solution), obtain the pH value of the sample solution by comparing the color with the standard colorimetric series.

Buffer capacity is a quantitative measure of the ability of the buffer solution to resist changes in pH. It depends on concentrations and the ratio [B$^-$] to [HB]. If the ratio [B$^-$] to [HB] is the same, the buffer capacity is directly proportional to the concentration. If the concentration is the same, the buffer capacity is largest when the ratio [B$^-$] to [HB] is 1 : 1.

III Apparatus and Reagents

Colorimetric tubes (10 mL×10), Mohr measuring pipets (10 mL×4, 5 mL×1), beakers (100 mL×4), test tubes (6), rubber pipet bulb and wash bottle.

K_2HPO_4 solution (0.2 mol · L^{-1}), KH_2PO_4 solution (0.2 mol · L^{-1}), NaOH solution (0.2 mol · L^{-1}), HCl solution (0.2 mol · L^{-1}), bromthymol blue indicator, extensive pH indicator and methyl orange indicator.

IV Procedure

1. Preparation of the Standard Colorimetric Series

The table below summarizes the preparation of the standard colorimetric series. Pipet 0.2 mol · L^{-1} KH_2PO_4 solution and 0.2 mol · L^{-1} K_2HPO_4 solution into each colorimetric tube, add 4 drops of bromthymol blue indicator respectively. Mix the solutions thoroughly, observe the color of each tube and calculate the pH of buffer solutions.

No.	I	II	III	IV	V	VI	VII	VIII	IX
$0.2\ mol \cdot L^{-1}KH_2PO_4/mL$	1.00	2.00	3.00	4.00	5.00	6.00	7.00	8.00	9.00
$0.2\ mol \cdot L^{-1}K_2HPO_4/mL$	9.00	8.00	7.00	6.00	5.00	4.00	3.00	2.00	1.00
Bromthymol blue/drops	4	4	4	4	4	4	4	4	4
Theoretical value of pH				.					
Measured value of pH									

2. Preparation of a Buffer Solution

Calculate the volumes of $0.2\ mol \cdot L^{-1}\ NaOH$ solution and $0.2\ mol \cdot L^{-1}$ KH_2PO_4 solution ($pK_a = 7.40$) required for preparing 30 mL of a pH 7.21 buffer solution.

According to the results of calculation, pipet the NaOH solution and KH_2PO_4 solution into a 50 mL beaker, and mix the solution well. Pipet 10.00 mL of the prepared buffer solution into a colorimetric tube, add 4 drops of bromthymol blue indicator, measure the pH value of the solution by comparing color with the standard colorimetric series.

3. Properties of Buffer Solutions

Measure out the solutions according to the table below, and observe the color change before or after adding acid, base and distilled water. Explain the reason.

No.	Reagent	Extensive pH indicator	Phenomenon	Add	Phenomenon	Reason
I	Prepared buffer solution, 2 mL	4 drops		2 drops of H_2O		
II	Prepared buffer solution, 2 mL	4 drops		2 drops of HCl		
III	Prepared buffer solution, 2 mL	4 drops		2 drops of NaOH		
IV	H_2O, 2mL	4 drops		2 drops of HCl		
V	H_2O, 2mL	4 drops		2 drops of NaOH		

4. Buffer Capacity

(1) The relationship between buffer capacity and the ratio $[B^-]$ to $[HB]$.

According to the table below, pipet $0.2\ mol \cdot L^{-1}\ KH_2PO_4$ solution and 0.2 $mol \cdot L^{-1}\ K_2HPO_4$ solution into a colorimetric tube, and add 1 drop of methyl orange indicator respectively. Mix the solutions thoroughly, and observe the color of each tube. Add 0.2 mol $\cdot$ L^{-1} HCl solution drop by drop respectively until the color of the solution just changes, record the drops of the HCl solution used. Account for the reason.

No.	0.2 mol $\cdot$ L^{-1} KH$_2$PO$_4$/mL	0.2 mol $\cdot$ L^{-1} K$_2$HPO$_4$/mL	Methyl orange	Color	The drops of HCl solution used	Reason
I	2.00	2.00	1 drop			
II	3.00	1.00	1 drop			

(2) The relationship between buffer capacity and concentrations.

According to the table below, pipet 0.2 mol $\cdot$ L^{-1} KH$_2$PO$_4$ solution and 0.2 mol $\cdot$ L^{-1} K$_2$HPO$_4$ solution and distilled water into a colorimetric tube, and add 1 drop of methyl orange indicator respectively. Mix the solutions thoroughly, and observe the color of each tube. Add 0.2 mol $\cdot$ L^{-1} HCl solution drop by drop respectively until the color of the solution just changes, record the amount of the HCl solution used. Account for the reason.

No.	0.2 mol $\cdot$ L^{-1} KH$_2$PO$_4$/mL	0.2 mol $\cdot$ L^{-1} K$_2$HPO$_4$/mL	H$_2$O/mL	Methyl orange	Color	The drops of HCl solution used	Reason
I	2.00	2.00	0.00	1 drop			
II	0.50	0.50	3.00	1 drop			

V Question

Does NaHCO$_3$ solution have buffer capacity? Why?

Experiment 15 Oxidation-Reduction Reaction and Electrode Potential

I Learning Objectives

(1) Understand the relationship between oxidation-reduction (redox) reaction and electrode potential.

(2) Qualitatively compare the electrode potential of redox couple.

(3) Understand the effect of concentration and acidity on redox reaction.

Ⅱ Principles

An oxidation-reduction reaction, or redox reaction, is one in which electrons are transferred from one species to another. An oxidant is a species that oxidizes another species, and it is itself reduced. Similarly, a reductant is a species that reduces another species, and it is itself oxidized. Electrode potentials are useful in determining the strengths of oxidant and reductant. For any half-cell reaction:

$$p\text{Ox} + ne^- \rightleftharpoons q\text{Red}$$

$$\varphi(\text{Ox/Red}) = \varphi^{\ominus}(\text{Ox/Red}) + \frac{RT}{nF}\ln\frac{(c_{\text{Ox}})^p}{(c_{\text{Red}})^q}$$

This is the Nernst equation for the electrode. n is the number of electrons involved in the half-cell reaction. c_{Ox} refers to the concentration of oxidized form and c_{Red} refers to the concentration of reduced form.

The strongest oxidants are the oxidized species with the largest (most positive) φ values. The strongest reductants are the reduced species with the smallest (most negative) φ values.

In a redox reaction, the stronger oxidant takes electrons from the stronger reductant, yielding the weaker reductant and weaker oxidant. Thus, the oxidation state of redox couple with the larger electrode potential can oxidize the reduction state of redox couple with the lower electrode potential. In other words, we can estimate the direction of the redox reaction in accordance with their electrode potential.

The relatively magnitude of electrode potential is affected by concentration, pH and temperature etc. , according to Nernst equation. Consequently, they will affect the direction, rate and product of the redox reaction.

The strength of oxidant and reductant is relative. Such as H_2O_2: if it reacts with a strong oxidant, it will unfold reducing property; when it reacts with a strong reductant, it is an oxidant.

When a metal is immersed in a solution of its ion, an electromotive force (voltage) develops between the ion-metal interface. If this half-cell is connected via a salt bridge to another half-cell comprising a different metal, the voltage and current will flow between the two cells. A typical cell would look like the Figure 2-3.

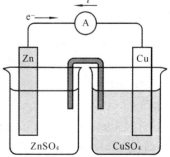

Figure **2**-3   A copper-zinc cell

The half-cell reactions that would occur with such a cell would be:

$$Cu^{2+}(aq)+2e^- \Longrightarrow Cu(s) \quad \varphi^{\ominus}(Cu^{2+}/Cu)=0.34 \text{ V}$$
$$Zn(s)-2e^- \Longrightarrow Zn^{2+}(aq) \quad \varphi^{\ominus}(Zn^{2+}/Zn)=-0.76 \text{ V}$$

If the concentrations of all ions were 1 mol $\cdot$ L^{-1}, this cell would produce a potential (voltage) of about 1.1 V. If the concentration of either the Zn^{2+} or Cu^{2+} is changed, the voltage will also change. It has been found that the voltage is related to the concentration by the following equation:

$$E_{cell}=E_{cell}^{\ominus}-\frac{RT}{nF}\ln Q \text{ or } E_{cell}=E_{cell}^{\ominus}-\frac{2.303RT}{nF}\lg Q(\text{the Nernst equation for the cell})$$

The variables E_{cell}, $E_{cell}^{\ominus}$, and n are the calculated cell electromotive force (emf), the standard emf, and the number of electrons transferred, respectively. The variable Q takes the same form as the equilibrium constant.

III Apparatus and Reagents

Test tubes (10), test tube racks, dropping bottles, salt bridge, beakers (50 mL×2) and voltmeter.

ZnSO$_4$ solution (0.1 mol $\cdot$ L^{-1}), CuSO$_4$ solution (0.1 mol $\cdot$ L^{-1}), KMnO$_4$ solution (0.01 mol $\cdot$ L^{-1}), KI solution (0.1 mol $\cdot$ L^{-1}), KBr solution (0.1 mol $\cdot$ L^{-1}), FeCl$_3$ solution (0.1 mol $\cdot$ L^{-1}), FeSO$_4$ solution (0.1 mol $\cdot$ L^{-1}), KSCN solution (0.1 mol $\cdot$ L^{-1}), H$_2$O$_2$ solution (0.1 mol $\cdot$ L^{-1}), Br$_2$ water (saturated solution), I$_2$ water (saturated solution), H$_2$SO$_4$ solution (1.0 mol $\cdot$ L^{-1}), HAc solution (6 mol $\cdot$ L^{-1}), NaOH solution (6 mol $\cdot$ L^{-1}), Na$_2$SO$_3$(AR,s), Na$_2$SO$_3$ solution (0.1 mol $\cdot$ L^{-1}), NH$_3$ $\cdot$ H$_2$O(concentrated solution), distilled water, CCl$_4$, zinc strip and copper strip.

IV Procedure

1. The Nernst Equation and a Copper-Zinc Cell

(1) Assemble the apparatus as Figure 2-3.

(2) Fill the beaker two-thirds full with 0.1 mol $\cdot$ L^{-1} ZnSO$_4$ solution and place a clean strip of zinc into it. The zinc strip should be connected to the negative terminal of the voltmeter.

(3) Place about 30 mL of 0.1 mol $\cdot$ L^{-1} CuSO$_4$ solution in a 50 mL beaker and place a clean strip of copper into it. Connect the copper strip to the positive terminal of the voltmeter.

(4) A salt bridge filled with an inert electrolyte (such as 1 mol $\cdot$ L^{-1} Na$_2$SO$_4$

solution) may be used. A salt bridge consists of a U-tube filled with the electrolyte and stoppered with cotton or glass wool plugs. Insert one leg of the U-tube into the beaker with the zinc metal and zinc solution. Insert the other leg into the beaker with the copper metal and copper solution.

(5) After the voltage stabilizes, take a reading.

(6) Take out the salt bridge, and then add concentrated $NH_3 \cdot H_2O$ dropwise into the beaker with the copper metal and copper solution until a deep purple-blue color remains (due to $[Cu(NH_3)_4]^{2+}$). Repeat steps (4) and (5). Record the voltage.

(7) Take out the salt bridge, and then add concentrated $NH_3 \cdot H_2O$ dropwise into the beaker with the zinc metal and zinc solution until a transparent liquid remains (due to $[Zn(NH_3)_4]^{2+}$). Repeat steps (4) and (5). Record the voltage.

2. Relationship between Electrode Potential and Redox Reaction

(1) Qualitatively compare with electrode potential.

To two test tubes add 2 drops of $0.1 \ mol \cdot L^{-1}$ $FeCl_3$ solution and 20 drops of CCl_4. Then to one test tube add 10 drops of $0.1 \ mol \cdot L^{-1}$ KI solution and the other add 10 drops of $0.1 \ mol \cdot L^{-1}$ KBr solution, shake the test tubes sufficiently. Observe the color change in CCl_4 layer and explain the phenomenon. Write down their reaction equation.

To two test tubes add 10 drops of bromine water and 10 drops of iodine water, respectively. Add 10 drops of $0.1 \ mol \cdot L^{-1}$ $FeSO_4$ solution in each tube, shake, and then add 5 drops of $0.1 \ mol \cdot L^{-1}$ KSCN solution. Observe the color change and record the phenomenon. Explain it.

Compare with the electrode potentials of I_2/I^-, Br_2/Br^- and Fe^{3+}/Fe^{2+}. Point out the strongest oxidant and reductant among these redox couple. Deduce the relationship between electrode potentials and redox reactions.

(2) Relativity of redox.

Oxidation of H_2O_2: To a test tube add 10 drops of $0.1 \ mol \cdot L^{-1}$ KI solution, and then add 3 drops of $1.0 \ mol \cdot L^{-1}$ H_2SO_4 solution, 2 drops of $0.1 \ mol \cdot L^{-1}$ H_2O_2 solution and 20 drops of CCl_4, shake the tube. Record the observation and explain the change with the reaction equation.

Reduction of H_2O_2: To a test tube add 5 drops of $0.01 \ mol \cdot L^{-1}$ $KMnO_4$ solution, and then add 3 drops of $1.0 \ mol \cdot L^{-1}$ H_2SO_4 solution, shake. Now add $0.1 \ mol \cdot L^{-1}$ H_2O_2 solution dropwise with stirring. Record the observation and write the reaction equation.

Conclude when H_2O_2 can be used as an oxidant or a reductant and indicate its oxidized product or reduced product with redox reaction equation.

3. The Effect of pH on Redox Reaction

(1) To two test tubes add 10 drops of $0.1 \, \text{mol} \cdot \text{L}^{-1}$ KBr solution. To one test tube add 5 drops of $1.0 \, \text{mol} \cdot \text{L}^{-1} \, H_2SO_4$ solution and the other add 5 drops of $6.0 \, \text{mol} \cdot \text{L}^{-1} \, \text{HAc}$ solution, shake the test tubes sufficiently. Then to each tube add 1 drop of $0.01 \, \text{mol} \cdot \text{L}^{-1} \, KMnO_4$ solution. Compare the rate of reaction and explain it.

(2) To three test tubes add 10 drops of $0.1 \, \text{mol} \cdot \text{L}^{-1} \, Na_2SO_3$ solution. To one test tube add 10 drops of $1.0 \, \text{mol} \cdot \text{L}^{-1} \, H_2SO_4$ solution, to the second one add 10 drops of distilled water, and to the third one add 10 drops of $6.0 \, \text{mol} \cdot \text{L}^{-1} \, \text{NaOH}$ solution, shake them all. Then add 5 drops of $0.01 \, \text{mol} \cdot \text{L}^{-1} \, KMnO_4$ solution into each tube. Record the observation and write the reaction equation.

(3) To a test tube add 10 drops of $0.1 \, \text{mol} \cdot \text{L}^{-1} \, \text{KI}$ solution, and then add 2 drops of $0.1 \, \text{mol} \cdot \text{L}^{-1} \, KIO_3$ solution, shake. Now add $1 \, \text{mol} \cdot \text{L}^{-1} \, H_2SO_4$ solution dropwise with stirring. What sign of a reaction do you observe? Then add $1 \, \text{mol} \cdot \text{L}^{-1}$ NaOH dropwise with stirring. What happens? Write the reaction equation.

(4) To two dry test tubes add a portion of the crystal MnO_2. Then to one test tube add 20 drops of $2 \, \text{mol} \cdot \text{L}^{-1}$ HCl solution and the other add 20 drops of concentrated hydrochloric acid solution. Hang a piece of moist potassium iodide starch test paper near the mouth of the tube and heat the test tubes respectively. Record the observation and write the reaction equation.

V Questions

(1) What factors will affect the electrode potential?

(2) Can we get a conclusion that the larger the cell electromotive force, the higher the reaction rate?

(3) What is the role of the salt bridge?

Experiment 16　Preparation and Properties of Coordination Compounds

I Learning Objectives

(1) Learn the preparation of coordination compounds.

(2) Understand the differences between coordination compounds and simple compounds.

(3) Know the stability of coordination compounds and the factors that will influence the stability of coordination compounds. (The coordination equilibrium is affected by complexant, solubility, pH and redox reaction.)

(4) Learn the chelating effect.

II Principles

Coordination compounds are an important class of inorganic substances that contain a metal ion to which other ions or molecules are attached by means of coordinate covalent bonds. The ions or molecules that are bonded to the metal ion are called ligands. The central metal ion and attached ligands form a complex ion, or complex. The simplest complexes are the hydrated cations of the transition metals.

In this experiment, you will prepare tetraamminecoper (II) sulfate monohydrate, $[Cu(NH_3)_4]SO_4 \cdot H_2O$, from a reaction of $CuSO_4 \cdot 5H_2O$, in the crystalline state this compound is composed of tetraaquacopper (II) complex ions, $[Cu(H_2O)_4]$ $SO_4 \cdot H_2O$. If the reaction is carried out with high concentrations of copper(II) and ammonia present, the sulfate salt of the complex can be precipitated by the addition of ethanol to an aqueous solution of copper sulfate and ammonia. The chemical reaction described above is

$$[Cu(H_2O)_4]SO_4 \cdot H_2O(aq) + 4NH_3(aq) \rightleftharpoons [Cu(NH_3)_4]SO_4 \cdot H_2O(aq) + 4H_2O(l)$$

This is a single replacement reaction in which NH_3 molecules replace the water molecules originally bonded to the copper(II) ion.

The aqueous copper(II) ion forms a complex ion with ammonia by reacting with NH_3 in steps. The equilibria and the corresponding equilibrium constants are as follows.

$$Cu^{2+} + 4NH_3 \rightleftharpoons [Cu(NH_3)_4]^{2+}$$

$$K_s = \frac{[[Cu(NH_3)_4]^{2+}]}{[Cu^{2+}][NH_3]^4}$$

The larger the K_s is, the more stable the complex ion is, for ions of the same coordination number.

Le Chatelier's principle predicts that when a stress is applied to an equilibrium mixture, the equilibrium will shift to relieve the stress. Stresses include temperature changes, pressure changes, and changes in the concentrations of species in the mixture. For example, increasing the concentration of a complexant, NH_3, drives the reaction above forward.

The formation of complexes can have a large effect on the solubility of a compound in water. Silver chloride is only very weakly soluble in water, but addition of ammonia (NH_3) to the solution allows the complex ion $[Ag(NH_3)_2]^+$ to form:

$$AgCl(s) + 2NH_3(aq) \rightleftharpoons [Ag(NH_3)_2]^+(aq) + Cl^-(aq)$$

This greatly increases the solubility of the silver chloride. This process relies heavily on solubility and precipitation processes governed by solubility equilibria (with equilibrium constants known as K_{sp}) as well as complex formation equilibria (with equilibrium constants represented by K_s). Note that the smaller K_s and K_{sp} are, the more unstable the corresponding complex ion is.

The least stable oxidation state for cobalt is $+3$, except in the presence of strong complexing ligands.

$$Co^{3+} + e^- \rightleftharpoons Co^{2+} \quad \varphi^\ominus(Co^{3+}/Co^{2+}) = 1.81 \text{ V}$$

As can be seen from the above half-equation, cobalt (Ⅲ) ions are powerful oxidizing agents, being reduced to cobalt (Ⅱ) ions. Strong complexing agents, such as ammonia (or nitrile ions) allow the cobalt (Ⅱ) ions to be readily oxidized to cobalt (Ⅲ).

$$[Co(NH_3)_6]^{2+}(aq) - e^- \rightleftharpoons [Co(NH_3)_6]^{3+}(aq)$$
$$\varphi^\ominus([Co(NH_3)_6]^{3+}/[Co(NH_3)_6]^{2+}) = 0.13 \text{ V}$$

The stability of metal complexes depends on the metal ion and the ligand. In general the stability of metal complexes increases if the central ion increases in charge, decreases in size, and increases in electron affinity. Several characteristics of the ligand are known to influence the stability of metal complexes: ① basicity of the ligand; ② the number of metal-chelate rings per ligand; ③ the size of the chelate ring; ④ steric effects; ⑤ resonance effects; ⑥ the ligand atom. Since coordination compounds are formed as a result of acid-base reactions where the metal ion is the acid and the ligand is the base, it follows that generally the more basic ligand will tend to form the more stable complex. The size of the chelate ring is likewise an important factor. For saturated ligands such as dimethylglyoxime, five-membered rings are the most stable for chelates containing the more double bonds.

III Apparatus and Reagents

Analytical balance (0.01 g), beakers (50 mL×2), stirring rod, test tubes (10) and Buchner funnel.

$CuSO_4 \cdot 5H_2O$ (AR,s), HCl solution (1 mol $\cdot$ L^{-1}, 6 mol $\cdot$ L^{-1}), $NH_3 \cdot H_2O$ solution (2 mol $\cdot$ L^{-1}, concentrated solution), NaOH solution (1 mol $\cdot$ L^{-1}), Na_2CO_3 solution (0.1 mol $\cdot$ L^{-1}), Na_2S solution (0.1 mol $\cdot$ L^{-1}), $BaCl_2$ solution (0.1 mol $\cdot$ L^{-1}), $(NH_4)_2S$ solution (0.1 mol $\cdot$ L^{-1}), $(NH_4)_2C_2O_4$ solution (0.1 mol $\cdot$ L^{-1}), $FeCl_3$ solution (0.1 mol $\cdot$ L^{-1}), KSCN solution (1 mol $\cdot$ L^{-1}), NaBr solution (0.1 mol $\cdot$ L^{-1}), Na_2H_2Y solution (EDTA, 0.1 mol $\cdot$ L^{-1}), $Na_2S_2O_3$ solution (0.1 mol $\cdot$ L^{-1}), $AgNO_3$ solution (0.1 mol $\cdot$ L^{-1}), $CuSO_4$ solution (0.1 mol $\cdot$ L^{-1}), $CoCl_2$ solution (0.5 mol $\cdot$ L^{-1}), $NiCl_2$ solution (0.1 mol $\cdot$ L^{-1}), ethanol solution (95%), H_2O_2 solution (30%), dimethylglyoxime solution (1%), pH test paper and red litmus paper.

IV Procedure

1. Preparation and Analysis of Tetraamminecopper(II) Sulfate Monohydrate

(1) Preparation of $[Cu(NH_3)_4]SO_4 \cdot H_2O$.

Weigh about 2.5 g of $CuSO_4 \cdot 5H_2O$ into a clean 50 mL beaker. Add 10 mL of distilled water to the solid in the beaker. Stir with a glass stirring rod until the solid completely dissolves. Slowly add 5 mL of concentrated $NH_3 \cdot H_2O$ solution to the solution in the beaker. Stir the reaction mixture after each 1-2 mL addition of $NH_3 \cdot H_2O$ solution. Add, in a slow, dropwise manner, with continual stirring, 15 mL of ethanol to the beaker. The ammine complex salt should precipitate as deep purple-blue crystals. Cool the mixture in an ice water bath for about 15 min, and then isolate the product by suction filtration. Rinse the product on the funnel with a small amount of ethanol, and then spread it out on a watch glass to dry. (Store it in a desiccator over anhydrous calcium chloride until your next lab period.) Weigh the product for calculation of the percent yield.

(2) Analysis of $[Cu(NH_3)_4]SO_4 \cdot H_2O$.

Dissolve a portion of the crystal in several drops of distilled water, add excess 1 mol $\cdot$ L^{-1} HCl solution dropwise, observe and record the color change of the solution. Then add excess concentrated $NH_3 \cdot H_2O$ solution and observe the color change. Discuss the formation of $[Cu(NH_3)_4]SO_4 \cdot H_2O$.

Dissolve a portion of the crystal in several drops of distilled water, and then divide the solution into three tubes. To one test tube add $0.1 \ mol \cdot L^{-1} \ Na_2CO_3$ solution and observe whether there are $Cu_2(OH)_2CO_3$ precipitated from the solution. To the second one add $0.1 \ mol \cdot L^{-1} \ Na_2S$ solution and observe whether there are CuS precipitated from the solution. To the third one add $0.1 \ mol \cdot L^{-1}$ $BaCl_2$ solution and observe whether there are $BaSO_4$ precipitated from the solution.

Smell a portion of dried crystal to determine whether there is the odor of NH_3, and then put it in a dry test tube. Hang a piece of moist pH test paper or red litmus paper near the mouth of the tube and heat the crystal. Record the observation and write the reaction equation.

Conclude that whether NH_3 takes part in composing the coordination compound and whether the bond between NH_3 and Cu^{2+} is stable.

2. Complex Ions and Solubilities

(1) To two test tubes add 5 drops of $0.1 \ mol \cdot L^{-1} \ (NH_4)_2S$ solution and 5 drops of $0.1 \ mol \cdot L^{-1} \ (NH_4)_2C_2O_4$ solution, respectively. Add 5 drops of 0.1 $mol \cdot L^{-1} \ CuSO_4$ solution into each tube and observe whether there are precipitates formed from the solution. Add 10 drops of $6 \ mol \cdot L^{-1} \ NH_3 \cdot H_2O$ solution to the each precipitate above. What happens? Write the reaction equation.

Compare with K_{sp} of CuS and CuC_2O_4. Interpret your results in terms of solubility constants.

(2) To two test tubes add 10 drops of $0.1 \ mol \cdot L^{-1} \ AgNO_3$ solution. To one test tube add $0.1 \ mol \cdot L^{-1} \ Na_2S_2O_3$ solution dropwise until the precipitate forms. Continue to add excess $Na_2S_2O_3$ solution and observe the phenomenon. To the other add $2 \ mol \cdot L^{-1} \ NH_3 \cdot H_2O$ solution dropwise until the precipitate forms. Continue to add excess $NH_3 \cdot H_2O$ solution until the precipitate dissolves. Then to each tube add $0.1 \ mol \cdot L^{-1} \ NaBr$ solution. What happens? Write the reaction equation.

Compare with K_s of $[Ag(NH_3)_2]^+$ and $[Ag(S_2O_3)_2]^{3-}$. Interpret your results in terms of complex formation constants.

3. Effect of a Change in pH on the Coordination Equilibrium

Add 4-5 drops of $0.1 \ mol \cdot L^{-1} \ FeCl_3$ solution to 1 mL of $1 \ mol \cdot L^{-1} \ KSCN$ solution. Then divide the solution into two test tubes. To one test tube add several drops of $1 \ mol \cdot L^{-1} \ HCl$ solution and the other add several drops of $1 \ mol \cdot L^{-1}$ NaOH solution. Shake the test tubes sufficiently and observe the color change. Discuss the stability of $[Fe(SCN)_6]^{3-}$ in acidic and alkaline solution.

4. Complex Ions and Redox Reactions

(1) Add 4-5 drops of 30% H_2O_2 solution to 4-5 drops of $CoCl_2$ solution, observe and record the phenomenon. Can H_2O_2 solution oxidize Co^{2+} to brown Co^{3+}?

(2) Add excess concentrated $NH_3 \cdot H_2O$ solution to 4-5 drops of $CoCl_2$ solution until the precipitate dissolves. Observe the color change. Add H_2O_2 solution to see whether the color will change. Acidify the solution with 6 mol $\cdot$ L^{-1} HCl solution, observe and record the color change. Explain the effect of formation of complex ion on the reduction of Co^{2+}.

5. Chelating Effect

(1) To a test tube add 10 drops of $[Fe(SCN)_6]^{3-}$ solution from Step 3, and then add 0.1 mol $\cdot$ L^{-1} EDTA solution dropwise with stirring. Record the observation and write the reaction equation.

(2) Dissolve a portion of the crystal $[Cu(NH_3)_4]SO_4 \cdot H_2O$ in several drops of distilled water, and add 0.1 mol $\cdot$ L^{-1} EDTA solution dropwise with stirring. Record the observation and write the reaction equation.

(3) Add 2 drops of 0.1 mol $\cdot$ L^{-1} $NiCl_2$ solution to a test tube, and then add 1 drop of 2 mol $\cdot$ L^{-1} $NH_3 \cdot H_2O$ solution. What happens? Now add 2 drops of 1% dimethylglyoxime solution. What happens then? Write the reaction equation.

V Questions

(1) How to prove that $[Cu(NH_3)_4]^{2+}$ is formed in the experiment?

(2) How to judge the relative stability of various coordination compounds? What factors will influence the stability of coordination compounds?

(3) Compare the similarity and difference between chelant and complexant.

Experiment 17   Transition Metals

I Learning Objectives

(1) Know the oxidation-reduction properties of the transition metals (chromium, manganese, iron, cobalt, nickel, copper, silver, zinc, cadmium, and mercury).

(2) Know the preparation and properties of hydroxides of iron(Ⅱ), cobalt(Ⅱ), nickel(Ⅱ), manganese(Ⅱ), iron(Ⅲ), cobalt(Ⅲ) and nickel(Ⅲ).

(3) Know how to prepare the complexes of transition metal (chromium, manganese, iron, cobalt, nickel, copper, silver, zinc, cadmium, and mercury).

Ⅱ Principles

1. Chromium Chemistry

(1) $Cr(OH)_3$ is amphoteric. It will react with excess hydroxide ion to give the green $[Cr(OH)_4]^-$, which is then oxidized by warming it with H_2O_2 solution. You eventually get a bright yellow solution containing chromate(Ⅵ) ions. The equation for the oxidation stage is

$$2[Cr(OH)_4]^- + 4H_2O_2 \rightleftharpoons 2CrO_4^{2-} + 8H_2O$$

(2) The chromate-dichromate equilibrium.

The yellow chromate ion and orange dichromate ion are in equilibrium, with the chromate ion predominating in base and the dichromate ion in acid. Addition of hydrogen(hydronium) ion to chromate ion solution will drive the equilibrium towards dichromate:

$$2CrO_4^{2-}(aq) + 2H^+(aq) \rightleftharpoons Cr_2O_7^{2-}(aq) + H_2O(l)$$

Addition of hydroxide ion to dichromate ion solution will drive the equilibrium towards chromate:

$$Cr_2O_7^{2-}(aq) + 2OH^-(aq) \rightleftharpoons 2CrO_4^{2-}(aq) + H_2O(l)$$

Barium chromate is insoluble while barium dichromate is soluble. Addition of barium ion to dichromate ion solution usually results in the formation of barium chromate:

$$H_2O(l) + 2Ba^{2+}(aq) + Cr_2O_7^{2-}(aq) \rightleftharpoons 2BaCrO_4(s, yellow) + 2H^+(aq)$$

(3) Dichromate ion as an oxidizing agent.

Potassium dichromate(Ⅵ) solution acidified with dilute sulfuric acid is used to oxidize ethanol, CH_3CH_2OH, to acetic acid, CH_3COOH.

$$2Cr_2O_7^{2-} + 3C_2H_5OH + 16H^+ \rightleftharpoons 4Cr^{3+}(green) + 3CH_3COOH + 11H_2O$$

2. Manganese Chemistry

Addition of hydroxide ion to the manganese(Ⅱ) ion solution results in the formation of a precipitate of white manganese(Ⅱ) hydroxide. Manganese(Ⅱ) is very easily oxidized under alkaline conditions. Oxygen in the air oxidizes the manganese(Ⅱ) hydroxide to manganese(Ⅳ) hydroxide oxide.

$$Mn^{2+} + 2OH^- \rightleftharpoons Mn(OH)_2(white)$$

$$2Mn(OH)_2 + O_2 = 2MnO(OH)_2 (reddish\ brown)$$

In acidic solution manganese(Ⅱ) ion is stable. But in the presence of the strongest oxidants, such as $NaBiO_3$, PbO_2, and $S_2O_8^{2-}$, it will convert to the intense purple permanganate ion. This is a specific test for manganese(Ⅱ) ion.

$$2Mn^{2+} + 5NaBiO_3(s) + 14H^+ = 2MnO_4^- + 5Bi^{3+} + 5Na^+ + 7H_2O$$

Manganate ions in basic or weak basic solution are disproportionate to give permanganate ions and a precipitate of manganese(Ⅳ) oxide.

$$3MnO_4^{2-} + 2H_2O = 2MnO_4^- + MnO_2 + 4OH^-$$

The most common manganese(Ⅶ) compound is the permanganate(Ⅶ) ion, MnO_4^-, which is a very intense purple color. It is a powerful oxidizing agent. Manganese(Ⅶ) in the form of the permanganate ion, can be reduced to manganese (Ⅵ), manganese(Ⅳ), and manganese(Ⅱ) by the hydrogen sulfite(acidic solution) and sulfite(basic solution) ions. The product depends upon the pH of the solution. Under very strongly alkaline conditions, the dark green manganate(Ⅵ) ion is the product.

$$MnO_4^-(aq) + e^- = MnO_4^{2-}(aq)$$

In approximately neutral solution, a deep brown precipitate of manganese(Ⅳ) oxide forms.

$$MnO_4^-(aq) + 2H_2O(l) + 3e^- = MnO_2(s) + 4OH^-(aq)$$

In acidic solution the almost colorless manganese(Ⅱ) ion is the product.

$$MnO_4^-(aq) + 8H^+(aq) + 5e^- = Mn^{2+}(aq) + 4H_2O(l)$$

3. Chemistry of Iron, Cobalt and Nickel

(1) Reaction of iron(Ⅱ) ion with hydroxide ion.

Addition of hydroxide ion to the green iron(Ⅱ) chloride solution results in the formation of a precipitate of white iron(Ⅱ) hydroxide. Iron(Ⅱ) is very easily oxidized under alkaline conditions. Oxygen in the air oxidizes the iron(Ⅱ) hydroxide to iron(Ⅲ) hydroxide.

$$Fe^{2+}(aq) + 2OH^-(aq) = Fe(OH)_2(s)$$
$$4Fe(OH)_2(s) + O_2(g) + 2H_2O(l) = 4Fe(OH)_3(s)$$

In the presence of concentrated base from the NaOH, iron(Ⅱ) hydroxide reacts to give a stable and soluble iron(Ⅱ) complex, $[Fe(OH)_6]^{4-}$.

(2) Reaction of cobalt(Ⅱ) ion with hydroxide ion.

Addition of hydroxide ion to the pink cobalt(Ⅱ) chloride solution first results in the formation of a precipitate of blue cobalt(Ⅱ) hydroxide chloride, warming with excess hydroxide ion gives the pink cobalt(Ⅱ) hydroxide which upon standing converts to brown cobalt(Ⅲ) hydroxide.

$$Co^{2+}(aq)+OH^-(aq)+Cl^-(aq)\!=\!\!=\!Co(OH)Cl(s)$$
$$Co(OH)Cl(s)+OH^-(aq)\!=\!\!=\!Co(OH)_2(s)+Cl^-(aq)$$
$$4Co(OH)_2(s)+O_2(g)+2H_2O(l)\!=\!\!=\!4Co(OH)_3(s)$$

(3) Reaction of nickel(Ⅱ) ion with hydroxide ion.

Pale green nickel(Ⅱ) ion reacts with hydroxide ion to give a gelatinous pale green precipitate of nickel(Ⅱ) hydroxide.

$$Ni^{2+}(aq)+2OH^-(aq)\!=\!\!=\!Ni(OH)_2(s)$$

Pale green precipitate of nickel(Ⅱ) hydroxide reduces Br_2 in basic solution to Br^-, itself being oxidized to a precipitate of deep black precipitate of nickel(Ⅲ) hydroxide.

$$2Ni^{2+}+6OH^-+Br_2\!=\!\!=\!2Ni(OH)_3+2Br^-$$

(4) Reactions of cobalt(Ⅲ) hydroxide, nickel(Ⅲ) hydroxide, and iron(Ⅲ) hydroxide with hydrochloric acid.

When hydrochloric acid (HCl) is added to $Co(OH)_3$ or $Ni(OH)_3$, the corresponding ion with +3 charge is not obtained because it is extraordinary unstable to oxidize Cl^- to Cl_2.

$$2M^{3+}+2Cl^-\!=\!\!=\!2M^{2+}+Cl_2(M\!=\!Co,Ni)$$
$$4M^{3+}+2H_2O\!=\!\!=\!4M^{2+}+4H^++O_2$$

But only $Fe(OH)_3$ proceeds the neutralized reaction when HCl is added.

$$Fe(OH)_3+3HCl\!=\!\!=\!FeCl_3+3H_2O$$

(5) Reactions of iron(Ⅱ), iron(Ⅲ), nickel(Ⅱ) and cobalt(Ⅱ) ions with ammonia solution.

Addition of ammonia to the iron(Ⅱ) and iron(Ⅲ) ions results in the formation of a precipitate of white iron(Ⅱ) hydroxide and brown-red iron(Ⅲ) hydroxide, respectively.

Addition of ammonia to the green nickel(Ⅱ) ion results in the formation of the blue hexaamminenickel(Ⅱ) ion.

Cobalt(Ⅱ) ion reacts with a small amount of ammonia to give the precipitate. That precipitate dissolves if you add an excess of ammonia. The hexaamminecobalt(Ⅱ) complex is very easily oxidized to the corresponding cobalt(Ⅲ) complex.

$$4[Co(NH_3)_6]^{2+}(brown\text{-}red)+O_2+2H_2O\!=\!\!=\!4[Co(NH_3)_6]^{3+}(bule\text{-}purple)+4OH^-$$

4. Copper, Silver, Zinc, Cadmium and Mercury

In the presence of the excess ammonia, copper(Ⅱ), silver, zinc(Ⅱ) and cadmium(Ⅱ) ions react to form the corresponding ammonia complex.

Mercury(Ⅱ) chloride reacts with aqueous ammonia to form a white precipitate of mercury aminochloride.

$$HgCl_2 + 2NH_3 = HgNH_2Cl \downarrow (white) + NH_4Cl$$

(1) The reaction of mercury(Ⅱ) with iodide ions.

Mercury(Ⅱ) iodide is obtained as a scarlet precipitate on addition of potassium iodide to a solution of mercury(Ⅱ) chloride. It dissolves readily in a solution of potassium iodide due to the formation of iodic complex.

$$HgI_2 (orange) + 2KI = K_2[HgI_4] (colorless)$$

(2) The reaction of copper(Ⅱ) ions with iodide ions.

Copper(Ⅱ) ions oxidize iodide ions to iodine, and in the process themselves are reduced to an off-white precipitate of copper(Ⅰ) iodide. But in the presence of excess iodide ions from the KI, this reacts to give a stable and soluble copper(Ⅰ) complex. You can get the white precipitate of copper(Ⅰ) iodide mentioned above by adding water to this solution.

$$2Cu^{2+} + 4I^- = 2CuI \downarrow + I_2$$

$$CuI + I^- = [CuI_2]^-$$

$$[CuI_2]^- \overset{dilute}{\rightleftharpoons} CuI \downarrow + I^-$$

Ⅲ Apparatus and Reagents

Centrifuge, beakers (100 mL×4), centrifuge tubes (2) and test tubes (10).

$(NH_4)_2Fe(SO_4)_2 \cdot 6H_2O$ (CP,s), $NaBiO_3$ (CP,s), MnO_2 (CP,s), NH_4Cl (AR, s), HCl solution (2 mol $\cdot$ L^{-1}, concentrated solution), HNO_3 solution (6 mol $\cdot$ L^{-1}), H_2SO_4 solution (3 mol $\cdot$ L^{-1}), HAc solution (2 mol $\cdot$ L^{-1}), NaOH solution (2 mol $\cdot$ L^{-1}, 6 mol $\cdot$ L^{-1}, 40%), $NH_3 \cdot H_2O$ solution (2 mol $\cdot$ L^{-1}, concentrated solution), $CoCl_2$ solution (0.1 mol $\cdot$ L^{-1}), $NiSO_4$ solution (0.1 mol $\cdot$ L^{-1}), $MnSO_4$ solution (0.1 mol $\cdot$ L^{-1}), $CrCl_3$ solution (0.1 mol $\cdot$ L^{-1}), $FeCl_3$ solution (0.1 mol $\cdot$ L^{-1}), $K_2Cr_2O_7$ solution (0.1 mol $\cdot$ L^{-1}), $KMnO_4$ solution (0.01 mol $\cdot$ L^{-1}), Na_2SO_3 solution (0.1 mol $\cdot$ L^{-1}), $CoCl_2$ solution (0.5 mol $\cdot$ L^{-1}), $NiSO_4$ solution (0.5 mol $\cdot$ L^{-1}), NH_4Cl solution (1 mol $\cdot$ L^{-1}), H_2O_2 solution (3%), $CuSO_4$ solution (0.1 mol $\cdot$ L^{-1}), $AgNO_3$ solution (0.1 mol $\cdot$ L^{-1}), $ZnSO_4$ solution (0.1 mol $\cdot$ L^{-1}), $CdSO_4$ solution (0.1 mol $\cdot$ L^{-1}), $Hg(NO_3)_2$ solution (0.1 mol $\cdot$ L^{-1}), KI solution (0.1 mol $\cdot$ L^{-1}, 2 mol $\cdot$ L^{-1}), Br_2, ethanol solution (95%) and potassium iodide-starch test paper.

IV Procedure

1. Preparations and Properties of Hydroxides of Iron (II) , Cobalt (II) , Nickel (II) , Manganese(II) , Iron(III) , Cobalt(III)and Nickel(III)

(1) Preparation and property of iron(II) hydroxide. To a test tube add 1 mL of distilled water, 2 drops of 3 mol $\cdot$ L^{-1} H_2SO_4 solution. The solution in the test tube is boiled for a while. (Why?) After it cools a little amount of solid $(NH_4)_2Fe(SO_4)_2 \cdot 6H_2O$ is dissolved in it. Then 1 mL of 6 mol $\cdot$ L^{-1} NaOH solution boiled is quickly added to the Fe^{2+} solution. (Don't shake the tube). Note the color of the precipitate. Then divide the precipitate into three test tubes. To one test tube add several drops of 2 mol $\cdot$ L^{-1} HCl solution, to the second one add several drops of 40% NaOH solution, the third one stands in the air.

(2) Preparation and property of cobalt(II) hydroxide. React 0.1 mol $\cdot$ L^{-1} $CoCl_2$ solution with 2 mol $\cdot$ L^{-1} NaOH solution to form the precipitate $Co(OH)_2$. Then divide the precipitate into three test tubes. To one test tube add several drops of 2 mol $\cdot$ L^{-1} HCl solution, to the second one add several drops of 40% NaOH solution, the third one stands in the air.

(3) Preparation and property of nickel(II) hydroxide. React 0.1 mol $\cdot$ L^{-1} $NiSO_4$ solution with 2 mol $\cdot$ L^{-1} NaOH solution to form the precipitate $Ni(OH)_2$. Then divide the precipitate into three test tubes. To one test tube add several drops of 2 mol $\cdot$ L^{-1} HCl solution, to the second one add several drops of 40% NaOH solution, the third one stands in the air.

(4) Preparation and property of manganese (II) hydroxide. React 0.1 mol $\cdot$ L^{-1} $MnSO_4$ solution with 2 mol $\cdot$ L^{-1} NaOH solution to form the precipitate $Mn(OH)_2$. Then divide the precipitate into three test tubes. To one test tube add several drops of 2 mol $\cdot$ L^{-1} HCl solution, to the second one add several drops of 40% NaOH solution, the third one stands in the air.

(5) Preparation and property of chromium (III) hydroxide. React 0.1 mol $\cdot$ L^{-1} $CrCl_3$ solution with 2 mol $\cdot$ L^{-1} NaOH solution to form the precipitate $Cr(OH)_3$. Then divide the precipitate into three test tubes. To one test tube add several drops of 2 mol $\cdot$ L^{-1} HCl solution, to the second one add several drops of 40% NaOH solution, the third one stands in the air.

(6) Preparation and property of iron (III) hydroxide. React 0.1 mol $\cdot$ L^{-1} $FeCl_3$ solution with 2 mol $\cdot$ L^{-1} NaOH solution to form the precipitate $Fe(OH)_3$. Then divide the precipitate into three test tubes. To one test tube add several drops

of concentrated HCl solution and observe whether there is Cl_2 from the solution, to the second one add several drops of 2 mol $\cdot$ L^{-1} HCl solution and observe whether the precipitate dissolves, to the third one add several drops of 40% NaOH solution and observe whether the precipitate dissolves.

(7) Preparation and property of cobalt (Ⅲ) hydroxide. Several drops of bromine water are added to 5 drops of 0.1 mol $\cdot$ L^{-1} $CoCl_2$ solution before 5 drops of 6 mol $\cdot$ L^{-1} NaOH solution are added. Note the color of the precipitate. Add several drops of concentrated HCl solution to the precipitate and observe whether there is Cl_2 from the solution.

(8) Preparation and property of nickel (Ⅲ) hydroxide. Several drops of bromine water are added to 5 drops of 0.1 mol $\cdot$ L^{-1} $NiSO_4$ solution before 5 drops of 6 mol $\cdot$ L^{-1} NaOH solution are added. Note the color of the precipitate. Add several drops of concentrated HCl solution to the precipitate and observe whether there is Cl_2 from the solution.

2. Reduction of Mn^{2+} and Cr^{3+}

(1) Add 2 mol $\cdot$ L^{-1} NaOH solution dropwise to a test tube containing 0.1 mol $\cdot$ L^{-1} $CrCl_3$ solution until the precipitate formed is redissolved. Then add several drops of 3% H_2O_2 solution and heat it. Observe the color change and write the reaction equation.

(2) Add a little amount of solid $NaBiO_3$ to a test tube containing 0.1 mol $\cdot$ L^{-1} $MnSO_4$ solution. Then add 6 mol $\cdot$ L^{-1} HNO_3 solution dropwise with stirring. Observe the color change and write the reaction equation.

3. Oxidation of $Cr_2O_7^{2-}$ and MnO_4^{-}

(1) Add several drops of 0.1 mol $\cdot$ L^{-1} $K_2Cr_2O_7$ solution and 3 mol $\cdot$ L^{-1} H_2SO_4 solution to a test tube. Then add several drops of 95% ethanol solution and heat it. Observe the color change and write the reaction equation.

(2) To three test tubes add several drops of 0.01 mol $\cdot$ L^{-1} $KMnO_4$ solution. To one test tube add several drops of 3 mol $\cdot$ L^{-1} H_2SO_4 solution, to the second one add several drops of distilled water, and to the third one add several drops of 6.0 mol $\cdot$ L^{-1} NaOH solution, shake them all. Then add several drops of 0.1 mol $\cdot$ L^{-1} Na_2SO_3 solution into each tube. Record the observation and write the reaction equation.

4. The Chromate-Dichromate Equilibrium

(1) Add 5 drops of 0.1 mol $\cdot$ L^{-1} $K_2Cr_2O_7$ solution to a test tube containing 2 drops of 2 mol $\cdot$ L^{-1} NaOH solution. What sign of a reaction do you observe? Then

add 2 drops of 0. 5 mol $\cdot$ L^{-1} BaCl$_2$ solution. What happens? Explain the reason.

(2) Add 5 drops of 0. 1 mol $\cdot$ L^{-1} K$_2$Cr$_2$O$_7$ solution to a test tube containing 2 drops of 2 mol $\cdot$ L^{-1} HAc solution. What sign of a reaction do you observe? Then add 2 drops of 0. 5 mol $\cdot$ L^{-1} BaCl$_2$ solution. What happens? Explain the reason.

5. Preparation of Mn (Ⅵ) Compounds

Heat a mixture of 10 drops of 0. 01 mol $\cdot$ L^{-1} KMnO$_4$ solution, 20 drops of 40% NaOH solution and a little amount of solid MnO$_2$ until it is boiled. The mixture is stirred before it stands without disturbance for a while. Centrifuge, decant and save the green supernatant(due to MnO$_4^{2-}$).

To two test tubes add several drops of the green supernatant. Then to one test tube add 3 mol $\cdot$ L^{-1} H$_2$SO$_4$ solution dropwise with stirring, record the observation and write the reaction equation. To the other one add a little amount of solid NH$_4$Cl, shake sufficiently and heat it. Record the observation and write the reaction equation.

Conclude the stability of MnO$_4^{2-}$ from these experiments.

6. Ammonia Complexes of Cobalt, Nickel, Copper, Silver, Zinc, Cadmium and Mercury

(1) Add several drops of 0. 5 mol $\cdot$ L^{-1} CoCl$_2$ solution and 1 mol $\cdot$ L^{-1} NH$_4$Cl solution to a test tube. Then add 2 mol $\cdot$ L^{-1} NH$_3$ $\cdot$ H$_2$O solution dropwise with stirring. What sign of a reaction do you observe? Continue to add excess concentrated NH$_3$ $\cdot$ H$_2$O solution and observe the phenomenon. Explain the reason.

(2) Add several drops of 0. 5 mol $\cdot$ L^{-1} NiSO$_4$ solution and 1 mol $\cdot$ L^{-1}NH$_4$Cl solution to a test tube. Then add 2 mol $\cdot$ L^{-1} NH$_3$ $\cdot$ H$_2$O solution dropwise with stirring. What sign of a reaction do you observe? Continue to add excess concentrated NH$_3$ $\cdot$ H$_2$O solution and observe the phenomenon. Then divide the solution into four tubes. To one test tube add several drops of 2 mol $\cdot$ L^{-1} NaOH solution and observe the phenomenon. To the second one add several drops of 3 mol $\cdot$ L^{-1} H$_2$SO$_4$ solution and observe the phenomenon. To the third one add several drops of distilled water and observe the phenomenon. To the fourth one heat it and observe the phenomenon.

Conclude the stability of [Ni(NH$_3$)$_4$]$^{2+}$ from these experiments.

(3) To five test tubes add several drops of 0. 1 mol $\cdot$ L^{-1} CuSO$_4$, AgNO$_3$, ZnSO$_4$, CdSO$_4$, and Hg(NO$_3$)$_2$ solutions, respectively. Add several drops of 2 mol $\cdot$ L^{-1} NH$_3$ $\cdot$ H$_2$O solution into each tube and observe the phenomenon. Continue to add excess concentrated NH$_3$ $\cdot$ H$_2$O solution and observe whether the precipitates dissolve.

7. Mercury Halides and Copper Halides

(1) Add several drops of 0.1 mol $\cdot$ L^{-1} CuSO$_4$ solution and 0.1 mol $\cdot$ L^{-1} KI solution to a centrifuge tube. Observe the color of the precipitate. Centrifuge any precipitate that forms, decant and save the precipitate. Then add 2 mol $\cdot$ L^{-1} KI solution dropwise to the precipitate and observe the phenomenon.

(2) Add several drops of 0.1 mol $\cdot$ L^{-1} KI solution to a test tube containing 2 drops of 0.1 mol $\cdot$ L^{-1} Hg(NO$_3$)$_2$ solution. Then add excess 2 mol $\cdot$ L^{-1} KI solution and observe the phenomenon.

V Questions

(1) Which experiments show that disproportionation of manganese takes place? What are the media?

(2) How do you separate the metal ions Fe^{3+}, Al^{3+}, and Cr^{3+} from their mixture?

Experiment 18   Spectrophotometric Determination of Protein in Peanut

I Learning Objectives

(1) Learn to determine protein in peanut.

(2) Learn to use 723N spectrophotometer.

II Principles

In a pH 2.5 buffer solution containing 0.050% emulsifier OP, protein forms a blue complex with arsenazo M. Its maximum absorption peak is 605 nm with molar absorptivity of 4.5×10^5 L $\cdot$ mol^{-1} $\cdot$ cm^{-1}. Lambert-Beer's law is obeyed in a range from 3.3 mg $\cdot$ L^{-1} to 254 mg $\cdot$ L^{-1}. The proposed method has been applied to the determination of protein in serum and peanut samples.

III Apparatus and Reagents

723N spectrophotometer, cuvettes(2.0 cm$\times$4), analytical balance(0.01 g), pH meter(PB-10), blender, centrifuge, colorimetric tubes(10 mL$\times$7), beakers(250 mL $\times$1,500 mL$\times$1), transfer pipets(2 mL$\times$1,1 mL$\times$1), Mohr measuring pipets(1 mL

×3),Buchner funnel,wash bottle,rubber pipet bulb,graduated cylinder(100 mL× 1) and volumetric flasks(100 mL×2).

Standard protein solution(1 g $\cdot$ L^{-1}),arsenazo M solution (5.0×10^{-4} mol $\cdot$ L^{-1}), KH_2PO_4 solution (5.0×10^{-3} mol $\cdot$ L^{-1}),emulsifier OP solution (0.050%),NaCl solution (1.0%),$C_3H_6O_3$ (lactic acid)-$C_3H_5O_3Na$ buffer solution(pH=2.5)and sample(peanut).

Ⅳ Procedure

1. Preparation of Peanut Sample

In a blender,macerate 25 g sample of peanut with 50 mL of the solution containing 1.0% NaCl and 5.0×10^{-3} mol $\cdot$ L^{-1} KH_2PO_4(pH=7.2). Pour the mixture into a beaker,and rinse the blender with distilled water. Add the washings to the extract.

Filter the mixture through cheesecloth to remove coarse material and then, using vacuum filtration,through a Buchner funnel,wash with 30 mL of 5.0×10^{-3} mol $\cdot$ L^{-1} KH_2PO_4 solution(pH=7.2). Transfer the extract to a 250 mL beaker, and dilute to 100 mL with distilled water. Centrifuge,decant,save the supernatant and store at 4 ℃ overnight.

2. Determination of Protein

The table below summarizes the preparation of the test solutions. Add 0.50 mL of the extract sample with Mohr measuring pipet, or standards, or blank (distilled water) to 10 mL colorimetric tubes. Add 2.00 mL of $C_3H_6O_3$-$C_3H_5O_3Na$ buffer solution(pH=2.5),1.00 mL of 0.050% emulsifier OP solution and 0.80 mL of arsenazo M solution ,and then dilute to the mark. After mixing,let stand for 15 min to allow the color to stabilize. Measure the absorbance at 605 nm against the blank.

Using samples 5,6,and 7,prepare a calibration curve by plotting absorbance vs. the concentration of protein for the standards,extrapolate a line until it crosses to x-axis, and then determine the concentration of protein in the peanut extract according to the point of intersection.

No.	1	2	3	4	5	6	7
$V(C_3H_6O_3$-$C_3H_5O_3Na$ buffer solution)/mL	2.00	2.00	2.00	2.00	2.00	2.00	2.00
V(emulsifier OP)/mL	1.00	1.00	1.00	1.00	1.00	1.00	1.00

continued

No.	1	2	3	4	5	6	7
V(arsenazo M)/mL	0.80	0.80	0.80	0.80	0.80	0.80	0.80
V(sample supernatant)/mL	0.00	0.50	0.50	0.50	0.50	0.50	0.50
V(standard protein solution)/mL	0.00	0.00	0.00	0.00	0.20	0.40	0.60
A(absorbance)							

Experiment 19   Determination of the Composition and the Stability Constant for an Iron(Ⅲ)-Sulfosalicylate Complex

Ⅰ Learning Objectives

(1) Learn to determine the composition and the stability constant for the complex by method of continuous variations of the concentration.

(2) Learn to use 723N spectrophotometer.

Ⅱ Principles

Absorbance is related to the cell width b through which the light passes and the concentration c of the absorbing substances by what is called Lambert-Beer's law:

$$A = \varepsilon bc$$

where ε is the molar absorptivity coefficient and is a constant characteristic of the absorbing substance and the particular wavelength of light used. If the light path length and the wavelength of the light are maintained constant, A is directly proportional to concentration. This law will be used for determining the composition of complex ions and the evaluation of equilibrium constants.

The method of continuous variations is simply and widely used for the spectrophotometric determination of complex composition. However, it is reliable only for solution conditions where a single complex species is formed. The method also can be used for determination of stability constant with systems that contain only one complex species. If the total analytical concentrations c_t of complexing reagent c_x and metal ion c_m is held constant and only their ratio is varied, then

$$c_x + c_m = c_t$$

$$x=\frac{c_x}{c_t}, \quad \frac{c_x}{c_t}+\frac{c_m}{c_t}=\frac{c_t}{c_t}, \quad 1-x=\frac{c_m}{c_t}$$

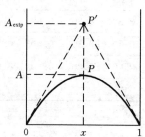

Figure 2-4　Continuous variations plot

A wavelength of light is selected where the complex absorbs strongly but the ligand and metal ions do not. A plot of the mole fraction of ligand in the mixture x vs. absorbance gives the triangular-shaped curve as shown in Figure 2-4. The legs of the triangle are extrapolated until they cross. The mole fraction at the point of intersection gives the composition of the complex, because here the ligand and metal are in proper relative concentration to give maximum complex formation for the complex ML_n, the reaction is

$$M+nL= ML_n$$

$$n=\frac{c_x}{c_m}=\frac{x}{1-x}$$

In the vicinity of maximum absorbance the actual curve may be observed to deviate somewhat from the extrapolated intersecting lines. The difference between the extrapolated values and the actual values of the absorbance can be used for calculation of stability constant. The extrapolated values (A_{extp}) on continuous variation plots correspond to the total absorbance of the complex if the complex formation is complete. Actually, the complex is slightly dissociated in this region, and the absorbance(A) reading is somewhat lower. The degree of ionization of the complex will be expressed as follows:

$$\alpha=\frac{A_{extp}-A}{A_{extp}}$$

For a 1 : 1 complex, you can write the stability constant, which corresponds to the reaction as follows:

$$ML \rightleftharpoons M + L$$

Starting concentrations　　　　　c　　　0　　　0

Equilibrium concentrations　　$c-c\alpha$　　$c\alpha$　　　$c\alpha$

$$K_s=\frac{[ML]}{[M][L]}=\frac{1-\alpha}{c\alpha^2}$$

where c is the concentration of the complex.

In this experiment, we will determine the composition and the stability constant for an iron(Ⅲ)-sulfosalicylate complex. The composition of this complex depends on pH. The iron(Ⅲ)-sulfosalicylate complex which contains one ligand is fuchsia in the pH range 2-3. The reaction is given:

$$Fe^{3+} + \ ^-O_3S-\!\!\!\!\bigcirc\!\!\!\!-OH \ (COOH) \rightleftharpoons \left[\ ^-O_3S-\!\!\!\!\bigcirc\!\!\!\!-O\!\!\diagdown\!\!\!\!\begin{array}{c}\\ C-O\end{array}\!\!\diagup Fe^+ \right] + 2H^+$$

It is red with two ligands in the pH range 4-9, and yellow with three ligands to the pH more than 10. In this experiment, we will select the pH range 2-3.

III Apparatus and Reagents

723N spectrophotometer, cuvettes (4), volumetric flasks (100 mL × 2), Mohr measuring pipets(10 mL×2), beakers(50 mL×11), rubber pipet bulb and medicine dropper.

$NH_4Fe(SO_4)_2$ solution (0.010 0 mol · L^{-1} ferric ammonium sulfate in 0.010 0 mol · L^{-1} $HClO_4$ solution), sulfosalicylic acid solution (0.010 0 mol · L^{-1} sulfosalicylic acid in 0.010 0 mol · L^{-1} $HClO_4$ solution) and $HClO_4$ solution (0.010 0 mol · L^{-1}).

IV Procedure

(1) Prepare 100 mL of 0.001 00 mol · L^{-1} sulfosalicylic acid solution. Transfer 10.00 mL of 0.010 0 mol · L^{-1} sulfosalicylic acid solution into a 100 mL volumetric flask with a Mohr measuring pipet and dilute the solution to 100 mL with 0.010 0 mol · L^{-1} $HClO_4$ solution.

Prepare 100 mL of 0.001 00 mol · L^{-1} ferric solution. Transfer 10.00 mL of 0.010 0 mol · L^{-1} ferric solution into a 100 mL volumetric flask with a Mohr measuring pipet and dilute the solution to 100 mL with 0.010 0 mol · L^{-1} $HClO_4$ solution.

(2) Prepare a series of solutions by mixing the indicated amount of 0.001 00 mol · L^{-1} sulfosalicylic acid solution (solution A)and 0.001 00 mol · L^{-1} ferric solution (solution B), respectively, into eleven 50 mL beakers with Mohr measuring pipets.

No.	1	2	3	4	5	6	7	8	9	10	11
V(solution A) /mL	10.00	9.00	8.00	7.00	6.00	5.00	4.00	3.00	2.00	1.00	0.00
V(solution B) /mL	0.00	1.00	2.00	3.00	4.00	5.00	6.00	7.00	8.00	9.00	10.00

continued

No.	1	2	3	4	5	6	7	8	9	10	11
The mole fraction of sulfosalicylic acid											
A(absorbance)											

(3) Determine the absorption spectrum for the solution with No. 6 over the spectral range from 400 nm to 620 nm, using distilled water as a blank. Next, measure the absorbance for each of the eleven solutions at the wavelength that corresponds to maximum absorption for the absorption spectrum, using distilled water as a blank. Plot the absorbance vs. the mole fraction of sulfosalicylic acid for the series of solutions that contain iron and sulfosalicylic acid. From this graph make a final conclusion concerning the composition of the iron(Ⅲ)-sulfosalicylate complex. Calculate the value of the stability constant.

V Question

Discuss how to evaluate the stability constant of a complex by a continuous variations plot. What are the limitations for using this method of evaluating a constant?

Experiment 20 Spectrophotometric Determination of Crystal Field Splitting Energy of $[Ti(H_2O)_6]^{3+}$

I Learning Objectives

(1) Learn to determine the crystal field splitting energy of $[Ti(H_2O)_6]^{3+}$.

(2) Learn to use 723N spectrophotometer.

II Principles

Complex ions containing transition metals are usually colored, whereas the similar ions from non-transition metals are not. That suggests that the partly filled d orbitals must be involved in generating the color in some way. Remember that transition metals are defined as having partly filled d orbitals.

For simplicity, you are going to look at the octahedral complexes which have six simple ligands arranged around the central metal ion.

When the ligands bond with the transition metal ion, there is repulsion between the electrons in the ligands and the electrons in the d orbitals of the metal ion. That raises the energy of the d orbitals.

However, because of the way the d orbitals are arranged in space, that doesn't raise all their energies by the same amount. Instead, it splits them into two groups.

The diagram shows the arrangement of the d electrons in a Ti^{3+} ion before and after six water molecules bond with it.

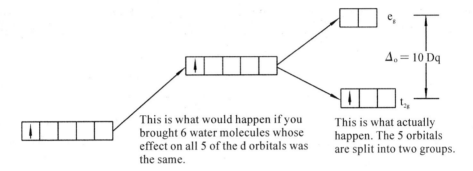

This is what would happen if you brought 6 water molecules whose effect on all 5 of the d orbitals was the same.

This is what actually happen. The 5 orbitals are split into two groups.

Whenever six ligands are arranged around a transition metal ion, the d orbitals are always split into two groups in this way — two with a higher energy than the other three.

An electron can move from one orbital to a higher-energy orbital by absorbing light that has exactly the same energy as the energy difference between the orbitals. For transition metals, this energy difference is often the crystal field splitting energy(Δ_o). Δ_o is related to wavelength by following formula:

$$\Delta_o = h\nu = \frac{hc}{\lambda}$$

Remember that if this wavelength of light is absorbed, you can't see it! What you see instead is a mixture of all the wavelengths that are not absorbed.

Ⅲ Apparatus and Reagents

723N spectrophotometer, cuvettes(4), volumetric flask(50 mL×1), beaker(50 mL×1), transfer pipet(5 mL × 1), rubber pipet bulb, wash bottle and medicine dropper.

TiCl$_3$ solution (15%) and HCl solution (2 mol · L^{-1}).

IV Procedure

1. Preparation of [Ti(H$_2$O)$_6$]$^{3+}$ Solution

Transfer 5.00 mL of 15% TiCl$_3$ solution into a 50 mL volumetric flask with a transfer pipet, and then dilute to the mark.

2. Absorption Spectra

Obtain a cuvette. Make sure it is clean inside and out. Rinse the cuvette in, with small amount of the blank. Then fill the cuvette about three-quarters full. Dry the outside of the cuvette carefully, and insert it into the sample compartment with its transparent sides aligned with the light path. Close the cover. Set the wavelength dial at 420 nm, and press 0.000Abs/100.0%T to set the absorbance of the blank to zero. Place Ti (Ⅲ) solution in your second cuvette and read the absorbance value on the LED. Continue this procedure at 10 nm intervals from 420 nm to 600 nm. Be sure to set the absorbance of the blank to zero after each change of wavelength. Again, measure and record A at 2 nm intervals in the vicinity of maximum absorbance.

λ/nm	
A	

V Question

What causes transition metal ions to absorb light from visible light (causing color) whereas non-transition metal ions do not? And why does the color vary so much from ion to ion?

Experiment 21　Measurement of Chloride Ion Content in Saline

I Learning Objectives

(1) Master the preparation and calibration methods of AgNO$_3$ standard solution.

(2) Familiar with the method and principle of determination of chloride ion by the Mohr method using K$_2$CrO$_4$ as indicator.

II　Principles

The Mohr method is a method of titrating Cl^- etc. in a neutral or weak alkaline solution with K_2CrO_4 as indicator and $AgNO_3$ standard solution as titrant. Since the solubility of AgCl precipitate is lower than that of Ag_2CrO_4, AgCl is precipitated first in the solution. At the endpoint, slightly excessive Ag^+ and K_2CrO_4 generate brick-red Ag_2CrO_4 precipitate, indicating the arrival of the end point. The main reaction formulas are as follows:

$$Ag^+ + Cl^- =\!\!=\!\!= AgCl \downarrow (white)$$
$$2Ag^+ + CrO_4^{2-} =\!\!=\!\!= Ag_2CrO_4 \downarrow (brick\text{-}red)$$

The optimal pH range for titration is between 6.5 and 10.5. If there are ammonium salts in the solution, the pH range should be controlled between 6.5 and 7.2. If there are more colored ions such as Cu^{2+}, Co^{2+} and Cr^{3+} in the solution, the observation of the endpoint will be affected. Any anion and cation that can react with Ag^+ or CrO_4^{2-} will interfere with the determination.

III　Apparatus and Reagents

Analytical balance (0.1 mg), acid burette (brown, 50 mL×1), pipet (25 mL ×1), beakers (500 mL×2), Erlenmeyer flasks (250 mL×3), volumetric flasks (250 mL×2), reagent bottle (brown), etc..

$AgNO_3$ (CP), NaCl (reference reagent, 500-600 ℃ burned to constant mass), K_2CrO_4 solution (5%), normal saline solution.

IV　Procedure

1.　Preparation of 0.02 mol · L^{-1}AgNO$_3$ Standard Solution

Weigh about 0.85 g $AgNO_3$ into a clean 500 mL beaker, dissolve it by adding 250 mL pure water. Transfer the solution into a brown reagent bottle, and then store it in the dark.

2.　Calibration of AgNO$_3$ Solution

Accurately weigh 0.25-0.3 g NaCl in a small beaker, and dissolve it by adding the appropriate volume of distilled water. Transfer the solution into a 250 mL volumetric flask, dilute to the mark and mix the solution thoroughly. Pipet 25.00 mL of this solution to a 250 mL Erlenmeyer flask, add 25 mL distilled water and 1.00 mL of 5% K_2CrO_4 solution, and titrate the sample with $AgNO_3$ standard solution to a brick red. Repeat the titration two more times. Then calculate the concentration of $AgNO_3$.

3. Sample Analysis

Transfer 25.00 mL of normal saline solution into a 250 mL volumetric flask, dilute to the mark and mix the solution thoroughly. Pipet 25.00 mL of the diluted saline solution to a 250 mL Erlenmeyer flask, add 25 mL distilled water and 1.00 mL of 5% K_2CrO_4 solution, and titrate the sample with $AgNO_3$ standard solution to a brick red. Repeat the titration two more times. Then calculate the content of sodium chloride in normal saline solution.

After the experiment, the burette containing the $AgNO_3$ solution is rinsed 2-3 times with distilled water, and then rinsed with tap water to avoid AgCl from remaining in the tube.

V Data

$$c(AgNO_3) = \frac{m(NaCl) \times 1\ 000}{M(NaCl) \times V} \times \frac{25.00}{250.00}$$

Calculate the content of sodium chloride in normal saline solution according to the following formula:

$$\rho(NaCl)(g/100\ mL) = \frac{c(AgNO_3) \times V \times M(NaCl)}{25.00} \times \frac{250.00}{25.00} \times 100$$

VI Questions

(1) Why should the pH of the solution be controlled within 6.5-10.5 for the determination of chlorine by the Mohr method?

(2) Can NaCl standard solution be used to titrate Ag^+ directly by the Mohr method?

Experiment 22　Measurement of Nitrite Concentration in Food

I Learning Objectives

(1) Learn to use 723N spectrophotometer.

(2) Learn to determine nitrite concentration in food.

II Principles

Nitrite is widely used as color fixatives and preservatives in meat products, but it can react with amine to produce carcinogenic nitrosamine. Therefore, nitrite concentration in food must be strictly monitored. After depositing protein and removing fat for food sample, the nitrite reacts with p-aminobenzene sulfonic acid to form diazonium salt, which is then coupled with naphthalene ethylenediamine hydrochloride to form a purple-red azo compound. The chemical reactions are as follows:

Diazotization:

Coupled reaction:

Ⅲ Apparatus and Reagents

723N spectrophotometer, cuvettes (1 cm × 4), volumetric flasks (50 mL × 7), electronic balance (0.01 g), beaker (50 mL × 1), Mohr measuring pipets (2.00 mL × 4), rubber pipet bulb, wash bottle, medicine dropper, etc..

Standard sodium nitrite solution (400 $\mu g \cdot mL^{-1}$, 10.00 $\mu g \cdot mL^{-1}$), naphthalene ethylenediamine hydrochloride solution (0.3%), p-aminobenzene sulfonic acid solution (1.0%).

Ⅳ Procedure

1. Pretreatment of Food Samples and Preparation of Test Solutions

Design them by yourself.

2. Preparation of Calibration Curve and Determination of Nitrite in Food

Transfer 0.30 mL, 0.60 mL, 0.90 mL, 1.20 mL and 1.50 mL of 10.00 $\mu g \cdot mL^{-1}$ standard $NaNO_2$ solution, respectively, into five 50 mL volumetric flasks with a Mohr measuring pipet. Add 30 mL of distilled water, 2.00 mL of 1.0% p-aminobenzene sulfonic acid solution and place for 3 min, and then add 2.00 mL of 0.3% naphthalene ethylenediamine hydrochloride solution, dilute to the mark, let stand for 15 min to allow the color to stabilize. Prepare a blank in the same way, omitting the standard sodium nitrite solution. Measure the absorbance for each of the five solutions at 538 nm against the blank. Prepare a calibration curve by plotting absorbance vs. the concentration of $NaNO_2$ for the standards, and then determine the concentration of $NaNO_2$ in food ($mg \cdot kg^{-1}$).

$V(NaNO_2)/mL$	0.00	0.30	0.60	0.90	1.20	1.50	Sample (25 mL)
$c(NaNO_2)/(\mu g \cdot mL^{-1})$							
Absorbance							

V Questions

(1) If the solution is red, is it indicates the solution absorbs or transmits for red light?

(2) Why nitrite concentration in the sample should be determined in time?

Experiment 23　Determination of Nitrate Content in Water Samples by Dual-Wavelength Spectrophotometry

I Learning Objectives

(1) Master the basic principles of dual-wavelength spectrophotometry for the determination of nitrate content.

(2) Familiar with the structure and operation of UV-Vis spectrophotometer.

II Principles

The dual-wavelength spectrophotometry can be used for determination when the absorption spectrum of a certain component interferes with the absorption spectrum of the component to be measured or the solution with a large background absorption is measured. In the presence of the nitrite (interfering component), the principle of the dual-wavelength absorption method for the determination of nitrate concentration is as follows (Figure 2-5).

According to the superposition principle of the absorbance, there are:

$$A_1 = A_1^a + A_1^b, \quad A_2 = A_2^a + A_2^b$$
$$\Delta A = A_1 - A_2 = A_1^a - A_2^a = (\varepsilon_1^a - \varepsilon_2^a)bc$$

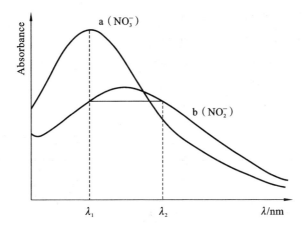

Figure 2-5 The principle of the dual-wavelength absorption method for
the determination of nitrate concentration

The above formula shows that the absorbance difference ΔA of nitrate at λ_1 and λ_2 is proportional to the concentration of nitrate, and irrelevant to the amount of nitrite. This can be used to eliminate the interference of nitrite.

Ⅲ Apparatus and Reagents

Ultraviolet-visible spectrophotometer, cuvettes (1 cm $\times$ 2), volumetric flasks (50 mL $\times$ 7), Mohr measuring pipets (5 mL $\times$ 2), small beaker, etc..

Standard $NaNO_3$ solution (1. 000 mg $\cdot$ mL^{-1}, 50. 00 μg $\cdot$ mL^{-1}), standard $NaNO_2$ solution (250. 0 μg $\cdot$ mL^{-1}, 5. 00 μg $\cdot$ mL^{-1}).

Ⅳ Procedure

1. Draw Absorption Spectrum Curve

Determine the absorption spectrum for 5. 00 μg $\cdot$ mL^{-1} standard $NaNO_2$ solution over the spectral range from 190-230 nm; use distilled water as a blank. Determine the absorption spectrum curve for 5. 00 μg $\cdot$ mL^{-1} standard $NaNO_3$ solution over the spectral range from 190-230 nm.

2. Select the Measuring Wavelengths λ_1 and λ_2

According to the drawn absorption spectrum curve, select the measuring wavelengths λ_1 and λ_2.

3. Preparation of the Series of Standard Solutions

Into each of six 50 mL volumetric flasks, pipet 0. 00 mL, 1. 00 mL, 2. 00 mL, 3. 00 mL, 4. 00 mL and 5. 00 mL of the 50. 00 μg $\cdot$ mL^{-1} standard $NaNO_3$ solution, respectively, and then dilute to the mark with distilled water.

4. Measurement of the Absorbance

Using distilled water as the reference solution, the absorbance of the standard solutions and the solutions to be tested at wavelengths λ_1 and λ_2 are measured. Plot the ΔA vs. the concentration of $NaNO_3$. From this graph, determine the concentration of the nitrate in sample solution.

V Data

$V(NaNO_3)/mL$	1.00	2.00	3.00	4.00	5.00	Solution to be tested
$c(NaNO_3)/(\mu g \cdot mL^{-1})$						
$A_1(\lambda_1)$						
$A_2(\lambda_2)$						
$\Delta A = A_1 - A_2$						

VI Questions

(1) What is the principle of wavelength selection for dual-wavelength spectrophotometry?

(2) What are the advantages of dual-wavelength spectrophotometry?

Experiment 24   Determination of Zinc in Human Hair by Flame Atomic Absorption Spectroscopy

I Learning Objectives

(1) Master basic principles of atomic absorption spectroscopy.

(2) Familiar with wet digestion technology for hair sample.

(3) Familiar with the structure and operation of atomic absorption spectrophotometer.

II Principles

The hair sample is digested by wet method and atomized by a flame atomizer. When the characteristic spectrum line of the measured element, radiated by the sharp-line light source (hollow cathode lamp), passes through the atomization zone of the flame, the gaseous atoms of the measured element absorb the spectrum line.

Under certain experimental conditions, the absorbance is proportional to the concentration of the measured component in the solution ($A = Kc$). The standard curve method can be used for quantitative analysis.

III Apparatus and Reagents

Atomic absorption spectrophotometer, zinc hollow cathode lamp, air compressor, acetylene cylinder, electronic balance (0.01 g), electric heating plate, Mohr measuring pipets (2 mL×2), volumetric flasks (50 mL×7, 25 mL×1), Erlenmeyer flask (50 mL×1), etc..

Standard zinc solution (1.000 mg • mL^{-1}, 50.00 μg • mL^{-1}), mixed acid (nitric acid : perchloric acid = 4 : 1), metallic zinc (GR), nitric acid (GR), perchloric acid (GR).

IV Procedure

1. Sample Pretreatment

Take 0.5 g hair of the human from 2 cm of the occipital scalp and cut into about 1 cm pieces. Wash the samples with a neutral detergent solution and keep stirring for 30 min. Then, wash with tap water until no foam appears, rinse several times with distilled water. Soak in absolute ethanol for 2 min and then place in a drying oven at 80 ℃ for 30 min until the ethanol evaporates to dryness. Dissolve 0.1-0.15 g samples in an Erlenmeyer flask with 2.0 mL mixed acid and heat on an electric heating plate until the solution turns transparent. Cool down, transfer the digestion solution to a 25 mL volumetric flask, dilute to the mark by purified water, shake well. Prepare the blank solution in the same way.

2. Preparation of Standard Solution

Into each of six 50 mL volumetric flasks, pipet 0.00 mL (blank), 0.30 mL, 0.60 mL, 0.90 mL, 1.20 mL and 1.50 mL of 50.00 μg • mL^{-1} standard zinc solution, respectively, and then dilute to the mark with 1% HNO_3 solution.

3. Instrument Adjustment and Operating Conditions

Detection wavelength: 213.9 nm. Spectral passband: 0.5 nm. Lamp current: 3.0 mA. Acetylene flow rate: 1.2 L • min^{-1}. Air flow rate: 6.0 L • min^{-1}. Preheat the instrument for 30 min.

4. Sample Measurement

Adjust the absorbance to zero with blank solution. Determine the absorbance of standard solutions from diluted to concentrated solutions. Under the same condition, determine the absorbance of blank solution and sample solution. Calculate the zinc concentration from the standard curve.

V Data

Standard curve is drawn with absorbance vs. standard concentration, and the result is calculated as follows:

$$\omega = \frac{(c-c_0)KV}{m_s} \times 10^{-6}$$

where ω is the content of zinc in hair ($\mu g \cdot g^{-1}$); V is the volume of the sample solution; K is the dilution ratio of the sample; c is the concentration of zinc in the sample solution ($\mu g \cdot mL^{-1}$); c_0 is the concentration of zinc in reagent blank ($\mu g \cdot mL^{-1}$); m_s is the mass of the hair sample (g).

VI Questions

(1) What is the practical significance of the determination of zinc in hair?

(2) How does the slit width affect the measurement? How to choose the slit width?

Experiment 25   Determination of Riboflavin in Milk by Fluorimetry

I Learning Objectives

(1) Learn the basic principles and measurement method of fluorescence spectrophotometry.

(2) Understand the experimental method for the determination of riboflavin in milk.

II Principles

Riboflavin (vitamin B_2) can emit fluoresces in neutral and weak acidic solutions. The content of riboflavin can be determined by measuring the fluorescence intensity of the solution. In order to eliminate the interference of stray light on the measurement, add acetate buffer solution (pH = 4.6) to precipitate protein and use sodium dithionite as a quenching agent. Determine the content of riboflavin in the sample by using the difference of the fluorescence intensity before and after adding the quenching agent.

III Apparatus and Reagents

Fluorometer, cuvette (1 cm $\times$ 1), volumetric flask (50 mL $\times$ 1), Mohr measuring pipets (5 mL$\times 3$), colorimetric tubes (10 mL$\times 7$), funnel, glass rod, small beaker, etc..

Standard vitamin B_2 solution (100.0 μg $\cdot$ mL^{-1}, 2.00 μg $\cdot$ mL^{-1}), HAc-NaAc buffer solution (pH$=4.6$), HCl solution (0.1 mol $\cdot$ L^{-1}), HAc solution (1%), $Na_2S_2O_4$. All reagents are analytically pure.

IV Procedure

1. Sample Handling

Accurately transfer 5.00 mL of milk into a 50 mL small beaker, add 10 mL of 0.1 mol $\cdot$ L^{-1} HCl solution, stir thoroughly, put it in the dark and let it stand for 10 min. Transfer the solution to a 50 mL volumetric flask, add 20 mL of HAc-NaAc buffer solution, and then dilute to the mark. After standing for several minutes, filter the mixture with rapid qualitative filter paper, discard the first 10 mL filtrate, and collect the subsequent filtrate for further determination.

2. Standard Curve Method

(1) Plotting the standard curve: Into each of six 10 mL colorimetric tubes, pipet 0.00 mL, 0.50 mL, 1.00 mL, 1.50 mL, 2.00 mL and 2.50 mL of 2.00 μg $\cdot$ mL^{-1} standard vitamin B_2 solution, respectively, and then dilute to the mark with 1% HAc solution. Selecte the excitation wavelength of 425 nm and fluorescence emission wavelength of 525 nm to measure the fluorescence intensity of the standard series. Draw the standard curve with $F-F_0$ vs. the concentration of vitamin B_2.

(2) Sample measurement: Pipet 5.00 mL of the sample filtrate into a 10 mL colorimetric tube and dilute to the mark with 1% HAc solution. Measure F_x under the same conditions as the standard curve. Calculate the concentration of vitamin B_2 in the sample from the standard curve.

3. Direct Comparison Method

(1) Preparation of 0.25 μg $\cdot$ mL^{-1} standard vitamin B_2 solution: Pipet 1.25 mL of 2.00 μg $\cdot$ mL^{-1} standard vitamin B_2 solution into a 10 mL colorimetric tube and dilute to the mark with 1% HAc solution.

(2) Measurement: Determine the fluorescence intensity of the 0.25 $\mu g \cdot mL^{-1}$ standard vitamin B_2 solution. Add about 10 mg $Na_2S_2O_4$ into the cuvette, shake, and measure the fluorescence intensity immediately. Then measure the fluorescence intensity of the sample filtrate before and after adding $Na_2S_2O_4$. Repeat the measurement two more times.

V Data

1. Standard Curve Method

V(standard vitamin B_2 solution)/mL	0.00	0.50	1.00	1.50	2.00	2.50	Sample solution
c(vitamin B_2)/($\mu g \cdot mL^{-1}$)							
F							

2. Direct Comparison Method

Calculate the vitamin B_2 concentration in the sample according to the following equation:

$$\omega(\mu g \cdot mL^{-1}) = \frac{(F_x - F_0') \times 0.25}{F_s - F_0} \times \frac{50.00}{5.00}$$

where F_x and F_s are fluorescence intensity of the sample and standard measured before adding $Na_2S_2O_4$, respectively; F_0' and F_0 are the fluorescence intensity of the sample and standard measured after adding $Na_2S_2O_4$, respectively.

VI Questions

(1) Describe the principles of this measurement.

(2) Can we measure the fluorescence spectrum and excitation spectrum of riboflavin with a fluorometer?

Experiment 26 The Inspection of the Perfermance of the Glass Electrode and the Determination of the pH Value of a Beverage

I Learning Objectives

(1) Understand the principle of measuring the pH value of a solution.

(2) Know the method for measuring pH value of a solution with a pH meter.

(3) Understand how to evaluate the electrode performance.

II Principles

The pH value of a solution can be determined by potentiometry. The glass electrode is used as indicator electrode, and the saturated calomel electrode is used as reference electrode:

(−) Ag, AgCl(s) | 0. 1 mol • L^{-1} HCl | glass membrane |H$^+$ (x mol • L^{-1}) ‖ KCl(saturated) | Hg$_2$Cl$_2$(s), Hg (+)

The electromotive force of the cell:

$$E = \varphi_+ - \varphi_- = K + \frac{2.303RT}{F}pH$$

Modern combined electrode is the combination of both reference electrode and glass electrode. When measuring pH value with a pH meter, the double measurement method can be used. First, calibrate pH meter with standard buffer solutions; then determine the electromotive force of the solution to be tested, which can be used to calculate the pH value of the solution:

$$E_s = K + \frac{2.303RT}{F}pH_s \quad E_x = K + \frac{2.303RT}{F}pH_x$$

Subtract these two equations to get the following equation:

$$E_s = E_x + \frac{2.303RT}{F}(pH_s - pH_x)$$

With one unit change of the pH value, the electromotive force of the battery is changed by $2.303RT/F$ volts. This value varies with the temperature. Therefore, there is a temperature compensation device on the pH meter to adjust the change caused by the temperature change. Theoretically, a good pH glass electrode should have a Nernst response. But in practice, there is a certain deviation between the actual corresponding slope of the electrode and the theoretical response slope.

III Apparatus and Reagents

pH meter, electrode (glass electrode and saturated calomel electrode (or a combined electrode)), analytical balance (0. 01 g), small beakers (10 mL×5).

Potassium hydrogen phthalate standard buffer solution (0. 05 mol • L^{-1}, pH= 4. 00), mixed phosphate standard buffer solution (KH$_2$PO$_4$ 0. 025 mol • L^{-1}, Na$_2$HPO$_4$ 0. 025 mol • L^{-1}, pH = 6. 86), borax standard buffer solution (0. 05 mol • L^{-1}, pH=9. 18).

IV Procedure

1. Calibration of pH Meter

Use the buffer solutions with pH = 6.86, pH = 4.00 and pH = 9.18 for calibration, respectively.

2. Determination of pH Value of Beverage Solution

Make a galvanic cell with the solution to be tested, the glass electrode as indicator electrode and the saturated calomel electrode as reference electrode, and then determine the pH of the solution.

3. The Performance of the pH Glass Electrode

Measurement of the electromotive forces of three different standard buffer solutions: Transfer pH 4.00 standard buffer solution into a 10 mL small beaker, immerse the electrode in the solution to measure the electromotive force of the cell. Record the electromotive force and clean the electrode. Measure the electromotive force of the standard buffer solutions (pH = 6.86 and pH = 9.18) in the same way. Plot the electromotive force vs. the pH value of the standard buffer solutions. From the diagram, inspect the linear relationship of the response of glass electrode to H^+ and calculate the actual slope of glass electrode.

V Question

Why do we use standard buffer solutions for calibration of the pH meter?

Experiment 27   Determination of Water Purity by Conductometry

I Learning Objectives

(1) Master the basic principles and experimental method of determining water purity by conductometry.

(2) Know the determination method of conductivity cell constant.

(3) Understand the structure of the conductivity meter.

II Principles

The conductivity κ (S · cm^{-1}) is related to the concentration of ions in the solution, migration speed, valence state and temperature etc. , can be used as a reference index of electrolyte content in water, also one of the comprehensive indexes for evaluating water quality. The relationship between conductance $G(S)$, conductivity (electrical conductance) and conductivity cell constant (θ) is as follows:

$$G = \kappa \frac{A}{l} = \frac{\kappa}{\theta}$$

where A (cm^2) is the electrode area; l (cm) is the distance between the electrodes; $\theta = \frac{l}{A}$ (cm^{-1}) is the conductivity cell constant. The theoretical conductivity of pure water is 5.48×10^{-2} μS $\cdot$ cm^{-1} at room temperature (25 ℃). Generally, the conductivity of experimental distilled water or deionized water should be less than 1 μS $\cdot$ cm^{-1}.

III Apparatus and Reagents

Conductivity meter, electrodes (platinum black electrode and platinum bright electrode), thermostatic water bath, volumetric flask (1 000 mL × 1), small beakers (50 mL × 7).

KCl standard solution (0.01 mol $\cdot$ L^{-1}): Accurately weigh 0.745 6 g KCl (Dried for 4 hours at 120 ℃) in a beaker, and dissolve it with pure water (conductivity <1 μS $\cdot$ cm^{-1}). Transfer it to a 1 000 mL volumetric flask and dilute to the mark. Store in a plastic bottle.

IV Procedure

1. Determination of the Constant of Conductivity cell (θ)

Put 30 mL of 0.01 mol $\cdot$ L^{-1} KCl standard solution into a 50 mL beaker, put in a constant temperature bath (25 ℃) and wait 15 min to reach thermal equilibrium. Wash the electrode with distilled water and dry before the measurement. Determine the conductance (G_{KCl}) by conductivity meter at 25 ℃. Record the conductivity of KCl solution, and find out the standard conductivity of 0.01 mol $\cdot$ L^{-1} KCl standard solution at 25 ℃. Calculate the cell constant.

2. Determination of the Electrical Conductivity of Deionized Water/ Distilled Water/Commercial Purified Water

Set the displayed constant value on the instrument to be consistent with the electrode conductivity cell constant by adjusting the constant compensation button.

Set the temperature value to be consistent with the solution temperature by adjusting the temperature compensation button. Put 30 mL deionized water/ distilled water/commercial purified water to three beakers (rinsed three times), respectively. Place a platinum bright electrode into it and choose the suitable range, and record the conductivity of the solution. Test three times and take the average value.

3. Determination of the Electrical Conductivity of Tap Water/Lake Water

Rinse the beaker with sample solution three times. Place a platinum black electrode into it and repeat step 2, record the conductivity of the solution.

V Questions

(1) Which kind of current should be chosen for conductivity meter, DC or AC? Why?

(2) Why do we measure the cell constant of the electrode? How to measure it?

Experiment 28　Determination of Fluorine Ion in Water by Fluoride Ion-Selective Electrode

I Learning Objectives

(1) Master the principle and method of fluoride ion-selective electrode.

(2) Know the standard curve method and standard addition method for the determination of fluoride ion in water samples.

II Principles

Fluoride ion-selective electrode is a kind of crystal membrane electrode. Its sensitive membrane is a lanthanum fluoride (LaF_3) single crystal membrane, which has a selective response to fluoride ions. The relationship between membrane potential and fluorine ion activity follows Nernst equation. In the process of the experiment, the fluoride ion-selective electrode and saturated calomel electrode (SCE) are employed as the indicator and reference electrodes, respectively. The electromotive force of the battery is linear with the logarithm of the activity of fluorine ion.

$$E = \varphi_{F^-} - \varphi_{ref} = K - 0.059 \lg a_{F^-}$$

When the ionic strength of the solution is stable:

$$E = K - 0.059 \lg c_{F^-}$$

Ⅲ Apparatus and Reagents

pH meter, fluoride ion-selective electrode and saturated calomel electrode (or composite electrode), electromagnetic stirrer, volumetric flasks (25 mL × 6), Mohr measuring pipets (2 mL×2, 10 mL×3), small beakers (50 mL×7), etc...

Fluorine standard solution (1.000 mg · mL^{-1}, 10.00 μg · mL^{-1}), total ionic strength adjustment buffer solution (dissolve 58 g NaCl, 57 mL glacial acetic acid, 3.4 g trisodium citrate pentahydrate in distilled water, adjust the pH to 5.0-5.5 by 10 mol · L^{-1} NaOH, dilute the solution with distilled water to 1000 mL). All the above reagents are analytical reagents (AR).

Ⅳ Procedure

1. Determination of Fluoride Concentration in Water Sample by Standard Curve Method

Transfer 0.40 mL, 0.60 mL, 1.00 mL, 1.50 mL and 2.00 mL of 10.00 μg · mL^{-1} fluorine standard solution, respectively, into five 25 mL volumetric flasks with Mohr measuring pipets. Add 10 mL total ionic strength adjustment buffer solution and then dilute to the mark with deionized water. Transfer the prepared standard solution series to small beakers according to the concentration from low to high. Place a cleaned electrode into it with magnetic stirring, record the electromotive force E. Draw a standard curve with the logarithm of the fluorine concentration as the abscissa (x-axis) and the electromotive force E as the ordinate (y-axis).

Pipet 10.00 mL sample solution into a 25 mL volumetric flask and add 10.00 mL total ionic strength adjustment buffer solution. Constant volume by deionized water and shake the volumetric flask sufficiently. Transfer the solution to a small beaker and place a cleaned electrode into it. Record the electromotive force E_x during magnetic stirring. Find out the fluoride ion concentration on the standard curve, and calculate the concentration of fluoride ion in water sample.

2. Determination of Fluoride Concentration in Water Sample by Standard Addition Method

Place 10.00 mL water in a small beaker, add 10.00 mL total ionic strength adjustment buffer solution. Place a cleaned electrode into it and record the electromotive force E_1 during magnetic stirring. Subsequently, add 0. 20 mL of 1. 000 mg • mL^{-1} fluorine standard solution and record the electromotive force E_2 during magnetic stirring. Calculate fluoride ion concentration by E_1 and E_2.

Compare the results of the two methods.

V Questions

(1) What is the role of total ionic strength adjustment buffer solution?

(2) The result measured by the above method is activity or concentration? Why?

Experiment 29　Determination of Benzene Series in Waste-Water by Gas Chromatography

I Learning Objectives

(1) Understand the structure and operation of gas chromatograph.

(2) Master the principles and experimental method of gas chromatography for the determination of benzene series.

(3) Understand the quantitative method of internal standard curve method.

II Principles

The retention time of benzene and benzene series in gas chromatography is different due to the different partition coefficients of benzene and benzene series in intermediate polarity stationary phase or non-polar stationary phases. The retention time of benzene series in the sample is used for qualitative analysis and the peak area is recorded for quantitative analysis.

III Apparatus and Reagents

Gas chromatograph (FID), capillary column (HP-1, DB-5 or OV1701, 30 m× 0. 25 mm×0. 25 μm), microsyringe (10 μL×1), volumetric flasks (10 mL×7), pipette and pipette tips, etc. .

Standard stock solution for benzene (100 μg • mL^{-1}): Measure appropriate amount of benzene, dissolve in carbon disulfide, dilute to 10. 00 mL, and shake well. Standard stock solution for toluene (100 μg • mL^{-1}): Measure appropriate amount of toluene, dissolve in carbon disulfide, dilute to 10. 00 mL, and shake well. Standard stock solution for ethylbenzene (100 μg · mL^{-1}): Measure appropriate amount of ethylbenzene, dissolve in carbon disulfide, dilute to 10 mL, and shake well. All the above reagents are chromatographically pure.

IV Procedure

1. GC Conditions

GC inlet temperature: 230 ℃. GC oven: 80 ℃. FID: 230 ℃. Carrier gas: N_2. Carrier gas flow rate: 2. 0 mL · min^{-1}. Hydrogen flow rate: 30 mL · min^{-1}. Air flow rate: 300 mL · min^{-1}. Auxiliary gas flow rate: 25 mL · min^{-1}. Split ratio: 10 : 1.

2. The Preparation of Standard Series

Pipet the standard stock solutions of benzene and toluene 0. 10 mL, 0. 20 mL, 0. 50 mL, 1. 00 mL and 2. 00 mL, respectively, into five 10 mL volumetric flasks, add 0. 50 mL of ethylbenzene standard stock solution to each flask, and dilute to mark with carbon disulfide. The concentration of benzene and toluene is 1. 00 μg · mL^{-1}, 2. 00 μg · mL^{-1}, 5. 00 μg · mL^{-1}, 10. 0 μg · mL^{-1}, 20. 0 μg · mL^{-1}, respectively, and the concentration of ethylbenzene is 5. 00 μg · mL^{-1}.

3. Preparation of Sample Solution

Transfer 25 mL of water sample into a 125 mL separatory funnel, add 5. 0 mL of carbon disulfide. Close the stopcock and shake the funnel, watching out for emulsions, place the separatory funnel back in the iron ring, allow the layers to separate, and then drain the bottom layer of carbon disulfide into a clean container. Pipet 1. 0 mL of extraction solution into a 10 mL volumetric flask, add 0. 50 mL of ethylbenzene standard stock solution, dilute to the mark with carbon disulfide, and shake well.

4. Retention Time of Standards

Prepare the standard solutions of 5. 00 μg · mL^{-1} benzene, 5. 00 μg · mL^{-1} toluene and 5. 00 μg · mL^{-1} ethylbenzene, respectively. Inject 0. 2 μL of each solution into the gas chromatograph to determine the retention time of benzene, toluene and ethylbenzene.

5. Internal Standard Curve Drawing

Inject 0. 2 μL of the prepared mixed standard series solution successively from low to high concentration, and calculate the ratio of peak area of benzene, toluene and ethylbenzene as the internal standard. Plot the internal standard curves of benzene and toluene, respectively, with the ratio of peak area as the ordinate and the concentration as the abscissa.

6. Determination of the Sample

Under the same chromatographic conditions, inject 0.2 μL of the sample solution and calculate the ratio of peak area of benzene as toluene and ethylbenzene as the internal standard. According to the ratio of the peak area of benzene, toluene and ethylbenzene in the sample solution, calculate the concentration of benzene and toluene from the standard curve of benzene and toluene internal standard, respectively. Calculate the concentration of benzene and toluene in the original water sample. Compare the retention time of each component in the sample with the standard solution, and use retention time for qualitative analysis.

V Questions

(1) What are the advantages of the internal standard curve method?

(2) Try to explain the peaking order of benzene, toluene and ethylbenzene.

Experiment 30　Determination of Pigments in Food by HPLC

I Learning Objectives

(1) Understand the basic structure and operation of high performance liquid chromatograph.

(2) Master the principles and experimental method of determining pigments in food by high performance liquid chromatography (HPLC).

II Principles

Tartrazine and sunset yellow are synthetic pigments allowed to be used in food in China. They can be used in fruit flavored water, fruit flavored powder, sherbet, soda, mixed wine, red and green silk, canned food and cake surface coloring, but the dosage is strictly limited. The structural formulas of tartrazine and sunset yellow are as follows:

Tartrazine   Sunset yellow

Tartrazine has two prominent peaks located within the UV-Vis spectrum (259 nm, 425 nm), whereas sunset yellow has three peaks within the UV-Vis region (238 nm, 315 nm, 476 nm), so they can be separated by high performance liquid chromatography and then be quantified by UV detector.

Ⅲ Apparatus and Reagents

High performance liquid chromatograph (UV detector), chromatographic column (C18 column, 150 mm × 4. 6 mm × 5 μm), microsyringe (100 μL × 1), analytical balance (0. 01 g), ultrasonic oscillator, volumetric flask (5 mL × 1), pipette and pipette tips, etc..

Citric acid solution: Weigh about 20 g of citric acid ($C_6H_8O_7 \cdot H_2O$), dilute to 100 mL by ddH_2O, dissolve and mix well.

Water (pH=6): Add citric acid solution to ddH_2O and adjust pH to 6.

Standard stock solutions of tartrazine and sunset yellow (1 mg · mL^{-1}): Weigh about 0. 1 g of tartrazine and sunset yellow (accurate to 0. 000 1 g) in a small beaker, respectively, and dissolve in water (pH = 6). Transfer it to a 100 mL volumetric flask, dilute to the mark and shake well.

Standard solutions of tartrazine and sunset yellow (50 μg · mL^{-1}): Dilute the standard stock solution 20 times with ddH_2O, and then filter through 0. 45 μm microporous membrane.

Ammonium acetate solution (0. 02 mol · L^{-1}): Weigh 1. 54 g of ammonium acetate, add ddH_2O to 1 000 mL, dissolve, and filter through 0. 45 μm microporous membrane.

Ⅳ Procedure

1. The Chromatographic Conditions

Chromatographic column: C18 column, 150 mm × 4. 6 mm × 5 μm. Sample size: 20 μL. Column temperature: 35 ℃. UV detection wavelength: 254 nm. Mobile phase: methanol-0. 02 mol $\cdot$ L^{-1} ammonium acetate solution (35 : 65). Flow rate: 1 mL $\cdot$ min^{-1}.

2. Sample Preparation

(1) Fruit juice drinks, fruit juice, fruit carbonated drinks, etc. : Accurately weigh 20-40 g of samples and put into a 100 mL beaker to remove carbon dioxide by ultrasound.

(2) Mixed wine: Accurately weigh 20-40 g of samples and put into a 100 mL beaker. Then add several pieces of small broken porcelain and heat to remove the ethanol.

(3) Hard candy, candied fruit, starch soft candy, etc. : Accurately weigh 5-10 g of crushed samples, put into a 100 mL beaker, add 30 mL of water and warm the solvent. If the pH of the sample solution is high, adjust the pH to about 6 with citric acid solution.

(4) Chocolate beans and colored icing products: Accurately weigh 5-10 g of samples, put into a 100 mL beaker, wash the pigment repeatedly with water until the chocolate is free of pigment, and combine the pigment rinsing solution as the sample solution.

3. Extraction of Pigment

Add citric acid to sample solution, adjust pH to 6, heat to 60 ℃, add 1 g of polyamide powder with a little water to make paste, and lead into sample solution; stir for a while, filter with G3 vertical melting funnel, wash with ddH$_2$O of 60 ℃ and pH$=$4 for 3-5 times, wash with methanol-formic acid mixture for 3-5 times, and then wash to neutral with water. Then desorb 3-5 times with ethanol-ammonia-water mixed solution until the pigment desorbed completely. Collect the desorbed solution, add acetic acid for neutralization, evaporate to near dry, add water solution, and constant volume to 5 mL. Filter the solution by 0. 45 μm microporous membrane.

4. Determination

Inject the sample extracts, the standard solutions of tartrazine and sunset yellow into the high performance liquid chromatograph, respectively. Compare the retention time of each component in the sample with the standard solution, and qualitatively analyze each component in the sample. According to the peak areas of tartrazine and sunset yellow in the sample solutions, the external standard peak area method is used for quantitative analysis.

Ⅴ Questions

(1) Why should the sample be filtered before injection?

(2) How to choose mobile phase and chromatographic column?

Experiment 31   Purification of Sodium Chloride

Ⅰ Learning Objectives

(1) Learn the manipulation of crystallization, filtration and evaporation.

(2) Use scientific knowledge to plan how to separate pure salt from raw salt.

Ⅱ Principles

Sodium chloride is soluble in aqueous solution, so the impurities in sodium chloride can be removed with the processes shown below.

(1) The insoluble impurities are removed by filtration.

(2) Some soluble impurities can be removed by precipitation basing on their chemical properties. For example, sulfate can be separated as $BaSO_4$ by $BaCl_2$ solution. Metal ions, such as Ca^{2+}, Mg^{2+}, Ba^{2+}, etc., can be removed as insoluble precipitates.

(3) Some low content soluble impurities, such as Br^-, I^-, and K^+, having different solubility from sodium chloride, can be removed by recrystallization. They will be retained in the mother liquor and moved away.

Ⅲ Apparatus and Reagents

Analytical balance(0.01 g), beaker(100 mL×1), hot plate, filter paper, filter flask, Buchner funnel, desiccator, centrifuge, wire gauze, evaporating dish, test tubes (6) and centrifuge tubes(4).

Raw salt(s), HCl solution (6 mol · L^{-1}), H_2SO_4 solution (3 mol · L^{-1}), $BaCl_2$ solution (1 mol · L^{-1})and Na_2CO_3 solution (saturated solution).

Ⅳ Procedure

(1) Weigh out 5.0 g of raw salt. Place it in a 100 mL beaker and add 20 mL of distilled water. Slowly heat the beaker and its contents until the salt dissolves.

Filter hot solution through filter paper. Discard the solids (sludge, sand carbonaceous deposit) and the paper. Save the filtrate for step (2).

(2) Heat the filtrate (from step (1)) to boiling. Add 0.8-1.3 mL of 1 mol $\cdot$ L^{-1} BaCl$_2$ solution with stirring until a large amount of the precipitates form. After about 5 min, remove the heater. Centrifuge any precipitate (that's the solid, BaSO$_4$) that forms, decant and save the supernatant (that's the liquid). Place several drops of the supernatant to a test tube, add several drops of 6 mol $\cdot$ L^{-1} HCl solution, and then add several drops of BaCl$_2$ solution. A white precipitate is BaSO$_4$ and shows that SO$_4^{2-}$ is present. If no precipitate forms, SO$_4^{2-}$ is absent.

(3) Heat the supernatant (from step (2)) to boiling. Add saturated Na$_2$CO$_3$ solution dropwise with stirring until no precipitate forms. Continue to add excess (0.2 mL) saturated Na$_2$CO$_3$ solution. Centrifuge, decant, and save the supernatant for step (4). Place several drops of the supernatant to a test tube, add several drops of 3 mol $\cdot$ L^{-1} H$_2$SO$_4$ solution. A white precipitate is BaSO$_4$ and shows that Ba^{2+} is present. If no precipitate forms, Ba^{2+} is absent.

(4) The supernatant (from step (3)) is put in an evaporating dish and adjust pH to between 2.0 and 3.0 by adding 6 mol $\cdot$ L^{-1} HCl solution dropwise. Then, place this on the hot plate and concentrate the solution until a thin crystal film appears on its surface. Allow the solution to cool to room temperature. Use a vacuum filtration setup to separate the crystal from the liquid. Wash the crystal with a little amount of distilled water. Slowly heat filtrate with stirring and reduce the heating level to keep the material at a gentle boil. When dry, cool down, weigh the dry crystal and calculate the yield.

(5) Determination of the purity of the product. To eight test tubes dissolve 0.5 g of the raw salt and the product with 1.5 mL of distilled water, respectively. Detect ions, such as SO$_4^{2-}$, Ca^{2+}, Mg^{2+}, and Ba^{2+}, in the raw salt and the product, respectively. Compare the results in the raw salt with the results in the product.

Ⅴ Questions

(1) What impurities are contained in raw salt? How to remove these impurities?

(2) How to remove the low content soluble impurities such as K$^+$, Br$^-$, I$^-$?

(3) To remove SO$_4^{2-}$, Ca^{2+}, Mg^{2+}, etc., as precipitate by addition of corresponding precipitators, what influences the result, heating or not heating? How to determine whether these ions are removed entirely?

(4) During the adjustment of pH of the solution with HCl solution, what can we deal with the excess HCl solution? Why should we adjust the solution to be weak acidic? Can we adjust the solution to be weak alkaline?

(5) Why, during the purification of NaCl, should the agents be added sequentially: $BaCl_2$, Na_2CO_3, and HCl? Can we change the order of agents?

Experiment 32　Synthesis of Ferrous Ammonium Sulfate

Ⅰ Learning Objectives

(1) Study the principles and methods of synthesis of Mohr's salt.
(2) Review the manipulation of crystallization, filtration and water bath.

Ⅱ Principles

The purpose of this experiment is to synthesize—that is, to prepare from other reagents—Mohr's salt, $FeSO_4 \cdot (NH_4)_2SO_4 \cdot 6H_2O$, as source of redox-stable ferrous ions. The color of Mohr's salt is pale green, due to the presence of hydrated Fe^{2+} ions in the crystal. The crystal is relatively stable in air. It must, however, be oxidized to the ferric state by potassium permanganate solution prior to using as a standard solution.

The crystal will be prepared by first preparing $FeSO_4$, and then mixing this with $(NH_4)_2SO_4$, to form $FeSO_4 \cdot (NH_4)_2SO_4 \cdot 6H_2O$.

$FeSO_4$ is obtained from metallic iron foil(95% Fe) by adding a stoichiometric amount of 3 mol $\cdot$ L^{-1} H_2SO_4 solution to metallic Fe. The solution is heated until the iron foil is completely dissolved.

$$Fe + H_2SO_4 = FeSO_4 + H_2 \uparrow$$

Subsequently, the solution containing the mixture of $FeSO_4$ and $(NH_4)_2SO_4$ is concentrated at 80 ℃ until a thin crystal film appears on its surface. Crystal of $FeSO_4 \cdot (NH_4)_2SO_4 \cdot 6H_2O$ forms.

$$FeSO_4 + (NH_4)_2SO_4 + 6H_2O = FeSO_4 \cdot (NH_4)_2SO_4 \cdot 6H_2O$$

Ⅲ Apparatus and Reagents

Analytical balance (0. 01 g), Erlenmeyer flasks (50 mL × 1, 15 mL × 1), volumetric flask (1 L×1), water bath, graduated cylinders(50 mL×1,10 mL×1), funnel, evaporating dish, hot plate, Buchner funnel, filter paper, filter flask, vacuum pump, beaker(250 mL×1), colorimetric tubes(25 mL×4), Mohr measuring pipets (1 mL×1, 2 mL×1, 5 mL×1) and stirring rod.

Na_2CO_3 solution (10%), H_2SO_4 solution (3 mol • L^{-1}), HCl solution (3 mol • L^{-1}), $(NH_4)_2SO_4$(s), KSCN solution (1 mol • L^{-1}), ethanol solution (95%), oxygen-free distilled water, iron foil, pH test paper, filter paper and standard Fe^{3+} solution (0. 1 g • L^{-1}, accurately weigh 0. 863 4 g of $NH_4Fe(SO_4)_2$ • $12H_2O$ into a clean 150 mL beaker, dissolve it by adding the appropriate amount of distilled water. Add 2. 5 mL of concentrated H_2SO_4 solution and transfer the solution into a 1 L volumetric flask with a stirring rod. Rinse the beaker with distilled water for two or three times and add the rinsing to the flask. When the distilled water is added nearly to the calibration mark, distilled water is added with a medicine dropper until the bottom of the meniscus reaches the calibration mark. Stopper the flask, and mix the solution well).

Ⅳ Procedure

1. Preparation of Degreased Iron Foil

Weigh out 2. 0 g of iron foil. Place it into a 50 mL Erlenmeyer flask and add 10 mL of 10% Na_2CO_3 solution. Slowly heat the flask and its contents to boiling, stir and reduce the temperature to keep the material at a gentle boil. After about 5 min, remove the heat, and slowly decant(pour off the liquid layer and retain the wet solid). Wash the iron foil by rinsing it with distilled water.

2. Preparation of $FeSO_4$ Solution

Add 10 mL of 3 mol • L^{-1} H_2SO_4 solution to the Erlenmeyer flask with the iron foil. Place the Erlenmeyer flask in water bath. If the iron foil is not fully submerged, carefully push it down with a stirring rod. The H_2SO_4 solution will begin to dissolve the iron, producing hydrogen gas. The reaction can produce minor spattering as hydrogen bubbles to the surface of the acid. Continue to stir and keep the temperature at 80 ℃. You will see some bubbles (hydrogen), some color change, and a decrease in the amount of solid. Over the course of 30 min, the hydrogen bubbles will gradually disappear.

Green crystal should have started forming in the solution and settling to the bottom. Add acidified water (pH between 2 and 4) enough to redissolve all the green crystal that has settled out. If the solution turns brown, add H_2SO_4 solution just enough to make it green again.

Filter hot solution through filter paper. Discard the solid and the paper. Save the filtrate. The filtrate is put in an evaporating dish.

If the pH is not kept low enough, ferrous sulfate will be oxidized to ferric sulfate on standing. Normally, atmospheric oxygen oxidizes Fe^{2+} to Fe^{3+} quite readily. This reaction is reversible, however, by lowering the pH. Below 4 or so, ferrous ion is heavily favored over ferric, with the concentration of Fe^{3+} becoming vanishingly small at pH 1-2. Aqueous $FeSO_4$ in this pH range is stable for days, even contacting with much air.

3. Preparation of $FeSO_4 \cdot (NH_4)_2SO_4 \cdot 6H_2O$

Add 4.75 g of $(NH_4)_2SO_4$ into the evaporating dish with freshly prepared $FeSO_4$ solution. Mix completely and adjust pH to between 1.0 and 2.0 by adding 3 $mol \cdot L^{-1}$ H_2SO_4 solution dropwise. Place this on the hot plate. Subsequently, the mixture of $FeSO_4$ and $(NH_4)_2SO_4$ is concentrated at 80 ℃ (heat the mixture to boiling(beware of bumping)) until a thin crystal film appears on its surface. The color of the solution may change to yellowish, but don't let this discourage you. On cooling it becomes green again.

Allow the solution to cool to room temperature. Now wait. You should see some crystal forms as the solution cools. The process is slow and the crystal will be quite small.

Use a vacuum filtration setup to separate the crystal from the liquid. Wash the crystal with 5 mL of 95% ethanol solution twice. Spread the crystal on a fresh filter paper and allow them to dry in the air. When dry, weigh the dry crystal and record the result.

4. Determination of the Purity of the Product

Transfer 0.50 mL, 1.00 mL, and 2.00 mL of the standard iron solution, respectively, into three 25 mL colorimetric tubes with a Mohr measuring pipet. Add 1.00 mL of 3 $mol \cdot L^{-1}$ H_2SO_4 solution and 1.00 mL of 1 $mol \cdot L^{-1}$ KSCN solution, and then dilute to the mark. The content of Fe^{3+} in the different solutions is shown below.

Grade Ⅰ:0.05 mg.

Grade Ⅱ:0.10 mg.

Grade Ⅲ:0.20 mg.

Prepare the sample in the same way, omitting the standard iron solution. Dissolve 1 g ferrous ammonium sulfate hexahydrate with 15.00 mL of distilled water in a 25 mL colorimetric tube. Add 1.00 mL of 3 $mol \cdot L^{-1}$ H_2SO_4 solution and 1.00 mL of 1 $mol \cdot L^{-1}$ KSCN solution, and then dilute to the mark. Compare the color with that of the series of standard solution to determine the purity grade of the product.

V Questions

(1) Between the iron foil and the H_2SO_4 solution in step 2, which one should be present in considerable excess?

(2) Why should we filter the solution while it is still hot when the reaction for ferrous sulfate is completed? Why do we need warm water to wash the filter residue?

(3) Why should the pH of the solution be kept at 1-2 during evaporation?

Experiment 33　Preparation and Properties of the Colloid

I Learning Objectives

(1) Learn to prepare the colloid.

(2) Review the properties of colloidal system.

II Principles

In this experiment, the colloid will be prepared by using condensation method. Condensation methods involve the formation of colloidal particles by causing smaller particles to aggregate. Condensation methods usually employ chemical reactions. A dark red colloidal suspension of iron(Ⅲ) hydroxide may be prepared by mixing a concentrated solution of iron(Ⅲ) chloride with hot water. A colloidal suspension of antimony(Ⅲ) sulfide is produced by the reaction of hydrogen sulfide with antimony potassium tartrate dissolved in water. Dialysis is the separation of a solution from a colloid(protein) by means of a semipermeable membrane. Such a membrane is called a dialyzing membrane. In this experiment, we will separate and sublimate the colloid by means of a dialyzing membrane.

Colloidal dispersions involve particles whose size is larger than those found in solutions but smaller than those in suspensions. When a strong beam of light passes through a liquid, the Tyndall effect is exhibited as the larger-size colloidal particles reflect and scatter the light smaller-size particles in solution do not. The Tyndall effect is one property that distinguishes colloidal dispersions from solutions.

One of the most important properties of dispersed colloidal particles is that they are usually electrically charged. When an iron(Ⅲ) hydroxide solution is placed in an electrolytic cell, the dispersed particles move to the negative electrode. This is good evidence that the iron (Ⅲ) hydroxide particles are positively charged. The charges on colloidal particles result from the adsorption of ions that exist in the dispersion medium. Most hydroxides of metals have positive charges, while most sulfides of metals form negatively charged colloidal dispersions. These electrically charged crystals repel one another, so aggregation to larger particles is prevented.

You might expect these very small crystals to aggregate into larger crystals when adding ions of opposite charge. The iron(Ⅲ) hydroxide solution can be made to aggregate by the addition of an ionic solution, particularly if the solution contains anions with multiple charges (such as phosphate ions, PO_4^{3-}). The iron (Ⅲ) hydroxide colloidal particles are positively charged, so the greater of the negative charge, the more effective is the coagulation. The order of effective in coagulating colloidal particles would be $Na_3PO_4 > MgSO_4 > NaCl$.

Ⅲ Apparatus and Reagents

U-tube, instrument for Tyndall effect, beakers (100 mL × 3, 500 mL × 1), graduated cylinders (10 mL × 1, 50 mL × 1), test tubes (10), medicine dropper, hot plate, wire gauze, electrophoresis apparatus, stirring rod and string.

$FeCl_3$ solution (2%), antimony potassium tartrate solution (0. 4%), $AgNO_3$ solution (0. 1 mol · L^{-1}), KSCN solution (0. 5 mol · L^{-1}), HCl solution (0. 000 1 mol · L^{-1}), NaCl solution (0. 005 mol · L^{-1}, 5%), $CaCl_2$ solution (0. 005 mol · L^{-1}), $AlCl_3$ solution (0. 005 mol · L^{-1}), hydrogen sulfide solution (saturated solution), $CuSO_4$ solution (2%), sugar and celloidin.

Ⅳ Procedure

1. Preparation of the Colloid

(1) Preparation of the iron (Ⅲ) hydroxide solution. Boil about 25 mL of distilled water in a 100 mL beaker. While the water is boiling, add 4 mL of 2% iron (Ⅲ) chloride solution dropwise with stirring, and continue boiling for 1-2 min. Colloidal iron(Ⅲ) hydroxide forms.

(2) Preparation of the antimony(Ⅲ) sulfide solution. Measure out about 20 mL of antimony potassium tartrate solution into a 100 mL beaker. Add H_2S

solution drop by drop until the solution changes orange.

2. Purification of the Colloid—Dialysis

(1) Preparation of the dialysis bag. Place about 10 mL of celloidin in a small beaker and swirl until celloidin wet all inside of beaker. Wait for a minute and then turn the beaker upside down. The material should be solid. Take out it and get a dialysis bag.

(2) Dialysis. Place the colloidal iron(Ⅲ) hydroxide in the dialysis bag. Be careful that none of the liquids contaminate the outside of the dialysis bag and close it tightly. If they do, wash off with distilled water. Suspend the dialysis bag in a beaker with distilled water for 10 min. Test the liquid outside of the dialysis bag for chloride ions($AgNO_3$ test) and iron(Ⅲ) ions(KSCN test). Record your results. Which substances passed through the membrane? What does this experiment tell you about the relative size of the particles in these liquids?

3. Properties of Colloidal System

(1) Tyndall effect. Take three test tubes and fill each one-third full with one of the following liquids: the colloidal iron(Ⅲ) hydroxide, the colloidal antimony(Ⅲ) sulfide, $CuSO_4$ solution. Shine a light through each test tube. Observe the Tyndall effect. Which liquids did not give the Tyndall effect?

(2) Electrical properties of colloidal particles. Place the colloidal antimony(Ⅲ) sulfide in a U-tube and in an electrophoresis apparatus. Observe the dispersed particles. Which electrode will they move to? Why?

(3) Coagulation. To 1 mL of Sb_2S_3 solution, add $0.005 \text{ mol} \cdot \text{L}^{-1}$ NaCl solution drop by drop. Swirl the test tube gently and continuously as you add the NaCl solution. When the precipitation begins to persist, record the drops you add. How about $0.005 \text{ mol} \cdot \text{L}^{-1}$ $CaCl_2$ solution or $0.005 \text{ mol} \cdot \text{L}^{-1}$ $AlCl_3$ solution instead of $0.005 \text{ mol} \cdot \text{L}^{-1}$ NaCl solution? Record the drops and compare them. Explain.

Add 2 mL of the iron(Ⅲ) hydroxide solution into a small test tube, and then add 2 mL of the Sb_2S_3 solution. Swirl the mixture. Record your observations. Explain.

Put 2 mL of the Sb_2S_3 solution into a small test tube. Heat the tube. Record your observations. Explain.

Ⅴ Data

1. Preparation of the Colloid

Observations: (1) _____

(2) _____

2. Dialysis

Observations: _____

Did the colloidal iron(Ⅲ) hydroxide diffuse through the membrane? Explain.

3. Properties of Colloidal System

(1) The Tyndall effect.

Sample: iron(Ⅲ) hydroxide Sb_2S_3 $CuSO_4$ solution

Observations: _____   _____   _____

(2) Electrical properties of colloidal particles.

Observations: _____

(3) Coagulation.

Volume of NaCl solution: _____ drops

Volume of $CaCl_2$ solution: _____ drops

Volume of $AlCl_3$ solution: _____ drops

Experiment 34   Preparation of Tin Dioxide Nanopowder by Hydrothermal Method

Ⅰ Learning Objectives

(1) Learn the principles of synthesizing tin dioxide nanopowder by hydrothermal method.

(2) Understand the influences of hydrothermal treating temperature and time, pH value of medium, concentration of reactant on the morphology and crystallization.

(3) Learn the analysis of the nanomaterial.

Ⅱ Principles

In the last decades, a little word attracted enormous attention, interest and investigation from all over the world—nano. What are nanoscience and nanotechnology? In fact, there are no exact definitions for them. The following is the definition of nanoscience and nanotechnology given by the US National Nanotechnology Initiative(NNI): nanoscience and nanotechnology are "research and technology development at the atomic, molecular and macromolecular levels in the length scale of 1-100 nm, to provide a fundamental understanding of phenomena and materials at the nanoscale and to create and use structures, devices and systems that have novel properties and functions because of their small and/or intermediate size". Simply saying, nanoscience tells us how to understand the basic theories and principles of nanoscale structures, devices and systems (1-100 nm); and nanotechnology tells us what to do and how to use these nanoscale materials.

Tin dioxide is one of the most important metal oxide semiconductor materials, and is extensively applied to ceramic, gas sensor and catalyst, etc.. Especially, scientists are interested in SnO_2 nanomaterials for their evident surface effect and pay much attention to their synthesis methods. There are several methods to be used for obtaining SnO_2 nanomaterials such as surfactant-mediated method, Sol-Gel method, chemical precipitation method, hydrolytic method, hydrothermal method, etc.. However, in order to avoid agglomeration and obtain smaller SnO_2 nanoparticles in size, many chemists and material chemists have made efforts to research on more efficient synthesis methods.

In this experiment, SnO_2 nanopowder is synthesized by hydrothermal method. The influences of hydrothermal treating temperature and time, pH value of medium, concentration of reactant on the morphology and crystallization are studied. The structure of as-prepared SnO_2 nanopowder is characterized by powder X-ray diffraction (XRD), transmission electron microscopy (TEM), scanning electron microscopy(SEM), and isoelectric point determination.

III Apparatus and Reagents

Autoclave(100 mL), drying oven with temperature control, motor stirrer, vacuum pump, pH meter(PB-10), beaker(100 mL×1), Buchner funnel, filter paper and filter flask.

$SnCl_4 \cdot 5H_2O(AR,s)$, $KOH(AR,s)$, $HAc(AR,l)$, $NH_4Ac(AR,s)$ and ethanol solution (95%).

IV Procedure

1. Preparation of Raw Material

Prepare 1. 0 mol $\cdot$ L^{-1} $SnCl_4$ solution and 10 mol $\cdot$ L^{-1} KOH solution with distilled water. Transfer 50 mL of 1. 0 mol $\cdot$ L^{-1} $SnCl_4$ solution into a 100 mL beaker, add 10 mol $\cdot$ L^{-1} KOH solution dropwise with stirring, adjust the pH to appropriate value, and save the solution for the following experiment. Record the state change with the pH.

2. Study the Influences of Hydrothermal Treating Temperature and Time, pH Value of Medium, Concentration of Reactant on the Morphology and Crystallization

Simply saying, hydrothermal synthesis is the procedure that molecular precursors, e. g. metal chlorides react with H_2O, and form metal oxide network via inorganic polymerization including hydrolysis and condensation reactions. Conventionally, hydrothermal process, in which water is the solvent, is broadly used for the synthesis of metal oxide bulk materials as well as nanoparticles. The reaction mechanisms of hydrolysis and condensation processes are shown as follows. Firstly, metal chloride hydrolyzes and an $Sn(OH)_4$ species is generated:

$$SnCl_4 + 4H_2O \Longrightarrow Sn(OH)_4 + 4HCl$$

In the second step, the hydroxy groups react with each other and an M—O—M network is then formed upon the propagation of the condensation reaction and results in the elimination of water.

$$nSn(OH)_4 \Longrightarrow nSnO_2 + 2nH_2O$$

The reaction mechanism of hydrothermal synthesis is rather simple. However, resulting from the high reactivity of the precursor towards hydrolysis, it has several disadvantages. For instance, the resulting products are often amorphous, which means that post thermal treatments are not avoidable to get crystalline material; the reaction parameters, such as temperature, pH, concentration of reactant and even the method of mixing, have to be carefully controlled to achieve the desired products and reproducibility.

(1) Temperature. The rate of hydrolysis and condensation increases with increasing the temperature. However, the higher temperature produces the growth of large crystals. Thus, in this experiment, the temperature is controlled in the temperature range of 120-160 ℃.

(2) pH value of medium. The appropriate pH values of medium determine the properties of the SnO_2 particles produced by hydrothermal method. At high acidity, the hydrolysis of $SnCl_4$ is restrained and the intermediate, $Sn(OH)_4$, is less, the number of the particle nucleation(SnO_2) is less. This lead to agglomeration and the particle size is larger. On the other hand, the hydrolysis of $SnCl_4$ will be more completely at low acidity and the number of the particle nucleation(SnO_2) is more. Thus, the number of residual Sn^{4+} is less and the crystal is difficult to grow continuously. According to the hydrolysis and growth processes, the acidity is controlled at $pH = 1.45$.

(3) Concentration of reactant. Consider the concentration of reactant alone, the

higher the concentration of reactant is, the lower the yield of SnO_2 nanopowder is. The main reason is that the higher the concentration of $SnCl_4$ solution is, the higher acidity of the solution is, and the hydrolysis of $SnCl_4$ is inhibited. The viscosity of reactant is higher at pH$=$1.45. It is too hard for stirring. In general, the concentration of $SnCl_4$ solution is 1 mol $\cdot$ L^{-1}.

3. Preparation of SnO₂ Nanopowder

Pour the raw material synthesized above into an autoclave, heat, keep the temperature at 120 ℃(or 140 ℃ or 160 ℃) for 2 h, and cool to room temperature. Open the autoclave and take out the product. Let it stand for settling, discard the supernatant. Use a vacuum filtration setup to separate the crystal from the liquid. Wash the crystal with 20 mL mixture of 10% HAc with 1 g NH_4Ac for several times until Cl^- and K^+ are absent. Then wash the crystal with 10 mL of 95% ethanol solution twice. Spread the crystal on a watch glass and dry at 80 ℃.

4. Analysis of the Product

(1) X-ray. Crystal structure is investigated by XRD.

(2) Particle size analysis. Size of nanoparticles is calculated from the width of the half-height of the main peak of the X-ray diffraction using Scherer's formula.

$$D_{hkl} = \frac{K \cdot \lambda}{\beta \cdot \cos\theta_{hkl}}$$

where D_{hkl} is average crystal size; K is a constant($K=0.9$); λ is the X-ray wavelength; β is the width of the half-height of the main peak of the X-ray diffraction; θ_{hkl} is diffraction angle.

Morphology of samples is observed by TEM and SEM with EDS analysis.

(3) Determination of the specific surface area. The specific surface is observed by BET method(Brunauer, Emmett and Teller, 1938). Then calculate the particle size.

(4) Determination of the isoelectric point. Detect the isoelectric point of SnO_2 nanopowder with microscopic electrophoresis apparatus.

V Data Interpretation

Conclude the influences of hydrothermal treating temperature and time, the pH value of medium, and concentration of reactant on the morphology, crystallization and the particle size.

VI Questions

(1) You can determine the particle size with XRD or TEM or BET method,

which method is better? Why?

(2) Hydrothermal method is not a normal inorganic synthetic method, what features are there?

(3) What factors will affect the particle size and the morphology?

Experiment 35　Determination of Trace Elements in Tea

Ⅰ Learning Objectives

(1) Learn how to determine trace elements in tea.

(2) Learn sample pretreatment techniques.

(3) Learn spectrophotometric determination of trace iron and complexometric titration of magnesium and calcium in tea.

Ⅱ Principles

Tea is a stimulant, a very mild stimulant, since it contains caffeine. It contains fewer milligrams of caffeine per equal-sized cup than does coffee, but more than cocoa. Tea contains small quantities of tannic compounds technically called polyphenols (not tannic acid used in tanning leather), vitamin A, B_2, C, D, K, and P, plus a number of minerals in trace amounts and also aromatic oils.

Tea belongs to organism, which mainly consists of C, H, O, N and trace elements such as Fe, Al, Mg, Ca, etc.. Before determining the trace elements, the tea sample must be treated by dry ashing. The object of dry ashing is to combust all of the organic materials and to prepare the sample for subsequent treatment using wet ashing or fusion techniques. This procedure involves heating a sample in an open dish or crucible in air, usually in a muffle furnace to control the temperature and flow of air. Ashes are the compounds that remain after a sample is burned, and consist mostly of metal oxides. After dissolving the inorganic residue in an appropriate volume of dilute hydrochloric acid, the quantitative analysis can be carried out.

Fe^{3+}, Al^{3+}, Ca^{2+}, and Mg^{2+} can be identified by following characteristic reactions:

$$Fe^{3+} + nKSCN(saturated) \longrightarrow Fe(SCN)_n^{3-n}(red) + nK^+$$

$$Al^{3+} + aluminon + OH^- \longrightarrow red\ flocculent\ precipitate$$

$$Mg^{2+} + azoviolet + OH^- \longrightarrow sky\ blue\ precipitate$$

$$Ca^{2+} + C_2O_4^{2-} \xrightarrow{HAc} CaC_2O_4\ (white\ precipitate)$$

Using the amphoteric nature of Al^{3+}, you can separate the Fe^{3+} and Al^{3+} with any excess hydroxide ion.

The complexometry can be used for quantitative analysis of Ca^{2+} and Mg^{2+}. The total amount of Ca^{2+} and Mg^{2+} can be determined under the following conditions: pH = 10, eriochrome black T as indicator, EDTA as standard solution. Ca^{2+} is analyzed separately after precipitating $Mg(OH)_2$ with strong base (pH>12.5).

Some metal ions, such as Fe^{3+} and Al^{3+}, interfere with this titration by causing indistinct endpoints, or by complexing with EDTA and/or the indicator more strongly than the metals of interest. You will look at an example of a chemical masking agent(triethanolamine) that is used to counteract such occurrences.

1, 10-phenanthroline (o-phenanthroline, o-Phen) reacts with ferrous ion to produce a deeply colored red complex:

$$Fe^{2+} + 3o\text{-Phen} \Longleftrightarrow Fe(o\text{-Phen})_3^{2+}$$

The molar absorptivity ε of the ferrous complex, $[(C_{12}H_8N_2)_3Fe]^{2+}$, is $1.10 \times 10^4\ L \cdot mol^{-1} \cdot cm^{-1}$ at the wavelength of maximum absorbance intensity, $\lambda_{max} = 508$ nm. This large value indicates that the complex absorbs very strongly. The intensity of the color is independent of pH in the range 2-9. In strongly acidic solutions, the complex does not form. On the other hand, in basic solutions, many metal compounds are insoluble. To determine the total iron in the sample, it must be completely in the ferrous state, and Fe^{2+} can readily be air-oxidized to the ferric state, Fe^{3+}. o-Phen will form a colored complex with Fe^{3+}, but its spectrum is different from that of the ferrous complex and the color is not as intense. Thus, one could not determine the total iron present by making measurements at only one wavelength. Hence, a mild reducing agent is added before the color is developed in order to provide a measure of the total iron present in solution. Hydroxylamine, as its hydrochloride salt, can be used. The reaction is

$$2Fe^{3+} + 2NH_2OH \cdot HCl \Longleftrightarrow 2Fe^{2+} + N_2 \uparrow + 2H_2O + 4H^+ + 2Cl^-$$

Ⅲ Apparatus and Reagents

723N spectrophotometer, cuvettes(4), analytical balances(0.01 g, 0.1 mg), hot plate, mortar, evaporating dish, weighing bottle, filter paper, funnel, test tube, centrifuge, centrifuge tubes, beaker(150 mL×1), graduated cylinders(20 mL×1, 10 mL×2,5 mL×1),water bath,Geiser buret(50 mL×1),Erlenmeyer flasks(250 mL ×3),volumetric flasks(250 mL×2,50 mL×8),transfer pipets(25 mL×1,5 mL× 3),Mohr measuring pipet(10 mL×1),wash bottle,medicine dropper,rubber pipet bulb,stirring rod and watch glass.

Eriochrome black T indicator,HCl solution (6 mol · L^{-1}), HAc solution (2 mol · L^{-1}),NaOH solution (6 mol · L^{-1}),$(NH_4)_2C_2O_4$ solution (0. 25 mol · L^{-1}), EDTA solution (0.01 mol · L^{-1}, standardized), KSCN solution (saturated solution), iron (Ⅱ) standard solution (0. 10 mg · mL^{-1}), aluminon, azoviolet, triethanolamine solution (25%),NH_3-NH_4Cl buffer solution(pH = 10), HAc -NaAc buffer solution(pH = 4. 6), 1, 10-phenanthroline solution (0. 1%) and hydroxylamine solution (10%).

Ⅳ Procedure

1. Sample Preparation by Dry Ashing for the Determination of Various Elements in Tea

Weigh the amount of sample required(7-8 g of dry matter) into a crucible. Dry the tea in an oven for about 16 h(overnight) at 100-105 ℃. Place the tea in a mortar and grind it into powder with the pestle. Accurately weigh the tea and put it in an evaporating dish. Heat the tea in an open dish. Cool the ash down to near room temperature and add 10 mL of 6 mol · L^{-1} HCl solution with stirring(maybe there are insoluble proteins). Transfer the solution into a 150 mL beaker. Add 20 mL of distilled water and 10 mL of 6 mol · L^{-1} NaOH solution. The precipitate forms. After heating for 30 min,filter hot solution through filter paper. Wash the beaker and the precipitate with 100 mL of distilled water,decanting the supernatant through the filter. Then put the filtrate in a 250 mL volumetric flask,dilute to the mark and label #1(Ca^{2+} and Mg^{2+} sample).

Add 10 mL of 6 mol · L^{-1} HCl solution to redissolve the precipitate. Wash the filter paper and the precipitate with 100 mL of distilled water. Then put the filtrate in a 250 mL volumetric flask,dilute to the mark and label #2(Fe^{3+} and Al^{3+} sample).

2. Identification of Fe,Al,Ca,and Mg

Add 2 drops of #1 solution into a test tube,and then add 1 drop of azoviolet solution and 5 drops of 6 mol · L^{-1} NaOH solution. Observe the phenomenon. If no sky blue precipitate forms,Mg^{2+} is absent.

Add 2 drops of #1 solution into a test tube,and then add 2 drops of 2 mol · L^{-1} HAc solution and 2 drops of 0. 25 mol · L^{-1} $(NH_4)_2C_2O_4$ solution. Observe the phenomenon. A white precipitate is CaC_2O_4 and shows that Ca^{2+} is present.

Add 2 drops of #2 solution into a test tube, and then add 2 drops of saturated KSCN solution. Observe the phenomenon. This reaction confirms the presence of Fe^{3+}.

Add 1 mL of #2 solution into a centrifuge tube, and then add 6 mol $\cdot$ L^{-1} NaOH solution dropwise until a white precipitate dissolves. Centrifuge, decant the supernatant into a clean test tube, add 3-4 drops of aluminon solution, and then add several drops of 6 mol $\cdot$ L^{-1} NH_3 $\cdot$ H_2O solution. Slowly heat the tube with stirring and observe the phenomenon. A red flocculent precipitate confirms the presence of Al^{3+}.

3. Determination of Ca and Mg in Tea

Transfer 25.00 mL of #1 solution into a 250 mL Erlenmeyer flask. Add 5 mL of triethanolamine, 10 mL of pH=10 NH_3-NH_4Cl buffer solution, and 2 drops of eriochrome black T indicator and mix well. Titrate with the 0.02 mol $\cdot$ L^{-1} EDTA solution until the color changes from wine red to pure blue. Repeat the titration two more times. Using the volume of EDTA solution used, calculate the total amount of Ca and Mg as mg $\cdot$ L^{-1} of MgO equivalents.

4. Determination of Fe in Tea

(1) Into each of seven 50 mL volumetric flasks, pipet 0.00 mL, 1.00 mL, 2.00 mL, 3.00 mL, 4.00 mL, 5.00 mL and 6.00 mL of the standard iron solution, respectively.

(2) Obtain 2.50 mL of #2 solution and treat it in the same manner as the standards, as indicated below.

(3) Line all eight 50 mL volumetric flasks in this order: the blank, those with 1-6 mL of iron stock standard solution added, and #2 solution. To each flask (including the blank and the unknown), pipet in order as follows:

① 5 mL of hydroxylamine solution;

② 5 mL of 1,10-phenanthroline solution;

③ 5 mL of sodium acetate solution.

Note that the blank must have all the reagents in it except for any ferrous solution.

(4) Swirl each flask to mix the contents, and then carefully dilute each solution to the 50 mL mark and mix thoroughly.

(5) Allow the solutions to stand for 10 min to fully develop the color. Mix well again. Fill each of eight clean and dry 3 cm cuvettes about two-thirds full with each of the eight solutions, keeping them in same order.

(6) After scanning the spectrum, select the wavelength of maximum absorption

($\lambda_{max}=508$ nm) to use for the determination of iron with 1,10-phenanthroline. The blank is used as reference and measure the absorbance of each of the standard solutions and the unknown. Plot absorbance vs. the concentration of the standards. From the absorbance of the unknown, calculate the concentration of iron in the unknown in units of $mg \cdot L^{-1}$.

V Questions

(1) How to select the temperature for dry ashing?

(2) How do you separate the metal ions Fe^{3+}, Al^{3+}, Ca^{2+}, and Mg^{2+} from their mixture?

Experiment 36　Preparation of Zinc Gluconate and Complexometric Titration of Zinc with EDTA

I Learning Objectives

(1) Learn how to prepare zinc gluconate.

(2) Determine the amount of zinc present in zinc gluconate.

II Principles

Zinc is a naturally occurring mineral. Zinc is important for growth and health of body tissues. Zinc gluconate is used to treat and to prevent zinc deficiencies. Calcium gluconate reacts with equal molar zinc sulfate to produce zinc gluconate:

$$Ca(C_6H_{11}O_7)_2 + ZnSO_4 \Longrightarrow Zn(C_6H_{11}O_7)_2 + CaSO_4 \downarrow$$

The amount of zinc in solution will be determined through a titration procedure with a complexing agent, EDTA. You will determine the endpoint of the titration using an eriochrome black T indicator, and at that volume the moles of EDTA added will equal the moles of zinc in solution.

$$Zn^{2+} + H_2Y^{2-} \Longrightarrow ZnY^{2-} + 2H^+$$

III Apparatus and Reagents

Analytical balances(0.01 g, 0.1 mg), water bath, Buchner funnel, filter paper, filter flask, vacuum pump, Geiser buret(50 mL × 1), hot plate, evaporating dish, beaker(250 mL × 1) and graduated cylinders(20 mL × 1, 10 mL × 2, 5 mL × 1).

Calcium gluconate(AR,s),ZnSO$_4$ · 7H$_2$O(AR,s),ethanol solution (95%), NH$_3$-NH$_4$Cl buffer solution(pH=10),EDTA solution (0. 1 mol · L^{-1},standardized) and eriochrome black T indicator.

Ⅳ Procedure

1. Preparation of Zinc Gluconate, Zn(C$_6$H$_{11}$O$_7$)$_2$ · 3H$_2$O

Measure out 80 mL of distilled water to a 250 mL beaker,heat to 80-90 ℃, and then add 13. 4 g of ZnSO$_4$ · 7H$_2$O and dissolve it completely. Put the beaker in water bath and keep the temperature at 90 ℃, and add 20 g of calcium gluconate gradually with stirring. After about 20 min,filter hot solution through filter paper (double filter paper). Discard the solid(CaSO$_4$) and the paper. The filtrate is put in an evaporating dish.

Subsequently, the filtrate is concentrated at 80 ℃ until the crystal film appears. Allow the mixture to cool to room temperature. Add 20 mL of 95% ethanol solution with stirring. A lot of colloidal zinc gluconate is separated out. Decant the supernatant, add 20 mL of 95% ethanol solution with stirring. You should see some crystal forms. Use a vacuum filtration setup to separate the crystal from the liquid. Obtain the crude product.

Add 20 mL of distilled water to the beaker with the crude product,heat to 90 ℃ and dissolve it completely. Filter hot solution through a filter paper. Cool the solution to room temperature. Add 20 mL of 95% ethanol solution with stirring until the crystal forms. Again,use a vacuum filtration setup to separate the crystal from the liquid. Obtain the pure product and dry at 50 ℃.

2. Complexometric Titration of Zinc with EDTA

Accurately weigh about 0. 8 g(±0. 1 mg) of zinc gluconate into a 250 mL Erlenmeyer flask,dissolve it by adding 20 mL of distilled water(heat). Add 10 mL of pH=10 NH$_3$-NH$_4$Cl buffer solution,4 drops of eriochrome black T indicator and mix well. Titrate with the 0. 1 mol · L^{-1} EDTA solution until the color changes from magenta to pure blue. Repeat the titration two more times. From the titration volume and the mass of zinc gluconate,calculate the percentage of Zn.

$$w(\text{Zn}) = \frac{c(\text{EDTA}) \times V(\text{EDTA}) \times 65}{m(\text{sample}) \times 1\ 000} \times 100\%$$

Ⅴ Questions

(1) Why must we keep the temperature at 90 ℃ when zinc sulfate reacts with

calcium gluconate?

(2) Design flow chart of the preparation of zinc gluconate.

(3) You are given 0. 324 5 g of an unknown zinc ore to analyze with an EDTA titration. You dissolve this mass up into about 50 mL of an aqueous buffer solution, and then add 13. 65 mL of a 0. 205 2 mol · L^{-1} solution of EDTA to find an endpoint. What is the mass fraction of zinc in the unknown?

Experiment 37 Preparation and Analysis of Potassium Tris(oxalato)ferrate(Ⅲ) Trihydrate, $K_3[Fe(C_2O_4)_3] \cdot 3H_2O$

Ⅰ Learning Objectives

(1) Learn the operations such as synthesis, characterization and chemical analysis of coordination compounds.

(2) Review the manipulation of crystallization, filtration and water bath.

Ⅱ Principles

In this experiment you will prepare a coordination compound of iron, potassium tris(oxalato)ferrate(Ⅲ), $K_3[Fe(C_2O_4)_3]$. In this compound each oxalate ligand has two bonds to the iron(Ⅲ) ion, and hence this compound is an example of chelates.

It is of interest to compare the properties of chelating iron(Ⅲ) ion with that of the normal iron(Ⅲ) ion. The compound will be prepared by first preparing iron (Ⅱ) oxalate, $FeC_2O_4 \cdot 2H_2O$, and then oxidizing this with hydrogen peroxide, in the presence of potassium oxalate, to convert it to the ferric oxalate ion $[Fe(C_2O_4)_3]^{3-}$.

$$Fe^{2+} \xrightarrow{C_2O_4^{2-}} FeC_2O_4 \cdot 2H_2O \xrightarrow[K_2C_2O_4]{H_2O_2} \begin{array}{c} Fe(OH)_3 \\ K_3[Fe(C_2O_4)_3] \end{array} \xrightarrow{H_2C_2O_4} K_3[Fe(C_2O_4)_3]$$

$$FeSO_4 + H_2C_2O_4 + 2H_2O = FeC_2O_4 \cdot 2H_2O\downarrow + H_2SO_4$$

$$6FeC_2O_4 \cdot 2H_2O + 3H_2O_2 + 6K_2C_2O_4 = 4K_3[Fe(C_2O_4)_3] + 2Fe(OH)_3\downarrow + 12H_2O$$

$$2Fe(OH)_3 + 3H_2C_2O_4 + 3K_2C_2O_4 = 2K_3[Fe(C_2O_4)_3] + 6H_2O$$

Thus all the iron in the ferrous ammonium sulfate is converted to ferric oxalate, one-third of the ferric oxalate being formed from the iron(Ⅲ) hydroxide. Both H_2O_2 and $Fe(OH)_3$ are unstable to heat. Potassium tris(oxalato)ferrate(Ⅲ) is photosensitive, i. e. , it decomposes when exposed to light, reforming iron(Ⅱ) oxalate.

$$2K_3[Fe(C_2O_4)_3] \xrightarrow{\text{light}} 3K_2C_2O_4 + 2FeC_2O_4 + 2CO_2$$

The analysis of the $K_3[Fe(C_2O_4)_3] \cdot 3H_2O$ will use the redox reactions given below for the analysis of the oxalate and the iron, respectively. To save time and sample, you will first perform the oxalate analysis and then treat the titration solution with Zn to convert all of the Fe^{3+} present to Fe^{2+}. Titrating this solution with the standard MnO_4^- will allow you to determine the amount of iron present in the original compound.

$$5C_2O_4^{2-} + 2MnO_4^- + 16H^+ \Longrightarrow 10CO_2\uparrow + 2Mn^{2+} + 8H_2O$$
$$5Fe^{2+} + MnO_4^- + 8H^+ \Longrightarrow 5Fe^{3+} + Mn^{2+} + 4H_2O$$

Ⅲ Apparatus and Reagents

Analytical balances(0. 01 g, 0. 1 mg), beaker(100 mL×1), Buchner funnel, filter paper, filter flask, vacuum pump, evaporating dish, motor stirrer, Geiser buret (50 mL×1), volumetric flask(250 mL×1), transfer pipet(20 mL×1), Erlenmeyer flasks(250 mL×3), wash bottle, medicine dropper, rubber pipet bulb and stirring rod.

$FeSO_4 \cdot 7H_2O(AR,s)$, H_2SO_4 solution (1 mol $\cdot$ L^{-1}), $H_2C_2O_4$ solution (1 mol $\cdot$ L^{-1}), $K_2C_2O_4$ solution (saturated solution), H_2O_2 solution (3%), ethanol solution (95%), pH test paper, $Na_2C_2O_4$(AR,s), $KMnO_4$(AR,s), HCl solution (6 mol $\cdot$ L^{-1}) and Zn.

Ⅳ Procedure

1. Preparation of Potassium Tris(oxalato)ferrate(Ⅲ) Trihydrate, $K_3[Fe(C_2O_4)_3] \cdot 3H_2O$

(1) Preparation of $FeC_2O_4 \cdot 2H_2O$.

Add 4 drops of 3 mol $\cdot$ L^{-1} H_2SO_4 solution to 10 mL of warm water in a 250 mL beaker. Next add 2. 0 g of ferrous ammonium sulfate heptahydrate, $FeSO_4 \cdot 7H_2O$. When everything has been dissolved, add 10 mL of 1. 0 mol $\cdot$ L^{-1} oxalic acid($H_2C_2O_4$), and then heat the solution to boiling, stirring continuously.

(2) Preparation of potassium tris(oxalato)ferrate(Ⅲ)trihydrate, $K_3[Fe(C_2O_4)_3] \cdot 3H_2O$.

Allow the yellow precipitate—the solid in the beaker—to settle, and then decant the liquid. Wash the precipitate with distilled water, and then decant the liquid after the precipitate has again settled. Throw away the liquid(wash it down the drain with lots of water) and keep the solid.

Add 5 mL of saturated, aqueous potassium oxalate ($K_2C_2O_4$) to the washed solid precipitate. Heat the solution to 40 ℃, and then add 10 mL of 3% hydrogen peroxide (H_2O_2), a few milliliters at a time, stirring continuously. (Wait a moment between additions and keep the temperature near 40 ℃.)

Ignoring any red-brown precipitate ($Fe(OH)_3$) that may form, heat the solution to boiling, and add 5 mL of 1.0 mol · L^{-1} oxalic acid solution. Add another 3 mL of the oxalic acid solution dropwise, keeping the solution near boiling.

Filter the hot solution into a 100 mL beaker as demonstrated by your instructor. Add 10 mL of ethanol solution and warm to dissolve any crystal that may form. Set aside in the dark to crystallize. Filter and wash the crystal on the Buchner funnel with 95% ethanol solution and finally with acetone. Dry in the air and weigh.

2. Analysis of the $K_3[Fe(C_2O_4)_3] \cdot 3H_2O$

(1) Determination of oxalate in potassium tris(oxalato)ferrate(Ⅲ) trihydrate.

The iron(Ⅲ) complex is first decomposed in hot acid solution and the free oxalic acid is titrated against 0.01 mol · L^{-1} potassium permanganate standard solution. No indicator is required.

In duplicate, weigh accurately about 0.1 g of the potassium tris(oxalato)ferrate (Ⅲ) complex previously prepared. Boil the sample with 50 mL of 1 mol · L^{-1} H_2SO_4 solution in an Erlenmeyer flask. Allow the solution to cool to about 60 ℃ and titrate slowly with the potassium permanganate solution provided (which you will need to standardize). Continue until the warm solution retains a slight pink color after standing for about 30 s.

Calculate the percentage by mass of oxalate in the complex, compare this with the theoretical value and thus obtain the percentage purity of the complex.

(2) Determination of iron in potassium tris(oxalato)ferrate(Ⅲ) trihydrate.

Take your faintly-purple sample from the oxalate analysis above, and set it on a hot plate in the hood(there may be a small amount of brown precipitate forming at this point, do not be concerned). Gently heat it until it almost boils and add approximately 100 mg of Zn to the hot solution. Cover the flask with a watch glass and continue heating until the yellow color(from Fe^{3+}) disappears(Fe^{2+} is colorless in solution). While you are waiting, set up a gravity filtration with fluted filter paper(ask your instructor to demonstrate how to flute filter paper, if you are unsure). Quickly filter the hot and colorless solution into another Erlenmeyer flask, again using a folded paper towel to handle the hot flask. It is important that this filtration be done quickly to minimize the amount of Fe^{2+} that is reoxidized to

Fe^{3+} by O_2 in the air. Rinse the funnel with several small(approximately 5 mL total volume) portions of distilled water. Titrate this solution with the potassium permanganate solution in your buret until the first faint trace of a persistent pink color. Record the volume of potassium permanganate solution used. Repeat this procedure after each oxalate determination(at least three times).

V Question

Ferrous ammonium sulfate is used as the starting material rather than the use of ferrous sulfate. Explain.

Experiment 38   Titration of an Eggshell

Complexometric Titration of an Eggshell

I Principles

The eggshell consists of about 94%-97% of $CaCO_3$ and the other 3% is organic matter and egg pigment.

There are many sources of calcium from biological samples. Sources include seashells,eggshells and bone. Starting with a biological sample,you will prepare a solution of calcium ions which you will analyze, using HCl solution. You can determine the Ca^{2+} content in an eggshell by titration with EDTA solution. The reaction takes place at pH=10. The chemical reaction described above is shown by

$$Ca^{2+}(aq)+H_2Y^{2-}(aq)\Longleftrightarrow[CaY]^{2-}(aq)+2H^+(aq) \qquad (pH=10)$$

II Apparatus and Reagents

Analytical balances(0. 01 g, 0. 1 mg), beaker(100 mL×1), Buchner funnel, Geiser buret(50 mL×1), volumetric flask(250 mL×1), transfer pipet(25 mL×1), Erlenmeyer flasks(250 mL×3), wash bottle, medicine dropper and rubber pipet bulb.

HCl solution (6 mol · L^{-1}), eriochrome black T indicator, triethanolamine aqueous solution (1 : 2), NH_3-NH_4Cl buffer solution(pH=10) and EDTA solution (0. 01 mol · L^{-1}, standardized).

III Procedure

Eggshells will be provided to you in class. Typically you will find that a membrane is attached to the inside surface of the shell. Carefully peel away small pieces of the shell from the membrane until you have obtained about 1.25 g of shell. Find the mass of the shell pieces you will use accurately to four decimal places. Place the shell in a glass mortar and grind it with a glass pestle. Using medicine dropper(or dropper bottle) add 6 mol $\cdot$ L^{-1} HCl solution dropwise until all bubbling has ceased. (This might takes as much as 5 mL of HCl solution.) Quantatively transfer the mixture to a clean 250 mL volumetric flask and dilute to the mark with deionized water(if the bubbling appears, add 2-3 drops of 95% ethanol solution). Stopper the flask and mix its contents well.

Transfer 25.00 mL of this solution into a 250 mL Erlenmeyer flask. Add 20 mL of distilled water, 5 mL of triethanolamine, 10 mL of pH $=10$ NH$_3$-NH$_4$Cl buffer solution and 2 drops of eriochrome black T indicator, and mix well. Titrate with 0.01 mol $\cdot$ L^{-1} EDTA solution until the color changes from wine red to pure blue. Repeat the titration two more times. Using the volume of EDTA solution used, calculate the total amount of Ca and Mg as mass concentration (mg $\cdot$ L^{-1}) of CaO equivalents.

Acid-Base Titration of an Eggshell

I Principles

Determine the percent calcium carbonate in the entire eggshell. The reaction taking place is

$$CaCO_3 + 2H^+ \Longrightarrow Ca^{2+} + CO_2\uparrow + H_2O$$

CaCO$_3$ has consumed a portion of the acid. Our job is to figure out exactly how much HCl solution is consumed by titrating the acid left over with our standard base. "Back-titrate" the excess acid in the mixture with the NaOH standard solution.

$$HCl + NaOH \Longrightarrow H_2O + NaCl$$

II Apparatus and Reagents

Analytical balances(0.01 g, 0.1 mg), Geiser buret(50 mL$\times$1), Mohr buret(50 mL$\times$1), Erlenmeyer flasks(250 mL $\times$ 3), graduated cylinder(50 mL $\times$ 1), wash bottle, rubber pipet bulb, mortar (with pestle), reagent bottles(500 mL$\times$2) and beaker(500 mL$\times$1).

Concentrated HCl(AR, l), NaOH(AR, s) and phenolphthalein indicator.

III Procedure

Bring 3 or 4 eggshells from home. Boil them to remove a protein membrane on inside surface of shell. Cool and peel membrane away. Place all of the shell in the beaker and dry the shell in the oven overnight. Take out the eggshell from the oven and cool to room temperature. Place the eggshell in a mortar and grind it into a powder with the pestle. Weigh accurately about 0.3 g of the eggshell and place it into a 250 mL Erlenmeyer flask. Transfer exactly 40.00 mL of 1.0 mol $\cdot$ L^{-1} HCl standard solution into this flask. Warm the mixture over a low flame until all of the crystals have dissolved. Cool the solution down to near room temperature and add 2 drops of phenolphthalein indicator. Stir the solution for a few minutes and then titrate this mixture with NaOH standard solution to a pink color. Record the amount of NaOH solution added. Determine the number of moles of HCl left in solution. Determine the moles of calcium carbonate in the mixture. Determine the percent calcium carbonate in the entire eggshell.

Redox Titration of an Eggshell

I Principles

Hydrochloric acid reacts with calcium carbonate to produce water, carbon dioxide and calcium chloride. Calcium is determined by oxalate precipitation and the redox titration procedure.

$$Ca^{2+} + C_2O_4^{2-} = CaC_2O_4\downarrow$$
$$CaC_2O_4 + H_2SO_4 = CaSO_4 + H_2C_2O_4$$
$$5H_2C_2O_4 + 2MnO_4^- + 6H^+ = 10CO_2 + 2Mn^{2+} + 8H_2O$$

II Apparatus and Reagents

Analytical balance(0.1 mg), desiccator, weighing bottle, Geiser buret(50 mL $\times$ 1), Erlenmeyer flasks(250 mL $\times$ 3), beakers(250 mL $\times$ 2), graduated cylinders(100 mL $\times$ 1, 10 mL $\times$ 1), reagent bottle(500 mL $\times$ 1), Buchner funnel, filter paper, filter flask, vacuum pump, wash bottle, medicine dropper, rubber pipet bulb, stirring rod and watch glass.

KMnO$_4$ solution (0.01 mol $\cdot$ L^{-1}), (NH$_4$)$_2$C$_2$O$_4$ solution (5%), NH$_3$ $\cdot$ H$_2$O solution (10%), HCl solution (concentrated, 1 : 1), H$_2$SO$_4$ solution (1 mol $\cdot$ L^{-1}), methyl orange indicator(0.2%) and AgNO$_3$ solution (0.1 mol $\cdot$ L^{-1}).

III Procedure

Weigh accurately about 0.025 g of the eggshell and place it into a 250 mL beaker. Add 3 mL of 1 : 1 HCl solution and 20 mL of distilled water, heat and dissolve it. If there are insoluble proteins, filter the solution through a suction filter equipped with "fast" filter paper. The filtrate is put in a clean beaker. Add 50 mL of 5% $(NH_4)_2C_2O_4$ solution until the precipitate forms. Add concentrated HCl solution dropwise and dissolve the precipitate completely. Heat to 70-80 ℃, add 2 drops of methyl orange indicator, and then add 10% ammonia solution with stirring until the color changes from red to yellow and a pungent gas, NH_3, forms. Set aside to precipitate. Filter and wash the precipitate on the Buchner funnel with distilled water until Cl^- is absent. Put the filter paper and the precipitate into the beaker used. Add 50 mL of 1 mol · L^{-1} H_2SO_4 solution to redissolve the precipitate. Wash the filter paper and the precipitate with distilled water, and then dilute to 100 mL. Heat to 70-80 ℃. Titrate slowly with $KMnO_4$ standard solution to a faint pink. Put the filter paper into the beaker again. Continue to titrate with $KMnO_4$ standard solution to a faint pink and the color should persist for at least 30 s. Repeat the titration two more times. Calculate the content of Ca as mass concentration (mg · L^{-1}) of CaO equivalents.

Experiment 39　Synthesis of Cobalt(Ⅲ) Coordination Compounds

Ⅰ Learning Objectives

(1) Study the principles and methods of synthesis of coordination compounds.

(2) Learn the manipulation of rubbing, filtration and activation of activated charcoal.

Ⅱ Principles

In this experiment you will prepare the complex ion of cobalt(Ⅲ) by making use of reaction in which a ligand replaces another ligand on the central ion. The reaction will usually be carried out in water solution, in which the metallic cation will initially be present in the simple hydrated form, addition of a reagent containing a ligand will result in an exchange reaction.

$$[Co(H_2O)_6]^{2+}(aq) + 6NH_3(aq) \longrightarrow [Co(NH_3)_6]^{2+}(aq) + 6H_2O$$

The rate of this reaction involving complex ion formation reaction is very slow. The reaction obeys the law of chemical equilibrium and can thus be readily controlled as to direction by changing conditions of the reaction. The reaction proceeds to the right in the presence of NH_3 with moderate concentrations. The complex ion($[Co(NH_3)_6]^{2+}$) is labile. It can be oxidized readily. In this experiment, you will use hydrogen peroxide to oxidize the complex ion to $[Co(NH_3)_6]^{3+}$. Its color is golden. But under this condition, we can get other two products: $[Co(NH_3)_5Cl]Cl_2$ and $[Co(NH_3)_5(H_2O)]Cl_3$. Alteration of reaction conditions, perhaps by the addition of a catalyst, may raise the relative rate of formation of $[Co(NH_3)_6]Cl_3$. In your experiment you will use a catalyst, activated charcoal, in the preparation of the complex.

$$2[Co(NH_3)_6]^{2+} + H_2O_2 + 2H^+ \rightleftharpoons 2[Co(NH_3)_6]^{3+} + 2H_2O$$

Ⅲ Apparatus and Reagents

Buchner funnel, mortar, buret and water bath.

$CoCl_2 \cdot 6H_2O(AR, s)$, $NH_4Cl(AR, s)$, $NH_3 \cdot H_2O$ solution (15 mol $\cdot$ L^{-1}), H_2O_2 solution (30%), HCl solution (12 mol $\cdot$ L^{-1}) and activated charcoal.

Ⅳ Procedure

1. Synthesis of Hexaamminecobalt(Ⅲ) chloride

Weigh 8 g sample of cobalt(Ⅱ) chloride(milled), put it into a 100 mL beaker. Add 6.0 g of NH_4Cl, 0.5 g of activated charcoal and 10 mL of distilled water. Heat the solution to the boiling point, stirring the solution completely.

Cool the beaker with water, and slowly add 20 mL of 15 mol $\cdot$ L^{-1} $NH_3 \cdot H_2O$ solution. Cool to below 10 ℃. Stir until well mixed and then add 3 mL of 30% H_2O_2 solution drop by drop with stirring.

When the bubbling no longer appears, place the 100 mL beaker in constant temperature water bath at about 60 ℃. Leave the beaker in the water bath for 20 min, holding the temperature of the bath at (60 $\pm$ 5) ℃. Stir the mixture occasionally.

Remove the 100 mL beaker from the water bath and put it into the ice bath. Cool for about 5 min, stirring to promote crystallization of the crude product. Set up a Buchner funnel with suction, filter the mixture through the filter paper in the funnel. Transfer the filtrate to a 100 mL beaker and add 5 mL of 12 mol $\cdot$ L^{-1} HCl solution slowly. Place the beaker in an ice bath and stir for several minutes to promote formation of the golden crystal of $[Co(NH_3)_6]Cl_3$. Separate the crystal by filtration through the Buchner funnel. Turn the suction off, add 10 mL of 95% ethanol solution, and let stand for about 10 s. Turn the suction on and pull off the ethanol, which should carry with it much of the water and HCl remaining on the crystal. Draw air through the crystal for several minutes. Transfer the product to a piece of weighed filter paper. Let it dry for several more minutes and weigh it on the paper. Calculate the yield such as

$$\text{Yield} = \frac{m(\text{product})}{m(\text{CoCl}_2 \cdot 6\text{H}_2\text{O})} \times \frac{M(\text{CoCl}_2 \cdot 6\text{H}_2\text{O})}{M(\text{CoCl}_3 \cdot 6\text{NH}_3)} \times 100\%$$

2. Synthesis of [Co(NH₃)₅Cl]Cl₂

In a fume hood, dissolve 1 g of ammonium chloride in 9 mL of concentrated aqueous ammonia in a 100 mL Erlenmeyer flask. (The combination of NH_4Cl and NH_3(aq) guarantees a large excess of the NH_3 ligand.) Stir the ammonium chloride solution vigorously while adding 2 g of finely divided $CoCl_2 \cdot 6H_2O$ in small portions. A yellow-pink precipitate of the hexaammine Co(Ⅱ) salt forms on slight warming as the reddish starting material dissolves. Any air oxidation that occurs during this exothermic stage is ignored since the solution is going to be fully oxidized by adding H_2O_2.

Slowly add 2 mL of 30% H_2O_2 solution to the brown Co slurry, using a buret. An addition rate of about 2 drops per second is usually sufficient, but care should be taken to avoid excessive effervescence (if the reaction shows sign of excessive effervescence, stopping the stirring momentarily will usually prevent overflow of the solution).

You should notice that all the Co(Ⅱ) ammine dissolves to form a deep red solution. (This corresponds to the formation of the pentaammineaquacobalt(Ⅲ) salt.) When the effervescence has virtually ceased, cautiously add 6 mL of concentrated HCl solution in small portions, with continuous stirring. This operation needs to be carried out in a fume hood since fume of ammonium chloride will be produced during the neutralization. After this point the reaction may be removed from the hood. A purple product should then precipitate from the hot reaction mixture leaving a pale green-blue supernatant.

While occasionally stirring, use a steam bath or hot plate to heat the solution to 60 ℃. Hold the temperature between 55 ℃ and 65 ℃ for 15 min. This incubation period is necessary to allow complete displacement of all aqua ligands.

Collect the purple product by filtration. The mother liquor may be discarded.

When the product has been drained well, it is washed with 4 mL of ice-cold deionized water in small portions, followed by 5 mL of ice-cold 95% ethanol solution (the solution must be cold to prevent undue loss of product by redissolving). Transfer the product to a crucible and dry in an oven at 100 ℃ for one hour. This helps complete the conversion of any remaining pentaammineaquacobalt(Ⅲ) salt. Submit your sample to the demonstrator.

Experiment 40 Determination of Fe in Water Sample

Ⅰ Learning Objectives

(1) Learn to determine Fe in water sample by Lambert-Beer's law.

(2) Learn to get absorption spectra.

(3) Learn to use 723N spectrophotometer.

Ⅱ Principles

According to the Lambert-Beer's law, there is a linear relationship between the absorbance and the concentration. For absorbance, the desired equation is

$$A = \varepsilon bc \quad \text{or} \quad A = abc$$

here c is the concentration of the solution; ε is the molar absorptivity coefficient and is a constant characteristic of the absorbing substance and the particular wavelength of light used; b is the cell width. If the cell width and the wavelength of the light are maintained constant, A is directly proportional to concentration. Prepare a calibration curve by plotting absorbance vs. the concentration of the standard solution. From the calibration curve, determine the concentration of unknown solution.

The first step in such an analysis is to determine the optimum wavelength to use in the analysis. A graphical plot of absorbance vs. wavelength is referred to as an absorption spectrum. These are prepared by measuring the light absorbed by a solution with different known wavelength. By referring to your plots of absorbance vs. wavelength, select λ_{max} at which to study absorbance as a function of concentration.

Several contaminants in various types of water samples can be determined by using spectrophotometric method, and one of these is iron. One widely used iron complex is the orange-red iron(Ⅱ)-o-phenanthroline complex($\lg K_s = 21.3$). Like most complexation reactions, the metal ion must compete with H_3O^+, so that, in strongly acidic solutions, the complex does not form. On the other hand, in basic solutions, many metal compounds are insoluble. For these reasons, the Fe (II) complex is quite stable in the pH range 3-9. The reaction is given:

o-phenanthroline

Most iron will exist as Fe(III) in water samples so that reduction to Fe(II) must be carried out prior to measurement. This is accomplished in this procedure by the addition of hydroxylamine. The reaction is given:

$$2Fe^{3+} + 2NH_2OH \cdot HCl \Longrightarrow 2Fe^{2+} + N_2\uparrow + 2H_2O + 4H^+ + 2Cl^-$$

A similar procedure may be used for the determination of Fe in blood serum.

III Apparatus and Reagents

723N spectrophotometer, volumetric flasks (50 mL $\times$ 7), cuvettes (4), Mohr measuring pipets(1 mL $\times$ 1, 2 mL $\times$ 2, 5 mL $\times$ 1, 10 mL $\times$ 1), rubber pipet bulb and medicine dropper.

Ferrous ammonium sulfate (iron standard solution, 2×10^{-3} mol $\cdot$ L^{-1}), o-phenanthroline solution (8×10^{-3} mol $\cdot$ L^{-1}), hydroxylamine hydrochloride solution (1.5 mol $\cdot$ L^{-1}), sodium acetate solution (1 mol $\cdot$ L^{-1}) and sample solution(about 2.0×10^{-4} mol $\cdot$ L^{-1}).

IV Procedure

1. Absorption Spectra

(1) Transfer 3. 00 mL of the iron standard solution into a 50 mL volumetric flask with a Mohr measuring pipet. Add 1. 00 mL of hydroxylamine solution, 2. 00 mL of o-phenanthroline solution and 5. 00 mL of sodium acetate solution, and then dilute to the mark. Prepare the blank in the same way, omitting the iron standard solution.

(2) Obtain a cuvette. Make sure it is clean inside and out. Rinse the cuvette inside, with a small amount of the blank. Then fill the cuvette about three-quarters full. Dry the outside of the cuvette carefully, and insert it into the sample compartment with its transparent sides aligned with the light path. Close the

cover. Set the wavelength dial at 450 nm, and press 0.000Abs/100.0%T to set the absorbance of the blank to zero. Place Fe(Ⅱ) solution in your second cuvette and read the absorbance value on the LED. Continue this procedure at 10 nm intervals from 450 nm to 560 nm. Be sure to set the absorbance of the blank to zero after each change of wavelength. Again, measure and record A at 2 nm intervals in the vicinity of maximum absorbance.

2. Determination of Fe in a Water Sample

(1) Preparation of calibration curve. Transfer 1.00 mL, 2.00 mL, 3.00 mL, 4.00 mL and 5.00 mL of the iron standard solution, respectively, into five 50 mL volumetric flasks with a Mohr measuring pipet. Add 1.00 mL of hydroxylamine solution, 2.00 mL of o-phenanthroline solution and 5.00 mL of sodium acetate solution, and then dilute to the mark. Prepare the blank in the same way, omitting the iron standard solution. Transfer the standards and blank to clean cuvettes, and measure the absorbance for each of the five solutions at the wavelength that corresponds to maximum absorption for the absorption spectrum, using the blank as reference. Prepare a calibration curve by plotting absorbance vs. the concentration of Fe.

(2) Determination of Fe. With a Mohr measuring pipet, transfer 2.00 mL of the sample solution to a 50 mL volumetric flask. Add 1.00 mL of hydroxylamine solution, 2.00 mL of o-phenanthroline solution and 5.00 mL of sodium acetate solution, and then dilute to the mark. Transfer the sample diluted to a clean cuvette, and measure the absorbance using the blank as reference. From the calibration curve, determine the concentration of Fe(Ⅱ) in the sample solution.

Ⅴ Data

1. Absorption Spectra

λ/nm	
A	

2. Determination of Fe in Water Sample

No.	Ⅰ (blank)	Ⅱ	Ⅲ	Ⅳ	Ⅴ	Ⅵ	Ⅶ (sample)
$V(Fe^{2+})$/mL	0.00	1.00	2.00	3.00	4.00	5.00	2.00
V(hydroxylamine)/mL	1.00	1.00	1.00	1.00	1.00	1.00	1.00

continued

No.	I (blank)	II	III	IV	V	VI	VII (sample)
V(o-phenanthroline)/mL	2.00	2.00	2.00	2.00	2.00	2.00	2.00
V(NaAc)/mL	5.00	5.00	5.00	5.00	5.00	5.00	5.00
c/(mmol · L^{-1})							

VI Questions

(1) By referring to your Fe (II) absorption spectrum suggest a desirable wavelength for analyzing Fe (II) complex solutions that have a concentration between 0.016 mmol · L^{-1} and 0.080 mmol · L^{-1}. Explain briefly why this same wavelength might be undesirable for the determination of a Fe (II) complex solution with a concentration greater than 0.080 mmol · L^{-1} or less than 0.016 mmol · L^{-1}.

(2) When a solution is red in color, does the solution absorb or transmit red light strongly?

Experiment 41 Determination of Vitamin C in Juices

I Learning Objectives

(1) Learn to determine the concentration of vitamin C in juices.

(2) Review the knowledge of titrimetric analysis and spectrophotometry.

II Principles

Vitamin C (ascorbic acid) is an antioxidant that is essential for human nutrition. Vitamin C deficiency can lead to a disease called scurvy, which is characterized by abnormalities in the bones and teeth. Many fruits and vegetables contain vitamin C, but cooking destroys the vitamin, so raw citrus fruits and their juices are the main source of vitamin C for most people.

Due to the clinical significance of vitamin C, it is essential to be able to detect and quantify its presence in various biological materials. Analytical methods have been developed to determine the amount of vitamin C in foods and in biological fluids such as blood and urine. Vitamin C may be assayed by titration with iodine, reaction with 2, 4-dinitrophenylhydrazine (DNPH), or titration with the redox indicator 2,6-dichlorophenolindophenol(DCIP) in acid solution.

Vitamin C can be determined in food by use of an redox reaction. The redox reaction is preferable to an acid-base titration because a number of other species in juice can act as acids, but relatively few interfere with the oxidation of vitamin C by iodine. The iodine is reduced by the vitamin C to form iodide. The endpoint is indicated by the reaction of iodine with starch suspension, which produces a blue-black product. As long as vitamin C is present, the iodine is quickly converted to iodide ion, and no blue-black iodine-starch product is observed. However, when all the vitamin C has been oxidized, the excess iodine(in equilibrium with iodine) reacts with starch to form the expected blue-black color.

In alkaline medium, vitamin C can be oxidized to dehydroascorbic acid, which reacts with 2, 4-dinitrophenylhydrazine to form a red osazone. Its maximum absorption peak appears at 500 nm and the resulting red color is measured photometrically.

III Apparatus and Reagents

723N spectrophotometer, cuvettes(4), analytical balances(0. 01 g,0. 1 mg), hot plate, blender, filter paper, funnel, test tubes(6), beaker(100 mL×1), water bath, Geiser buret(50 mL×1), Erlenmeyer flasks(250 mL×3), volumetric flasks(250 mL ×1,100 mL×8), transfer pipets(25 mL×1, 10 mL×2), Mohr measuring pipet (5 mL×1), wash bottle, medicine dropper and rubber pipet bulb.

Juice, starch indicator, standard iodine solution (0. 01 mol · L^{-1}, standardized), $H_2C_2O_4$ solution (1%), activated charcoal, thiourea solution (2%), 2, 4-dinitrophenylhydrazine solution (2%), H_2SO_4 solution (85%) and standard dehydroascorbic acid solution (20 μg · mL^{-1}).

IV Procedure

1. Iodometric Titration

Blend a 100 g sample of juice. Filter the juice through cheesecloth to remove pulp and seeds. Quantitatively transfer 10. 00 mL of the filtrate to a 250 mL volumetric flask and adjust the pH to 3. 0 by adding several drops of 6 mol · L^{-1} HCl solution. Add 2 mL of starch indicator. Titrate directly with standardized iodine solution. Repeat the titration two more times. Calculate the concentration of vitamin C in juice.

2. Spectrophotometric Method

(1) Preparation of the sample. Blend a 100 g of the juice with 100 g of 1% oxalic acid solution. Strain the mixture. Wash the filter with a few milliliters of 1% oxalic acid solution. Add 1% oxalic acid solution to make a final solution of 100 mL in a volumetric flask.

(2) Treatment by oxidation. Transfer 25. 00 mL of the filtrate above into a clean 100 mL beaker, add 2 g of activated charcoal with stirring(1 min), and filter the solution through filter paper. Add 10 mL of 2% thiourea solution and mix thoroughly.

(3) Direct method for dehydroascorbic acid. After filtration, transfer 4. 00 mL of extract into three test tubes, respectively. Use one as blank, to each of the other two, 1. 00 mL of 2% 2, 4-dinitrophenylhydrazine in approximately 85% H_2SO_4 solution is added. All test tubes are held at (37 ± 0.5) ℃ for 3 h, and then cooled in ice water bath. To each of the three test tubes, while in the ice water bath, 5. 00 mL of 85% H_2SO_4 solution is added from a buret, drop by drop within one minute. (H_2SO_4 solution, not grease, should be used for lubricating the stop-cock of the buret.) Finally 1 mL of 2% 2, 4-dinitrophenylhydrazine solution is placed in the blank test tube. The test tubes are shaken thoroughly in the ice water, removed to a rack, and wiped dry after 30 min. The blank is used as reference and measure the absorbance of the solutions at 605 nm.

(4) Preparation of calibration curve. To prepare the dehydroascorbic acid standard, 5. 00 mL, 10. 00 mL, 20. 00 mL, 25. 00 mL, 40. 00 mL, 50. 00 mL and 60. 00 mL of 20 $\mu g \cdot mL^{-1}$ dehydroascorbic acid are transfered to seven 100 mL volumetric flasks, respectively. Standards of appropriate concentrations are made by diluting with 1% thiourea containing 1 $\mu g \cdot mL^{-1}$, 2 $\mu g \cdot mL^{-1}$, 4 $\mu g \cdot mL^{-1}$, 5 $\mu g \cdot mL^{-1}$, 8 $\mu g \cdot mL^{-1}$, 10 $\mu g \cdot mL^{-1}$, and 12 $\mu g \cdot mL^{-1}$ of dehydroascorbic acid, respectively.

V Question

Compare iodometric titration with 2, 4-dinitrophenylhydrazine method for determination of vitamin C.

Experiment 42   Determination of Some Elements in Plant

Ⅰ Learning Objectives

(1) Learn how to separate and identify Ca, Mg, Fe, Al, P, and I in plant.

(2) Learn sample pretreatment techniques.

(3) Review the properties of some elements and compounds.

Ⅱ Principles

The essential mineral elements are nitrogen, phosphorus, potassium, calcium, magnesium, sulfur, boron, chlorine, iron, manganese, zinc, copper, molybdenum, and nickel. In addition to the essential mineral elements are the beneficial elements which promote plant growth in many plant species but are not absolutely necessary for completion of the plant life cycle, or fail to meet Arnon and Stout's criteria on other grounds. Recognized beneficial elements are silicon, sodium, cobalt, and selenium. Other elements that have been proposed as candidates for essential or beneficial elements include chromium, vanadium, and titanium, although strong evidence is lacking at this time.

Before determining some elements, the plant must be treated by dry ashing.

Calcium is measured by turbidity after oxalate precipitation. Magnesium is determined by combination with azoviolet. Aluminum is determined by combination with aluminon. Iron(Ⅲ) ion reacts with thiocyanate ion to give a deep red color of the thiocyanato complex. Thiocyanate is a sensitive test for iron(Ⅲ) only — iron (Ⅱ) does not cause a color change. Both iron(Ⅱ) and iron(Ⅲ) ions form very stable complexes with the cyanide ion (in fact, iron is used to complex waste cyanides to render them less toxic). The ferrocyanide($[Fe(CN)_6]^{2-}$) reacts with iron(Ⅲ) to form an intensely blue pigment $KFe[Fe(CN)_6]$. Inorganic phosphorus was measured by reaction with ammonium molybdate to form a colored phosphomolybdate complex. Iodine is measured using chlorine water (or bromine water), which oxidizes iodide ion to iodine, which shows a rose color in the layer of CCl_4.

$$Ca^{2+} + C_2O_4^{2-} \xrightarrow{HAc} CaC_2O_4 \text{ (white precipitate)}$$

$$Mg^{2+} + azoviolet + OH^- \longrightarrow sky \text{ blue precipitate}$$

$$Al^{3+} + aluminon + OH^- \longrightarrow red\ flocculent\ precipitate$$
$$Fe^{3+} + K_4[Fe(CN)_6] = KFe[Fe(CN)_6](blue) + 3K^+$$
$$Fe^{3+} + nKSCN(saturated) = Fe(SCN)_n^{3-n}(red) + nK^+$$
$$HPO_4^{2-} + 3NH_4^+ + 12MoO_4^{2-} + 23H^+ = (NH_4)_3[P(Mo_3O_{10})_4] \cdot 6H_2O(yellow) + 6H_2O$$
$$2I^- + Cl_2(Br_2) = I_2 + 2Cl^-(Br^-)(rose\ in\ CCl_4)$$

Ⅲ Apparatus and Reagents

Analytical balance (0.01 g), hot plate, mortar, evaporating dish, weighing bottle, filter paper, funnel, test tube, centrifuge, centrifuge tube, beaker (150 mL × 1), graduated cylinders (20 mL × 1, 10 mL × 2, 5 mL × 1), water bath, wash bottle, medicine dropper and watch glass.

HCl solution (6 mol · L^{-1}), HAc solution (2 mol · L^{-1}), NaOH solution (6 mol · L^{-1}), $(NH_4)_2C_2O_4$ solution (0.25 mol · L^{-1}), KSCN solution (saturated solution), aluminon, azoviolet, $K_4[Fe(CN)_6]$ solution (0.1 mol · L^{-1}), $(NH_4)_2MoO_4$ solution (1%), HNO_3 solution (concentrated solution) and bromine water.

Ⅳ Procedure

1. Sample Preparation by Dry Ashing for the Identification of Various Elements in Plant

See experiment 35.

2. Identification of Fe, Al, Ca, Mg, P and I

Add 2 drops of the sample solution from step 1 into a test tube, and then add 1 drop of azoviolet and 5 drops of 6 mol · L^{-1} NaOH solution. Observe the phenomenon. If no sky blue precipitate forms, Mg^{2+} is absent.

Add 2 drops of the sample solution from step 1 into a test tube, and then add 2 drops of 2 mol · L^{-1} HAc solution and 2 drops of 0.25 mol · L^{-1} $(NH_4)_2C_2O_4$ solution. Observe the phenomenon. A white precipitate is CaC_2O_4 and shows that Ca^{2+} is present.

To the two test tubes, add 5 drops of the sample solution from step 1. To one test tube add 2 drops of 0.1 mol · L^{-1} KSCN solution and the other add 2 drops of 0.1 mol · L^{-1} $K_4[Fe(CN)_6]$ solution, and shake the test tubes sufficiently. Observe the phenomenon. These reactions confirm the presence of Fe^{3+}.

Add 1 mL of the sample solution from step 1 into a centrifuge tube, and then add 6 mol · L^{-1} NaOH solution dropwise until a white precipitate dissolves. Centrifuge, decant the supernatant into a clean test tube, add 3-4 drops of aluminon, and then add several drops of 6 mol · L^{-1} $NH_3 \cdot H_2O$ solution. Slowly heat the tube with stirring and observe the phenomenon. A red flocculent precipitate confirms the presence of Al^{3+}.

Add 1 mL of the sample solution from step 1 into a test tube, and then add 5 drops of 1% $(NH_4)_2MoO_4$ solution and 5 drops of concentrated HNO_3 solution. Observe the phenomenon.

Add 5 drops of the sample solution from step 1 and 20 drops of CCl_4 into a test tube, and then add 10 drops of bromine water. Observe the color change in CCl_4 layer and explain the phenomenon.

V Question

How to separate and identify P in tea?

附　　录

附录 A　元素相对原子质量表

元素			相对原子质量	元素			相对原子质量
符号(序数)	名称	英文名		符号(序数)	名称	英文名	
H(1)	氢	Hydrogen	1.007 94	Ni(28)	镍	Nickel	58.693 4
He(2)	氦	Helium	4.002 602	Cu(29)	铜	Copper	63.546
Li(3)	锂	Lithium	6.941	Zn(30)	锌	Zinc	65.409
Be(4)	铍	Beryllium	9.012 182	Ga(31)	镓	Gallium	69.723
B(5)	硼	Boron	10.811	Ge(32)	锗	Germanium	72.64
C(6)	碳	Carbon	12.010 7	As(33)	砷	Arsenic	74.921 60
N(7)	氮	Nitrogen	14.006 7	Se(34)	硒	Selenium	78.96
O(8)	氧	Oxygen	15.999 4	Br(35)	溴	Bromine	79.904
F(9)	氟	Fluorine	18.998 403 2	Kr(36)	氪	Krypton	83.798
Ne(10)	氖	Neon	20.179 7	Rb(37)	铷	Rubidium	85.467 8
Na(11)	钠	Sodium	22.989 770	Sr(38)	锶	Strontium	87.62
Mg(12)	镁	Magnesium	24.305 0	Y(39)	钇	Yttrium	88.905 85
Al(13)	铝	Aluminum	26.981 538	Zr(40)	锆	Zirconium	91.224
Si(14)	硅	Silicon	28.085 5	Nb(41)	铌	Niobium	92.906 38
P(15)	磷	Phosphorus	30.973 761	Mo(42)	钼	Molybdenum	95.94
S(16)	硫	Sulfur	32.065	Tc(43)	锝	Technetium	97.907
Cl(17)	氯	Chlorine	35.453	Ru(44)	钌	Ruthenium	101.07
Ar(18)	氩	Argon	39.948	Rh(45)	铑	Rhodium	102.905 50
K(19)	钾	Potassium	39.098 3	Pd(46)	钯	Palladium	106.42
Ca(20)	钙	Calcium	40.078	Ag(47)	银	Silver	107.868 2
Sc(21)	钪	Scandium	44.955 910	Cd(48)	镉	Cadmium	112.411
Ti(22)	钛	Titanium	47.867	In(49)	铟	Indium	114.818
V(23)	钒	Vanadium	50.941 5	Sn(50)	锡	Tin	118.710
Cr(24)	铬	Chromium	51.996 1	Sb(51)	锑	Antimony	121.760
Mn(25)	锰	Manganese	54.938 049	Te(52)	碲	Tellurium	127.60
Fe(26)	铁	Iron	55.845	I(53)	碘	Iodine	126.904 47
Co(27)	钴	Cobalt	58.933 200	Xe(54)	氙	Xenon	131.293

续表

符号(序数)	名称	英文名	相对原子质量	符号(序数)	名称	英文名	相对原子质量
	元 素				元 素		
Cs(55)	铯	Cesium	132.905 45	Bi(83)	铋	Bismuth	208.980 38
Ba(56)	钡	Barium	137.327	Po(84)	钋	Polonium	208.98
La(57)	镧	Lanthanum	138.905 5	At(85)	砹	Astatine	209.99
Ce(58)	铈	Cerium	140.116	Rn(86)	氡	Radon	222.02
Pr(59)	镨	Praseodymium	140.907 65	Fr(87)	钫	Francium	223.02
Nd(60)	钕	Neodymium	144.24	Ra(88)	镭	Radium	226.03
Pm(61)	钷	Promethium	144.91	Ac(89)	锕	Actinium	227.03
Sm(62)	钐	Samarium	150.36	Th(90)	钍	Thorium	232.038 1
Eu(63)	铕	Europium	151.964	Pa(91)	镤	Protactinium	231.035 88
Gd(64)	钆	Gadolinium	157.25	U(92)	铀	Uranium	238.028 91
Tb(65)	铽	Terbium	158.925 34	Np(93)	镎	Neptunium	237.05
Dy(66)	镝	Dysprosium	162.500	Pu(94)	钚	Plutonium	244.06
Ho(67)	钬	Holmium	164.930 32	Am(95)	镅	Americium	243.06
Er(68)	铒	Erbium	167.259	Cm(96)	锔	Curium	247.07
Tm(69)	铥	Thulium	168.934 21	Bk(97)	锫	Berkelium	247.07
Yb(70)	镱	Ytterbium	173.04	Cf(98)	锎	Californium	251.08
Lu(71)	镥	Lutetium	174.967	Es(99)	锿	Einsteinium	252.08
Hf(72)	铪	Hafnium	178.49	Fm(100)	镄	Fermium	257.10
Ta(73)	钽	Tantalum	180.9479	Md(101)	钔	Mendelevium	258.10
W(74)	钨	Tungsten	183.84	No(102)	锘	Nobelium	259.10
Re(75)	铼	Rhenium	186.207	Lr(103)	铹	Lawrencium	260.11
Os(76)	锇	Osmium	190.23	Rf(104)	𬬻	Rutherfordium	261.11
Ir(77)	铱	Iridium	192.217	Db(105)	𬭊	Dubnium	262.11
Pt(78)	铂	Platinum	195.078	Sg(106)	𬭳	Seaborgium	263.12
Au(79)	金	Gold	196.966 55	Bh(107)	𬭛	Bohrium	264.12
Hg(80)	汞	Mercury	200.59	Hs(108)	𬭶	Hassium	265.13
Tl(81)	铊	Thallium	204.383 3	Mt(109)	鿏	Meitnerium	266.13
Pb(82)	铅	Lead	207.2				

附录 B 常用指示剂

指示剂名称	变色范围pH 值	颜色变化	溶液配制方法
甲基紫(第一变色范围)	0.13～0.5	黄—绿	0.1%或 0.05%的水溶液

指示剂名称	变色范围 pH 值	颜色变化	溶液配制方法
苦味酸	0.0～1.3	无色—黄	0.1％水溶液
甲基绿	0.1～2.0	黄—绿—浅蓝	0.05％水溶液
孔雀绿 （第一变色范围）	0.13～2.0	黄—浅蓝—绿	0.1％水溶液
甲酚红 （第一变色范围）	0.2～1.8	红—黄	0.04 g 指示剂溶于 100 mL 50％乙醇中
甲基紫 （第二变色范围）	1.0～1.5	绿—蓝	0.1％水溶液
百里酚蓝 （麝香草酚蓝） （第一变色范围）	1.2～2.8	红—黄	0.1 g 指示剂溶于 100 mL 20％乙醇中
甲基紫 （第三变色范围）	2.0～3.0	蓝—紫	0.1％水溶液
茜素黄 R （第一变色范围）	1.9～3.3	红—黄	0.1％水溶液
二甲基黄	2.9～4.0	红—黄	0.1 g 或 0.01 g 指示剂溶于 100 mL 90％乙醇中
甲基橙	3.1～4.4	红—橙黄	0.1％水溶液
溴酚蓝	3.0～4.6	黄—蓝	0.1 g 指示剂溶于 100 mL 20％乙醇中
刚果红	3.0～5.2	蓝紫—红	0.1％水溶液
茜素红 S （第一变色范围）	3.7～5.2	黄—紫	0.1％水溶液
溴甲酚绿	3.8～5.4	黄—蓝	0.1 g 指示剂溶于 100 mL 20％乙醇中
甲基红	4.4～6.2	红—黄	0.1 g 或 0.2 g 指示剂溶于 100 mL 60％乙醇中
溴酚红	5.0～6.8	黄—红	0.1 g 或 0.04 g 指示剂溶于 100 mL 20％乙醇中
溴甲酚紫	5.2～6.8	黄—紫红	0.1 g 指示剂溶于 100 mL 20％乙醇中
溴百里酚蓝	6.0～7.6	黄—蓝	0.05 g 指示剂溶于 100 mL 20％乙醇中
中性红	6.8～8.0	红—亮黄	0.1 g 指示剂溶于 100 mL 60％乙醇中
酚红	6.8～8.0	黄—红	0.1 g 指示剂溶于 100 mL 20％乙醇中
甲酚红	7.2～8.8	亮黄—紫红	0.1 g 指示剂溶于 100 mL 50％乙醇中
百里酚蓝 （麝香草酚蓝） （第二变色范围）	8.0～9.0	黄—蓝	0.1 g 指示剂溶于 100 mL 20％乙醇中
酚酞	8.2～10.0	无色—紫红	0.1 g 指示剂溶于 100 mL 60％乙醇中

续表

指示剂名称	变色范围 pH 值	颜色变化	溶液配制方法
百里酚酞	9.4～10.6	无色—蓝	0.1 g 指示剂溶于 100 mL 90% 乙醇中
茜素红 S (第二变色范围)	10.0～12.0	紫—淡黄	0.1% 水溶液
茜素黄 R (第二变色范围)	10.1～12.1	黄—淡紫	0.1% 水溶液

附录 C　常用酸碱的相对密度和浓度

试剂名称	相对密度	含量/(%)	浓度/(mol·L^{-1})
盐酸	1.18～1.19	36～38	11.6～12.4
硝酸	1.39～1.40	65.0～68.0	14.4～15.2
硫酸	1.83～1.84	95～98	17.8～18.4
磷酸	1.69	85	14.6
高氯酸	1.68	70.0～72.0	11.7～12.0
冰乙酸	1.05	99.8(优级纯) 99.0(分析纯,化学纯)	17.4
氢氟酸	1.13	40	22.5
氢溴酸	1.49	47.0	8.6
氨水	0.88～0.90	25.0～28.0	13.3～14.8

附录 D　常用缓冲溶液的配制

缓冲溶液组成	pK_a	pH 值	缓冲溶液的配制方法
氨基乙酸-HCl	2.35(pK_{a1})	2.3	取 150 g 氨基乙酸溶于 100 mL 水中,加 80 mL 浓 HCl 溶液,稀释至 1 L
H$_3$PO$_4$-枸橼酸盐		2.5	取 113 g Na$_2$HPO$_4$·12H$_2$O 溶于 200 mL 水中,加 387 g 枸橼酸,溶解,过滤后,稀释至 1 L
一氯乙酸-NaOH	2.86	2.8	取 200 g 一氯乙酸溶于 200 mL 水中,加 40 g NaOH 溶解后,稀释至 1 L
邻苯二甲酸氢钾-HCl	2.95(pK_{a1})	2.9	取 500 g 邻苯二甲酸氢钾溶于 500 mL 水中,加 80 mL 浓 HCl 溶液,稀释至 1 L
甲酸-NaOH	3.76	3.7	取 95 g 甲酸和 40 g NaOH 于 500 mL 水中,溶解,稀释至 1 L

续表

缓冲溶液组成	pK_a	pH 值	缓冲溶液的配制方法
NH$_4$Ac-HAc		4.5	取 77 g NH$_4$Ac 溶于 200 mL 水中,加 59 mL 冰乙酸,稀释至 1 L
NH$_4$Ac-HAc		5.0	取 250 g NH$_4$Ac 溶于水中,加 25 mL 冰乙酸,稀释至 1 L
NH$_4$Ac-HAc		6.0	取 600 g NH$_4$Ac 溶于水中,加 20 mL 冰乙酸,稀释至 1 L
NaAc-HAc	4.74	4.7	取 83 g 无水 NaAc 溶于水中,加 60 mL 冰乙酸,稀释至 1 L
NaAc-HAc		5.0	取 160 g 无水 NaAc 溶于水中,加 60 mL 冰乙酸,稀释至 1 L
六次甲基四胺-HCl	5.15	5.4	取 40 g 六次甲基四胺溶于 200 mL 水中,加 10 mL 浓 HCl 溶液,稀释至 1 L
NaAc-Na$_2$HPO$_4$		8.0	取 50 g 无水 NaAc 和 50 g Na$_2$HPO$_4$ · 12H$_2$O 溶于水中,稀释至 1 L
Tris-HCl	8.21	8.2	取 25 g Tris 试剂溶于水中,加 8 mL 浓 HCl 溶液,稀释至 1 L
NH$_3$-NH$_4$Cl	9.26	9.2	取 54 g NH$_4$Cl 溶于水中,加 63 mL 浓氨水,稀释至 1 L
NH$_3$-NH$_4$Cl		9.5	取 54 g NH$_4$Cl 溶于水中,加 126 mL 浓氨水,稀释至 1 L
NH$_3$-NH$_4$Cl		10.0	取 54 g NH$_4$Cl 溶于水中,加 350 mL 浓氨水,稀释至 1 L

附录 E 常用一级标准物质的干燥条件和应用

一级标准物质		干燥后的组成	干燥条件	标定对象
名称	分子式			
碳酸氢钠	NaHCO$_3$	Na$_2$CO$_3$	270~300 ℃	酸
碳酸钠	Na$_2$CO$_3$ · 10H$_2$O	Na$_2$CO$_3$	270~300 ℃	酸
硼砂	Na$_2$B$_4$O$_7$ · 10H$_2$O	Na$_2$B$_4$O$_7$ · 10H$_2$O	放在含 NaCl 和蔗糖饱和溶液的干燥器中	酸
碳酸氢钾	KHCO$_3$	K$_2$CO$_3$	270~300 ℃	酸
草酸	H$_2$C$_2$O$_4$ · 2H$_2$O	H$_2$C$_2$O$_4$ · 2H$_2$O	室温空气干燥	碱或 KMnO$_4$
邻苯二甲酸氢钾	KHC$_8$H$_4$O$_4$	KHC$_8$H$_4$O$_4$	110~120 ℃	碱
重铬酸钾	K$_2$Cr$_2$O$_7$	K$_2$Cr$_2$O$_7$	140~150 ℃	还原剂
溴酸钾	KBrO$_3$	KBrO$_3$	130 ℃	还原剂

续表

一级标准物质		干燥后的组成	干燥条件	标定对象
名称	分子式			
碘酸钾	KIO_3	KIO_3	130 ℃	还原剂
铜	Cu	Cu	室温干燥器中保存	还原剂
三氧化二砷	As_2O_3	As_2O_3	同上	氧化剂
草酸钠	$Na_2C_2O_4$	$Na_2C_2O_4$	130 ℃	氧化剂
碳酸钙	$CaCO_3$	$CaCO_3$	110 ℃	EDTA
锌	Zn	Zn	室温干燥器中保存	EDTA
氧化锌	ZnO	ZnO	900~1000 ℃	EDTA
氯化钠	NaCl	NaCl	500~600 ℃	$AgNO_3$
氯化钾	KCl	KCl	500~600 ℃	$AgNO_3$
硝酸银	$AgNO_3$	$AgNO_3$	280~290 ℃	氯化物

附录 F　常用试剂的配制

1.2,4-二硝基苯肼溶液

(1) 在 15 mL 浓 H_2SO_4 溶液中,溶解 3 g 2,4-二硝基苯肼。另在 70 mL 95%乙醇溶液中加 20 mL 水。然后把硫酸苯肼倒入稀乙醇溶液中,搅动混合均匀即成橙红色溶液(若有沉淀应过滤)。

(2) 将 1.2 g 2,4-二硝基苯肼溶于 50 mL 30%高氯酸溶液中,配制好后储存于棕色瓶中。

2.饱和亚硫酸氢钠溶液

先配制 40%亚硫酸氢钠水溶液,然后在每 100 mL 的 40%亚硫酸氢钠水溶液中,加入 25 mL 不含醛的无水乙醇,溶液呈透明清亮状。

由于亚硫酸氢钠久置后易失去二氧化硫而变质,所以上述溶液也可按下法配制:将研细的碳酸钠晶体($Na_2CO_3 \cdot 10H_2O$)与水混合,水刚好覆盖粉末。然后在混合物中通入二氧化硫气体,至碳酸钠全部溶解,或将二氧化硫通入 1 份碳酸钠与 3 份水的混合物中,至碳酸钠全部溶解,配制好后密封放置,但不可放置太久,最好是用时新配。

3.饱和溴水

在磨口玻璃瓶内,将约 50 g 市售的 Br_2 注入 1 L 水中,在 2 h 内经常剧烈振摇,每次振摇后,微开磨口塞,使积聚的 Br_2 蒸气放出。在储存瓶底部总有过量的溴。将 Br_2 水倒入试剂瓶时剩余的 Br_2 应留于储存瓶中(倾倒 Br_2 或 Br_2 水时,应在通风橱中进行,应将凡士林涂在手上或戴上橡皮手套操作,以防被 Br_2 蒸气灼伤)。

4.淀粉-碘化钾试纸

取 3 g 可溶性淀粉,加入 25 mL 水,搅匀,倾入 225 mL 沸水中,再加入 1 g 碘化钾及 1 g 结晶硫酸钠,用水稀释到 500 mL。将滤纸片(条)浸渍,取出晾干,密封备用。

5.1% 淀粉溶液

将 1 g 可溶性淀粉溶于 5 mL 冷蒸馏水中,用力搅成稀浆状,然后倒入 94 mL 沸水中,即得透明胶体溶液,放冷备用。

6.碘溶液

(1)将 20 g KI 溶于 100 mL 蒸馏水中,然后加入 10 g 研细的碘粉,搅动使其全部溶解后溶液呈深红色。

(2)将 1 g KI 溶于 100 mL 蒸馏水中,然后加入 0.5 g 碘,加热溶解即得红色清亮溶液。

7.硫化钠溶液(1 mol · L^{-1})

称取 240 g $Na_2S · 9H_2O$、40 g NaOH 溶于适量水中,稀释至 1 L,混匀。

8.硫化铵溶液(3 mol · L^{-1})

将 H_2S 通入 200 mL 浓氨水中直至饱和,再加 200 mL 浓氨水,最后加水稀释至 1 L,混匀。

9.氯化亚锡溶液(0.25 mol · L^{-1})

称取 56.4 g $SnCl_2 · 2H_2O$ 溶于 100 mL 浓 HCl 溶液中,加水稀释至 1 L,在溶液中放几颗纯锡粒(亦可溶解于一定量的浓 HCl 溶液中配制)。

10.氯化铁溶液(0.5 mol · L^{-1})

称取 135.2 g $FeCl_3 · 6H_2O$ 溶于 100 mL 6 mol · L^{-1} HCl 溶液中,加水稀释至 1 L。

11.三氯化铬溶液(0.1 mol · L^{-1})

称取 26.7 g $CrCl_3 · 6H_2O$ 溶于 30 mL 6 mol · L^{-1} HCl 溶液中,加水稀释至 1 L。

12.硝酸铅溶液(0.25 mol · L^{-1})

称取 83 g $Pb(NO_3)_2$ 溶于少量水中,加入 15 mL 6 mol · L^{-1} HNO_3 溶液,用水稀释至 1 L。

13.硫酸亚铁溶液(0.25 mol · L^{-1})

称取 69.5 g $FeSO_4 · 7H_2O$ 溶于适量水中,加入 5 mL 18 mol · L^{-1} H_2SO_4 溶液,再加水稀释至 1 L,并放入小铁钉数枚。

14.Cl_2 水(0.25 mol · L^{-1})

将 Cl_2 通入水中至饱和为止(用时临时配制)。

15.铬黑 T(0.5%)

铬黑 T 与固体无水 Na_2SO_4 或 NaCl 以 1:100 的比例混合,研磨均匀,置于棕色瓶中,保存于干燥器内。

附录 G　化学手册简介

在工农业生产和科学实验工作中,经常需要了解各种物质的性质(如物质的状态、熔点、沸点、密度、溶解度、化学特性等)。为此,人们编辑了各种类型的手册(工具书),供有关人员查用。学会使用这些工具书,对培养分析问题和解决问题的能力是很重要的。这里介绍几种常用的手册。

《试剂手册》是 1963 年中国医药公司上海试剂采购供应站编写的,介绍了 4 000 多种化学试剂。每种都按中文、英文名称,分子式,分子量,主要物理化学性质,用途等分别阐述,并对常用试剂说明其用途和参考规格。

《化学分析手册》是丘星初编写的,由化学工业出版社出版,介绍了化学分析中应用到的一些基本知识,如化学分析的基本操作技术、实验室一般常识、化学分析知识、溶液和某些常用试剂的配制方法、定量分析中操作溶液的配制与标定、指示剂与试纸、化学分析中的有关计算等。书末还附有化学分析工作中经常要查阅的一些数据。

《无机化学试剂手册》是 1964 年由化工部图书编辑室将苏联卡尔亚金的 Чистые Хцмические Реактивы 一书翻译成中文而得的。它列举了 600 多种无机化合物的中、俄、拉丁、英、法文名词,并介绍了物理和化学性质及制备方法。

《简明化学手册》是 1957 年顾振军等人将苏联别列利曼的 Краткйи Справочник, химика 一书译成中文而得的。其主要内容有各种物质的物理和化学性质、与化学有关的资料和数据、实验室工作及化学分析等。共分十五章。

《苏联化学手册》是 1958 年由陶坤等将苏联的 Справогнцк Химика 一书翻译而得的。分Ⅰ、Ⅱ、Ⅲ册,共 3 000 多页,介绍了重要无机化合物、有机化合物的物理和化学性质及多方面常用的参考数据。

Handbook of Chemistry and Physics(《化学和物理手册》)一书由 C. D. Hodgman 等编写。它介绍了数学、物理、化学常用的参考资料和数据,逐年修改出版,1978 年出版了第 58 版。这是应用最广的手册。

Stability Constants of Metal-ion Complexes(《金属离子配合物的稳定常数》)一书由 L. G. Sillen 和 A. E. Martall 编写。1964 年出第 2 版,1972 年出补编本。本书不仅包括金属离子配合物的稳定常数,而且也包括有关金属离子和配体的水解常数、酸碱常数、溶解度、氧化还原平衡常数等。

Lang's Handbook of Chemistry(《兰氏化学手册》)一书由 J. A. Dean 编写。1973 年出第 11 版。这是较常用的化学手册,内容包括原子和分子结构、无机化学、分析化学、电化学、有机化学、光谱学、热力学性质、物理性质等方面的资料和数据。

Handbook of Analytical Chemistry(《分析化学手册》)一书是 1963 年由 L. Meites 主编的。这是一本分析化学的专业性手册,以表格的形式组织了大量与分析化学有关的数据和方法,并适当安排了一些理论说明与分析。

参 考 文 献

[1] 陈东红.医学化学实验[M].武汉:湖北科学技术出版社,2003.

[2] 周井炎.基础化学实验(上、下册)[M].武汉:华中科技大学出版社,2004.

[3] 方国女,王燕,周其镇.大学基础化学实验[M].2版.北京:化学工业出版社,
2005.

[4] 高丽华.基础化学实验[M].北京:化学工业出版社,2004.

[5] 郭伟强.大学化学基础实验[M].北京:科学出版社,2005.

[6] Lester R M, Robert S B. Chemical Principles in the Laboratory[M]. Second Edition. New York:Harper & Raw Publishers, 1978.

[7] Vlassis C G. A Laboratory Guide for Chemistry[M]. Philadelphia:The Williams & Wilkins Company, 1978.

[8] Steven M. Experiments in Basic Chemistry[M]. Third Edition. New York:John Wiley& Sons Inc. , 1994.

[9] Day R A, Underwood A L. Quantitative Analysis[M]. Sixth Edition. London:Prentice-Hall International Inc. , 1991.

[10] 朱明华.仪器分析[M].3版.北京:高等教育出版社,2000.

[11] Slowinski E J. Chemical Principles in the Laboratory[M]. Fifth Edition. New York:W. B. Saunders Company,2000.

[12] Kirk R E, Othmer D F. Encyclopedia of Chemical Technology[M]. Third Edition. New York:John Wiley& Sons Inc. , 1978.

[13] 分析化学手册编写组.分析化学手册(第一、二、四分册)[M].2版.北京:化学工业出版社,1997—1998.

[14] 樊行雪,方国女.大学化学原理及应用[M].2版.北京:化学工业出版社,
2004.

[15] 华东理工大学化学系,四川大学化工学院.分析化学[M].5版.北京:高等教育出版社,2003.

[16] 北京师范大学无机化学教研室.无机化学实验[M].2版.北京:高等教育出版社,1991.

[17] 柴田村治,寺田喜久雄.纸色谱法及其应用[M].王敬尊,译.北京:科学出版社,1978.

[18] 徐勉懿,方国春,潘祖亭,等.无机及分析化学实验[M].武汉:武汉大学出

版社,1991.

[19] 无锡轻工业学院,天津轻工业学院.食品分析[M].北京:轻工业出版社, 1983.

[20] 徐功骅,蔡作乾.大学化学实验[M].北京:清华大学出版社,1997.

[21] 胡立江,尤宏,郝素娥.工科大学化学实验[M].哈尔滨:哈尔滨工业大学出 版社,2003.

[22] 王克强,王捷,吴本芳.新编无机化学实验[M].上海:华东理工大学出版 社,2001.

[23] 甘孟瑜,曹渊.大学化学实验[M].3版.重庆:重庆大学出版社,2003.

[24] 国家药典委员会.中华人民共和国药典[M].北京:化学工业出版社,2000.

[25] 马全红,路春娥,吴敏,等.大学化学实验[M].南京:东南大学出版社, 2002.

[26] 天津大学无机化学教研组.大学化学实验[M].天津:天津大学出版社, 1998.

[27] 天津化工研究设计院.无机精细化学品手册[M].北京:化学工业出版社, 2001.

[28] Н. Г. Ключников.无机合成手册[M].申泮文,姚从工,译.北京:高等教 育出版社,1995.

[29] 王秋长,赵鸿喜,张守民,等.基础化学实验[M].北京:科学出版社,2003.

[30] 罗士平,陈若愚,朱建飞,等.基础化学实验[M].北京:化学工业出版社, 2004.